HEALTHCARE TECHNOLOGIES SERIES 58

# Technologies for Healthcare 4.0

## IET Book Series on e–Health Technologies

Book Series Editor: Professor Joel J.P.C. Rodrigues, College of Computer Science and Technology, China University of Petroleum (East China), Qingdao, China; Senac Faculty of Ceara', Fortaleza-CE, Brazil and Instituto de Telecomunicações, Portugal

Book Series Advisor: Professor Pranjal Chandra, School of Biochemical Engineering, Indian Institute of Technology (BHU), Varanasi, India

While the demographic shifts in populations display significant socio-economic challenges, they trigger opportunities for innovations in e-Health, m-Health, precision and personalized medicine, robotics, sensing, the Internet of things, cloud computing, big data, software defined networks, and network function virtualization. Their integration is however associated with many technological, ethical, legal, social, and security issues. This book series aims to disseminate recent advances for e-health technologies to improve healthcare and people's wellbeing.

## Could you be our next author?

Topics considered include intelligent e-Health systems, electronic health records, ICT-enabled personal health systems, mobile and cloud computing for e-Health, health monitoring, precision and personalized health, robotics for e-Health, security and privacy in e-Health, ambient assisted living, telemedicine, big data and IoT for e-Health, and more.

Proposals for coherently integrated international multi-authored edited or co-authored handbooks and research monographs will be considered for this book series. Each proposal will be reviewed by the book Series Editor with additional external reviews from independent reviewers.

To download our proposal form or find out more information about publishing with us, please visit https://www.theiet.org/publishing/publishing-with-iet-books/.

Please email your completed book proposal for the IET Book Series on e-Health Technologies to: Amber Thomas at athomas@theiet.org or author_support@theiet.org.

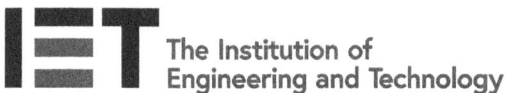

**IET** The Institution of Engineering and Technology

# Technologies for Healthcare 4.0

From AI and IoT to blockchain

Edited by
Karthik Ramamurthy, Suganthi Kulanthaivelu,
Kulandairaj Martin Sagayam, Soumi Dutta and Paryati

The Institution of Engineering and Technology

**British Library Cataloguing in Publication Data**
A catalogue record for this product is available from the British Library

**ISBN 978-1-83953-777-6 (hardback)**
**ISBN 978-1-83953-778-3 (PDF)**

Typeset in India by MPS Limited

Cover Image: OneForAll/E+ via Getty Images

# Contents

# About the editors

**Karthik Ramamurthy** completed his doctoral degree at the Vellore Institute of Technology Chennai and earned his Master's degree from MIT Campus of Anna University, India. Currently, he holds the position of senior assistant professor in the Centre for Cyber Physical Systems at Vellore Institute of Technology, Chennai. His areas of expertise encompass deep learning, computer vision, digital image processing, and medical image analysis. He has a notable publication record of approximately 70 papers in esteemed peer-reviewed journals and conferences. In addition, he actively serves as a reviewer for scholarly journals published by Elsevier, IEEE, Springer, and Nature.

**Suganthi Kulanthaivelu** is an associate professor in the School of Electronics Engineering, Vellore Institute of Technology, Chennai, India. She has 20 years of teaching and research experience in wireless sensor networks, Internet of Things applications, image processing, artificial intelligence, and industrial IoT. She has published more than 30 research papers in journals and conferences.

**Kulandairaj Martin Sagayam** is an assistant professor in the Department of ECE, Karunya University, India. His areas of interest include pattern recognition, artificial intelligence, and signal processing in imaging. He is an active member of the International Society of Promising Computer Engineers, Copernicus, the Scientific Engineering Research Corporation, the International Association of Computer Science and Information Technology, the International Association of Engineers, and the Indian Society of Electronics and Communication Engineering.

**Soumi Dutta** is an associate professor at the Institute of Engineering & Management, India. Her research interests are data mining, information retrieval, and image processing. She has published 30 papers, 5 book chapters, and 4 patents. She has delivered 27 keynote talks at various international conferences and has been awarded the Rashtriya Shiksha Ratna Award, InSc Research Education Excellence Award, and International Teacher Award (2020–2021) by the Ministry of MSME, Government of India. She is a member of several technical functional bodies such as ACM, IEEE, IFERP, MACUL, SDIWC, Internet Society, ICSES, ASR, AIDASCO, USERN, IRAN, and IAENG.

**Paryati** is an assistant professor at the National Development University "Veteran" Yogyakarta, Indonesia. Her research interests are genetic algorithms, artificial intelligence, expert systems, data mining, machine learning, deep learning systems, fuzzy logic, data analysis, and smart city information systems. She has published 28 papers, 4 book chapters, and 4 books. She is a member of many technical functional bodies.

*Chapter 1*

# Introduction to Healthcare 4.0

*R. Karthik[1], K. Suganthi[2], Kulandairaj Martin Sagayam[3], Soumi Dutta[4] and Paryati[5]*

## Abstract

The field of digital health aims to improve healthcare through the integration of digital technologies such as Internet of Things (IoT), EHRs, and telemedicine into clinical practice and patient care. Its goal is to provide healthcare providers with the tools and information needed to make better-informed decisions and deliver more personalized care. The increasing demand for hospital and healthcare management in India due to medical tourism, hygiene perception, and the need for efficient resource allocation highlights the importance of education and training in this field. Healthcare 4.0 is an emerging area that builds on digital health and aims to create an intelligent and interconnected healthcare system using emerging technologies such as artificial intelligence (AI), blockchain, and the Internet of Medical Things (IoMT) to transform the entire healthcare value chain. The main objective of Healthcare 4.0 is to improve patient outcomes, enhance the quality of care, and reduce costs by leveraging the power of these advanced technologies. This chapter discusses the recent trends, methodology, scope, and limitations in Healthcare 4.0. The potential scope of Healthcare 4.0 is vast and varied, ranging from personalized medicine, telemedicine, remote monitoring, and smart healthcare systems to drug discovery and development, clinical trials, and supply chain management.

**Keywords:** Healthcare 4.0; Internet of Things; Big data; Artificial intelligence

## 1.1 Introduction

Healthcare 4.0 has emerged to connect patients and healthcare professionals with organizations and treatment facilities. It incorporates core principles from Industry

[1]Centre for Cyber Physical Systems, Vellore Institute of Technology, Chennai, India
[2]School of Electronics Engineering, Vellore Institute of Technology, Chennai, India
[3]Department of Electronics and Communication Engineering, Karunya University, Coimbatore, India
[4]Department of Computer Applications, Institute of Engineering and Management, Kolkata, India
[5]National Development University "Veteran", Yogyakarta, Indonesia

4.0, enabling the transition from manufacturers to service providers [1]. This evolution aims to foster innovation and improve medical care delivery. Virtual reality (VR) has played a significant role in the advancement of healthcare technology during the fourth evolution of the industry. Healthcare 4.0 represents a new era characterized by the integration of cutting-edge technologies, including VR, artificial intelligence (AI), and Internet of Things (IoT) [2]. The primary goal is to enhance patient outcomes and experiences, optimize medical processes, and improve the overall efficiency of healthcare systems [3].

According to a report by Deloitte, Healthcare 4.0 can be defined as "a technology-enabled, data-driven, and patient-centric model of care delivery that emphasizes the use of emerging technologies to provide better quality care at lower costs" [4]. According to a report by Frost & Sullivan, Healthcare 4.0 is expected to revolutionize the healthcare industry by enabling remote patient monitoring, facilitating the use of predictive analytics to identify potential health risks, and enabling personalized treatments [5]. The report also notes that Healthcare 4.0 will improve patient engagement and empowerment by providing patients with access to their health information and enabling them to participate in their care. The goal of Healthcare 4.0 is to create a healthcare system that is more personalized, efficient, and effective, with a focus on prevention, early detection, and personalized treatment. Figure 1.1 presents the evolution of healthcare over the period, ranging from 1.0 to 4.0, including the range of technologies and techniques employed in each revolutionary stage.

Healthcare has undergone various transformations over the centuries with the aim of improving the delivery and quality of medical care. The first phase of healthcare, Healthcare 1.0, involved the traditional model of patient–clinician meetings where patients received consultations, testing, diagnosis, and follow-up plans from doctors [6]. In Healthcare 2.0, medical equipment development took the center stage, with an increased use of MRI scans, CT scans, pulse oximeters, arterial lines, and chest ducts. The introduction of information systems for clinical and operational processes marked Healthcare 3.0, which included Electronic Health or Medical Records (EHR or EMR), Computerized Provider Order Entry (CPOE),

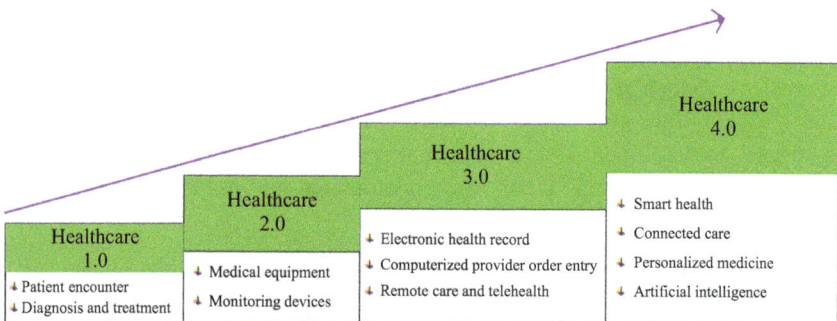

*Figure 1.1   Historical growth from Healthcare 1.0 to 4.0*

and electronic After Visit Summary (AVS). With the COVID-19 pandemic, tele-health and virtual appointments became more prevalent. In Healthcare 4.0, healthcare delivery aims to reach new heights with the use of medical robots, intelligent sensors, wearables, radio-frequency identification (RFID), cyber-physical system equipment, and IoT integrated with the cloud environment, big data analytics, and AI [7]. This approach aims to achieve resourceful and better fitness delivery, such as aggressive treatment, disease forecasting and avoidance, customized medicine, and advanced care for patients. The ultimate goal is to increase people's engagement, obtain more clinical data for proper treatment and care planning, and provide better healthcare services to patients.

One of the main benefits of Healthcare 4.0 is the ability to provide more per-sonalized and efficient healthcare services. With IoT-enabled devices, healthcare providers can remotely monitor patient health, reducing the need for hospital stays and lowering healthcare costs. Additionally, sensors placed on hospital staff can improve communication and coordination between different departments, opti-mizing the use of resources and advancing the overall functioning of the hospital [6]. The potential of Healthcare 4.0 is vast and can impact various aspects of the healthcare industry. Blockchain technology, for instance, has the potential to revolutionize data security and reduce administrative costs. The use of smart con-tracts can automate many administrative tasks, such as claims processing, and ensure that medical supply chains are transparent and accountable [8]. Healthcare 4.0 represents a new era in healthcare, characterized by the integration of advanced technologies and data-driven decision-making to improve patient outcomes, streamline processes, and enhance the efficiency of healthcare systems. The remainder of the chapter is as follows: Section 1.2 presents the recent trends in Healthcare 4.0 and their applications, followed by Section 1.3 which explains the methodology of Medical 4.0. Section 1.4 discusses the possible scope, opportu-nities, and challenges currently faced by Healthcare 4.0, and Section 1.5 comprises a conclusive summary of the report, its limitations, and avenues for future work.

## 1.2    Recent trends in Healthcare 4.0

Healthcare 4.0 is a concept that was inspired by the advancements of the Industrial Revolution 4.0, where technological improvements were utilized to optimize workflows in various industries to better serve their customers. The aim of Healthcare 4.0 is to facilitate the transformation of healthcare industries from being producers to becoming service providers [9]. This paradigm shift will enable clients to customize the services they use to suit their specific needs quickly and easily. Healthcare 4.0 can integrate the organization, therapeutic approaches, and tech-nology used with the patients and healthcare professionals, which is set to evolve into a patient-centric approach that shares data with industry players to promote cutting-edge technology and healthcare delivery ideas [10]. With the aid of the latest technologies, it intends to prioritize patient orientation and personal care services. The medical sector, from all around the world, is heavily engaged in the integration of medical delivery with precise medications and a lifestyle-based strategy for patient attendance and treatment. The development of Healthcare 4.0 will leverage emerging technologies such as IoT, AI, robots, and information security to streamline patient-centric care.

In Healthcare 4.0, the focus is on monitoring technological advancements that can provide accurate and reliable patient data essential for efficient therapy. This highlights the significance of instruments such as sensors, monitors, and other devices that can record and display data. IoT has emerged as a new development in medical technology, allowing for the creation of a customer-centric diagnostic model that can be used to closely monitor a patient's vital signs. Previously, IoT was only used for electronic equipment and appliances that enhance consumer lifestyles. The integration of medical domains with technological devices enables healthcare professionals to provide better treatment methods with precision. The use of equipment such as pulsometers and wearable devices is facilitating the promotion of patient self-care. IoT devices not only record data but also transmit it for analysis and effective medication, providing healthcare providers with a better understanding of various healthcare applications and diagnostics. VR has significantly advanced healthcare technology in the era of Healthcare 4.0. VR headsets enable patients to escape the clinical hospital environment and virtually explore new environments, simplifying their treatment moments. Additionally, VR has demonstrated efficient pain alleviation and improved vital signs in chronic pain patients, aiding doctors in developing diagnosis strategies. Patients can order VR headsets to monitor pain relief strategies at home through virtual treatment. VR has also changed how medical professionals learn and conduct practical investigations with reduced risks and errors [11].

AI is playing an increasingly tailored and sophisticated role in Healthcare 4.0. By enabling patients to express their mental state during therapy, AI is helping to improve diagnosis and keep doctors focused on each patient's needs. AI-based chatbots use preset questions to understand the patient's perspective and develop a more effective treatment plan. In the future, AI-based robots may even assist doctors with simple tasks, allowing them to focus on providing the best care possible [12]. In Healthcare 4.0, technology is being used to cater to the dietary preferences of patients in hospitals. The traditional practice of serving all patients at the same time can be frustrating for those who prefer to eat at different times. To address this issue, hospitals are using cutting-edge technology to better understand and accommodate patients' dietary needs. Many healthcare providers have started growing fresh veggies on-site to offer healthier meal options. Additionally, hospitals can use IoT to automate production operations and reduce the need for hiring a full gardening staff. IoT devices, such as wearable fitness bands, pulsometers, and digital thermometers, are empowering individuals to take care of their health. By allowing users to measure and record their health vitals, these devices enable remote communication with doctors when emergency diagnoses are required. As a result, traditional physical hospital spaces for routine check-ups or minor symptoms may become obsolete. This shift will impact future infrastructure and renovation of existing hospital facilities to prioritize patient care. Hospital-owned health-monitoring kiosks can serve as a streamlined infrastructure for healthcare services, with various monitoring systems integrated into a single dashboard. These kiosks can act as monitoring stations for the healthcare industry [13].

The advent of Healthcare 4.0 has brought about significant technological advancements that have transformed the healthcare industry. VR, AI, IoT devices, and other cutting-edge technologies have improved patient care, diagnosis, and treatment. Patients can now monitor their health vitals, receive treatment through VR, and communicate with doctors through AI chatbots. IoT devices and healthcare have streamlined healthcare services, while hospitals have begun growing fresh veggies to offer patients healthy and customized meals. Overall, the integration of technology in healthcare has revolutionized the industry, making healthcare services more efficient, patient-focused, and accessible to everyone.

## 1.3   Methodology

This section presents the methodology of a product under the Healthcare 4.0 regime. Healthcare 4.0 focuses on four new technologies: AI, blockchain, cloud computing, and IoT.

The methodology of Healthcare 4.0 focuses on the integration of advanced digital technologies and data analytics into the healthcare system to enhance the delivery of care. Figure 1.2 represents the structural workflow of a product implemented in Healthcare 4.0. The process begins with the initial step of data collection, which includes previous health reports, cloud platforms, big data repositories, and data handling stages. The collected data is then fed to the analysis phase where the patient record is stored in a smart system that includes the process of detection, analysis, and processing them accordingly. AI, blockchain, cloud computing, and IoT are the primary technologies employed in this process.

The next step involves the compilation of the processed data, which is then delivered to the end user. This step aims to provide more precise diagnoses, effective treatment plans, and better healthcare services to patients. The use of blockchain technology has gained significant attention in modern deployments, state-of-the-art applications, start-ups, and other innovative technologies in

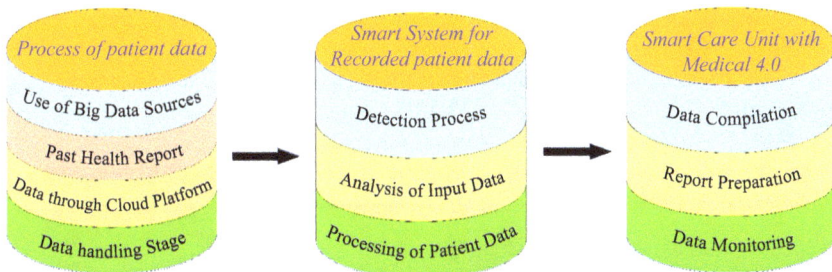

*Figure 1.2   Working procedure for implementation of Healthcare 4.0*

Healthcare 4.0. By leveraging blockchain technology, Healthcare 4.0 aims to enhance data security, reduce administrative costs, and promote health data interoperability.

The use of blockchain technology in Healthcare 4.0 has significant potential in enhancing data security, reducing administrative costs, and promoting the interoperability of health data. Decentralized ledger technology is particularly suitable for storing EHRs as data is distributed across a network of computers and protected by advanced cryptography, making it almost impossible for hackers to tamper with or steal the data. Smart contracts on the blockchain can also ensure that only authorized parties have access to specific patient data while still allowing for the easy sharing of information among doctors, hospitals, and insurance companies. Figure 1.3 presents the architectural overview of an EHR distribution system based on blockchain technology.

In addition to EHRs, blockchain technology is also being used to address other issues in the healthcare industry. For instance, the block-pharma platform is used by manufacturers, distributors, and hospitals to record and verify the authenticity of drugs. By creating an immutable record of a drug's journey from the manufacturer to the patient, the platform helps to decrease the number of counterfeit drugs in circulation, ultimately saving lives. Encrypgen is another example of a blockchain-based platform

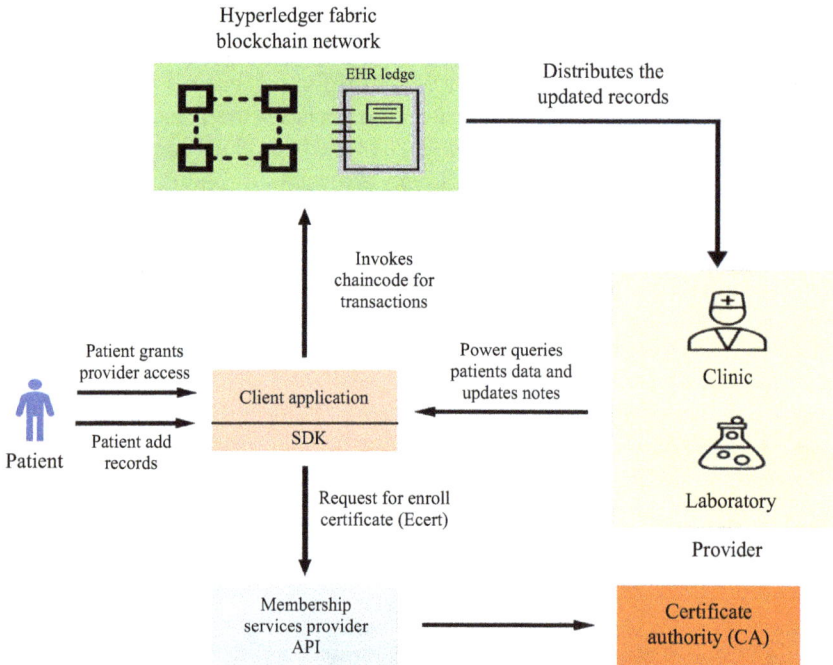

*Figure 1.3   Architectural overview of an EHR distribution system powered by blockchain*

that securely stores and shares genomic data, which can be used for research and personalized medicine.

Medical chain is yet another example of a blockchain-based platform that stores and shares health records, with the added feature of a telemedicine system to allow for remote consultations. The use of blockchain technology in healthcare is still in its early stages, but its potential to revolutionize the industry by improving the security and distribution of sensitive medical data cannot be underestimated. Additionally, it helps to maintain the balance between maintaining patient privacy and allowing for accessible, up-to-date medical records [14].

The healthcare payroll management system (HPMS) is one such example of an EHR distribution system. It is an important aspect of healthcare administration, and the integration of blockchain technology has the potential to revolutionize the system. Figure 1.3 depicts the four major participants involved in the system, namely patients, clinicians, laboratories, and system administrators. The system leverages blockchain technology to maintain secure and transparent EHRs that can be accessed by authorized parties in real time.

Patients play a crucial role in the HPMS by granting access to their EHRs via client applications or software development kit (SDK). They then request enrolment certification authority from membership service providers via application programming interface (API). Patients can add their records to the blockchain network by invoking the chain code for transactions. The smart contracts ensure that only authorized parties have access to specific patient data while maintaining patient privacy. Clinicians and laboratory technicians have the right to update the ledger, while patients are given special permission to add personal information to their records.

The second participant in the HPMS is the clinician. Clinicians are authorized users that are responsible for adding information to the patient's EHR, such as diagnoses, treatment plans, and medications. The clinician must have the appropriate credentials to access the system and can only access patient data for the patients that they are treating. The system ensures that only authorized clinicians can access patient data by using smart contracts on the blockchain.

The laboratory is the third participant in the HPMS. Laboratories are responsible for conducting various medical tests and providing the results to clinicians. Laboratories can also access the patient's EHR to update it with the results of the tests. Again, the laboratory technician must have the appropriate credentials to access the system and can only access patient data for the patients that they are testing. The system ensures that only authorized laboratory technicians can access patient data by using smart contracts on the blockchain.

The final participant in the HPMS is the system admin. The system admin is responsible for managing the overall system, including adding and removing users, ensuring the system is functioning correctly, and troubleshooting any issues that arise. The system admin has the highest level of access to the system and can access all patient data. The system ensures that only authorized system admins can access patient data by using smart contracts on the blockchain. The HPMS provides a secure and efficient platform for managing patient data while ensuring patient privacy and security.

The use of blockchain technology ensures that the created record is added to the blockchain network and remains an immutable ledger that cannot be changed or hacked. The updating rights are given only to clinicians and laboratory technicians. If the user wants to add personal information, they are given special permission to update the ledger. The actions are combined with the earlier hash with a timestamp that maintains the grid fully protected [15]. Therefore, the use of blockchain technology in HPMS has the potential to revolutionize the healthcare industry by improving the security and distribution of sensitive medical data.

## 1.4    Discussion

This section aims to explore the applications of various technologies in the healthcare industry and the potential opportunities that it presents. Furthermore, the final subsection of this discussion will address the current obstacles that Healthcare 4.0 faces and their possible solutions.

### 1.4.1    Scope of IoT

The IoT is a rapidly growing technology that is transforming various industries, including healthcare. The potential of IoT in healthcare is significant, as it has the capability to improve patient outcomes and enhance the quality of care by enabling remote monitoring, consistent treatment, and more efficient use of healthcare resources. According to a report by Grand View Research, the global IoT health-care market is expected to reach USD 534.3 billion by 2025 [16].

One of the most significant applications of IoT in healthcare is remote patient monitoring. IoT-enabled devices, such as wearables and sensors, can be used to collect and transmit patient health data in real time to healthcare providers. This technology can empower doctors to monitor patients remotely, reducing the need for hospital stays and lowering healthcare costs. Additionally, it can help doctors make more informed decisions about a patient's treatment and enable more seamless interactions between patients and healthcare specialists.

IoT-enabled devices also have the potential to improve the overall functioning of hospitals. For example, sensors placed on hospital staff can provide real-time information on their location, enabling better communication and coordination between different departments. This can optimize the use of resources and enhance the quality of care for patients. IoT devices can also facilitate quick and accurate processing of patient data, providing healthcare providers with real-time access to patient information and enabling the automatic transfer of data between different systems and devices.

Furthermore, IoT in healthcare can help healthcare providers to ensure that their patients follow their prescribed medical care. By providing real-time monitoring of patient health and activity, IoT-enabled devices such as wearables can help healthcare providers to ensure that patients are following their treatment plans and taking their medications as prescribed. IoT in healthcare can also help to improve patient outcomes by providing healthcare providers with more information about a patient's health and enabling them to take preventative measures to address health issues before they become serious [17].

IoT in healthcare has the potential to revolutionize the healthcare industry, enhance patient outcomes, and optimize the use of healthcare resources. Therefore, it is imperative for healthcare organizations to embrace this technology and harness its full potential.

## 1.4.2 Scope of big data

The use of big data analytics in the healthcare industry can revolutionize patient outcomes by providing a wealth of information on diseases, their progression, and their treatments. Big data analytics can facilitate the integration and analysis of data from multiple sources, such as wearable devices and EHRs, to identify patient conditions, predict outcomes, and identify potential obstacles to patient health. This has the potential to elevate evidence-based medicine to the next level and extend its reach globally, providing doctors with decision support systems. Predictive modeling and analysis of health-relevant big data are essential technological foundations for a true healthcare revolution [18].

One of the most significant benefits of big data analytics in healthcare is the ability to analyze vast amounts of data to uncover hidden patterns and insights. This can lead to the development of new treatments, identification of high-risk patients, and early intervention to prevent the onset of disease. For example, data analytics can help identify patients with high blood pressure, who are at risk for heart disease, and provide preventive measures such as lifestyle changes or medication [19]. Furthermore, big data analytics can enable doctors and researchers to conduct large-scale studies and clinical trials to evaluate the effectiveness of new treatments and drugs.

In addition, big data analytics can play a significant role in reducing healthcare costs. By analyzing patient data and identifying high-risk patients, doctors can intervene early and provide more effective treatments, thereby reducing the need for expensive hospital stays and procedures. Moreover, big data analytics can help healthcare providers to better allocate resources and optimize workflows, leading to improved operational efficiency and reduced costs.

## 1.4.3 Scope of AI

AI has emerged as a promising technology in the healthcare industry. AI has the potential to transform the way doctors diagnose, treat, and manage diseases by providing accurate and timely predictions. AI can analyze large amounts of data, such as EHRs and imaging studies, and identify patterns that can help doctors make informed decisions about patient care. AI can also be used for tasks such as image analysis, natural language processing, and robotic surgery, which can make healthcare processes more efficient and accurate [20].

A machine learning-based healthcare model can help identify various diseases in their early stages accurately. The model trains on a dataset of patient data like demographic data, medical history, lab results, imaging studies, and outcomes.

Once trained, the model can predict the likelihood of a patient having a specific disease based on patterns found in the data. This can allow doctors to make early diagnoses and informed decisions about patient care, leading to improved patient outcomes. Additionally, AI can predict a patient's response to a specific treatment, which can help doctors make more informed decisions about care.

However, there are challenges in implementing AI in healthcare. AI models require high-quality datasets, good feature engineering, and efficient algorithm selection. The interpretability and explainability of the models are important for trust and adoption in clinical practice [21]. Additionally, privacy concerns related to handling large amounts of patient data must be addressed. AI models should be developed with ethical considerations, such as ensuring that they are not biased and do not perpetuate health disparities. With these challenges in mind, AI has the potential to improve healthcare outcomes and revolutionize the healthcare industry.

The use of AI in healthcare has the potential to revolutionize the healthcare industry. AI can help doctors make early and accurate diagnoses, predict treatment outcomes, and make healthcare processes more efficient and accurate. However, challenges such as data quality, privacy concerns, and ethical considerations need to be addressed to ensure the responsible use of AI in healthcare. By addressing these challenges, AI can contribute to improved patient outcomes and advance the healthcare industry.

### 1.4.4   Scope of Healthcare 4.0 in industry

The healthcare industry has been slow to adopt new technologies, but with the rise of Industry 4.0, healthcare is poised to benefit from the integration of new digital technologies. Healthcare 4.0 is the new paradigm in healthcare that integrates the four design principles of Industry 4.0 to improve patient outcomes, reduce costs, and increase efficiency [22].

Interconnections are the first design principle of Industry 4.0, and it plays a critical role in Healthcare 4.0. Interconnectivity enables the seamless transfer of information between devices, sensors, and machines, allowing for the development of new medical devices and technologies. This can lead to better patient outcomes, increased efficiency, and cost savings. The ability of healthcare systems to interconnect also enables the use of real-time data to provide personalized care and predictive analysis for patients.

Information transparency is another critical design principle of Industry 4.0 that plays a crucial role in Healthcare 4.0. Healthcare generates vast amounts of data, and information transparency allows healthcare systems to collect and analyze this data to identify trends, improve decision-making, and reduce costs. By collecting and analyzing data, healthcare systems can identify inefficiencies, reduce waste, and improve outcomes.

Technical assistance is another important design principle of Industry 4.0, and it can be applied to Healthcare 4.0 to improve decision-making and problem-solving. Technical assistance includes the use of artificial intelligence, machine learning, and predictive analytics to identify trends, predict outcomes, and improve decision-making. These technologies can help healthcare professionals to make better decisions, reduce errors, and improve patient outcomes.

Finally, decentralized decisions are the fourth design principle of Industry 4.0 and play a critical role in Healthcare 4.0. Decentralized decisions enable autonomous environments and encourage operators at higher levels to make decisions. This can lead to improved efficiency, reduced costs, and better patient outcomes. By enabling autonomous decision-making, healthcare systems can reduce the time required for decision-making and reduce the risk of errors.

Healthcare 4.0 is the new paradigm in healthcare that integrates the design principles of Industry 4.0 to improve patient outcomes, reduce costs, and increase efficiency [23]. Interconnections, information transparency, technical assistance, and decentralized decisions are the four design principles of Industry 4.0 that can be applied to Healthcare 4.0 to drive innovation and progress in the healthcare industry. With the integration of new digital technologies, healthcare systems can improve patient care, reduce costs, and drive progress in the healthcare industry.

### 1.4.5  Challenges of Healthcare 4.0

The concept of a new industrial revolution was proposed several decades ago, specifically in the last decade of the 20th century, around 30 years after the third industrial revolution. While the previous transitions took a century to materialize, Industry 4.0 is rapidly emerging with the use of cyber-physical systems (CPSs) in smart factories, which is expected to enhance decision-making, engineering, and business processes, and optimize systems [24]. Various countries have launched initiatives aimed at improving their domestic productivity and industrial competitiveness. For example, the smart industry concept was introduced in the Netherlands in 2014, which involves three main pillars: providing knowledge and expertise in nine different sectors; establishing networks for public–private partnerships; and setting long-term agendas for improving industrial and technological conditions [25,26]. China launched the Made-in-China 2025 policy in 2015, which aims to become the most powerful manufacturing nation by 2049 through a three-phase plan [27]. South Korea also launched its initiative, Manufacturing Innovation 3.0, which aims to develop smart factories to achieve automation and sustainability in manufacturing processes [28]. Experts agree that Industry 4.0 is a transformative phenomenon with significant implications for various business sectors, including Healthcare, which accounts for more than 10% of the GDP in most developed countries and is projected to reach nearly $9 trillion in 2021 [29]. With rising healthcare costs, demand for more patient-centered services, and the need for more efficient physician practices, there is an urgent need to digitize healthcare systems. Industry 4.0 has expanded beyond manufacturing and automation to encompass the healthcare sector, giving rise to Healthcare 4.0. The objective of this concept is to enhance the processes within manufacturing units, improve the healthcare services offered, and address operational aspects of healthcare systems. As a result, its primary emphasis lies not only on the processes themselves but also on the beneficiaries. The implementation of Healthcare 4.0 solutions can yield several benefits, including enhanced surgical precision, expedited and secure storage of medical data, enhanced management of hospital resources, and reduced patient discomfort.

Based on a comprehensive research report by Market Research Future, it is projected that the global market will experience a compound growth rate of 18.2% and generate a revenue of 81.3 billion USD by 2030 [30]. In recent times, efforts have been made to establish a clear definition of Healthcare 4.0 and its association with Industry 4.0. Key technologies of Industry 4.0, such as cloud computing and the IoT, have been recognized as pertinent to the healthcare sector. However, the standardization of Healthcare 4.0 concepts and definitions remains incomplete [31]. While a few studies have provided a review of the current trends, challenges, and benefits of Healthcare 4.0, including aspects related to security, privacy, data requirements, and standardization [32–35], these works partially or fully overlook the framework of Healthcare 4.0, its emergence from Industry 4.0, the potential differences between Industry 4.0 and Healthcare 4.0 components, and the distinguishing characteristics of these components that give rise to opportunities and challenges. This literature mapping study seeks to fill this knowledge gap by precisely defining Industry 4.0, Healthcare 4.0, and their relationship, highlighting the significant applications of Industry 4.0 components in Healthcare 4.0, with a specific focus on data management, and identifying the benefits and obstacles associated with the adoption of Healthcare 4.0 solutions.

While the benefits of Healthcare 4.0 are many, some significant challenges must be addressed. One of the significant challenges faced by the healthcare industry is the management of vast amounts of data generated by various sources, including EHRs, medical imaging, and patient-generated data. The rapid growth of data poses a significant challenge to healthcare providers in terms of effective data management. Healthcare providers must invest in robust infrastructure that can manage and process large amounts of data effectively. This infrastructure must be equipped with tools and technologies that can analyze and make sense of the data to derive valuable insights that can be used for patient care and population health management. Data management is critical for healthcare providers to deliver accurate, timely, and high-quality care to patients, improve clinical outcomes, and reduce costs. The challenge of cybersecurity has also become more critical due to the increasing amount of sensitive data that is being stored digitally. Cyber threats such as data breaches, ransomware attacks, and other cyber-attacks pose a significant risk to the confidentiality, integrity, and availability of patient data. These threats can cause severe harm to both patients and healthcare providers, including financial losses, reputational damage, and even endangering patients' lives.

The adoption of new technologies and tools is essential to improve the quality and efficiency of healthcare services. However, the introduction of new technologies can also create challenges for healthcare providers, particularly with regard to workforce adaptability. As new technologies and tools are introduced, healthcare providers must ensure that their workforce is adequately trained and equipped to use them effectively. This requires significant investments in training and education, as well as the development of new roles and job functions. Interoperability is a key challenge in the implementation of Healthcare 4.0. The use of different technologies and software systems in healthcare organizations can hinder the ability to share and exchange data seamlessly between them. To address this issue, interoperability standards and protocols need to be developed and implemented. This requires collaboration among healthcare providers, technology vendors, and regulatory bodies to ensure that the systems are compatible and can communicate effectively. However, achieving interoperability is not a trivial task, as it requires significant investments in technology, resources, and policy. Healthcare providers must be willing to collaborate and invest in the necessary infrastructure and resources to achieve interoperability and realize the benefits of Healthcare 4.0.

The advent of Healthcare 4.0 has brought a new emphasis on patient empowerment and engagement. With the new technologies and tools, patients now have access to vast amounts of health information, and they are increasingly taking a more active role in managing their health. Healthcare providers must find ways to support this trend by providing patients with the necessary tools and information to make informed decisions about their health. This includes providing access to their medical records, as well as tools and resources that can help them monitor their health and track their progress. Additionally, healthcare providers must ensure that patients are actively involved in the care planning process and can communicate effectively with their healthcare team. This requires a shift in the traditional power dynamic between patients and healthcare providers and may require significant investments in patient education and engagement initiatives. The emergence of Healthcare 4.0 has opened up new possibilities for improving the quality and efficiency of healthcare services. However, there are various challenges that must be addressed to realize the full potential of these technologies. To overcome these challenges, significant investments are required in areas such as technology, training, and infrastructure. Despite all the challenges, addressing them will result in significant benefits in terms of improved healthcare outcomes, patient experience, and operational efficiencies.

## 1.5  Conclusion

Healthcare 4.0 is poised to transform the healthcare industry and enhance patient outcomes through the utilization of advanced technologies such as AI, big data analytics, IoT, robotics, and blockchain. The integration of these technologies can enable healthcare providers to offer more individualized care, strengthen disease management and prevention, and enhance overall patient outcomes. The use of recommendation systems in healthcare can make data-driven decisions to improve a patient's treatment and care, utilizing data collected from various sources. The distributed ledger technology of blockchain has the potential to revolutionize the healthcare industry by enhancing data security, reducing administrative costs, and streamlining supply chains. Its decentralized and immutable nature allows for the secure and transparent sharing of medical data among stakeholders and automates administrative tasks. Furthermore, blockchain has the potential to significantly improve healthcare systems' ability and accuracy. This framework can provide secure and effective access to medical data while protecting patient privacy. The framework's ability to meet the needs of patients, providers, and third parties and address privacy and security concerns in Healthcare 4.0 is evaluated.

The future of Healthcare 4.0 is likely to be shaped by continued investments in research and development, common standards and protocols for data sharing, and cybersecurity measures to protect patient data and ethical and responsible use of advanced technologies. By addressing these challenges and investing in developing and implementing Healthcare 4.0, we can work towards a future where healthcare is more personalized, efficient, and accessible to all.

# References

[1] Haleem A, Javaid M, Singh RP, and Suman R. Medical 4.0 technologies for healthcare: features, capabilities, and applications. *Internet of Things and Cyber-Physical Systems.* 2022.

[2] Naumann L, Babitsch B, and Hübner UH. eHealth policy processes from the stakeholders' viewpoint: a qualitative comparison between Austria, Switzerland, and Germany. In: *Health Policy and Technology* (vol. 10, issue 2, p. 100505), 2021. Elsevier BV. https://doi.org/10.1016/j.hlpt.2021.100505

[3] Li J and Carayon P. Health Care 4.0: a vision for smart and connected health care. In: *IISE Transactions on Healthcare Systems Engineering* (pp. 1–10), 2021. Informa UK Limited. https://doi.org/10.1080/24725579.2021.1884627

[4] Deloitte. Healthcare 4.0: How Technology Is Revolutionizing the Way We Care for Our Health. https://www2.deloitte.com/content/dam/Deloitte/lu/Documents/life-sciences-health-care/deloitte-lu-hc-40.pdf. Accessed May 11, 2023.

[5] Frost & Sullivan. Healthcare 4.0: Transforming the Future of Healthcare, 2020. https://www.frost.com/frost-perspectives/healthcare-40-transforming-the-future-of-healthcare/. Accessed May 11, 2023.

[6] Paul S, Riffat M, Yasir A, *et al.* Industry 4.0 applications for medical/healthcare services. *Journal of Sensor and Actuator Networks.* 2021;10(3):43.

[7] Sharma D, Singh Aujla G, and Bajaj R. Evolution from ancient medication to human-centered Healthcare 4.0: a review on health care recommender systems. *International Journal of Communication Systems.* 2019;36:e4058.

[8] Javaid M and Haleem A. Industry 4.0 applications in the medical field: a brief review. *Current Medicine Research and Practice.* 2019;9(3):102–109.

[9] Tortorella GL, Fogliatto FS, Mac Cawley Vergara A, Vassolo R, and Sawhney R. Healthcare 4.0: trends, challenges, and research directions. *Production Planning & Control.* 2019;31(15):1245–1260. doi:10.1080/09537287.2019.1702226.

[10] Al-Jaroodi J, Mohamed N, and Abukhousa E. Health 4.0: on the way to realizing the healthcare of the future. In: *IEEE Access.* 2020;8:211189–211210. doi:10.1109/ACCESS.2020.3038858.

[11] Chanchaichujit J, Tan A, Meng F, and Eaimkhong S. An introduction to Healthcare 4.0. In: *Healthcare 4.0.* Singapore: *Palgrave Pivot,* 2019. https://doi.org/10.1007/978-981-13-8114-0_1.

[12] Mohamed N and Al-Jaroodi J. The impact of industry 4.0 on healthcare system engineering. In: *2019 IEEE International Systems Conference (SysCon)*, Orlando, FL, 2019, pp. 1–7. doi:10.1109/SYSCON.2019.8836715.

[13] Mathew D, Shukla VK, Chaubey A, and Dutta S. Artificial intelligence: hope for future or hype by intellectuals? In: *2021 9th International Conference on Reliability, Infocom Technologies and Optimization (Trends and Future Directions) (ICRITO)*, pp. 1–6, 2021.

[14] Vora J, Nayyar A, Tanwar S, *et al.* BHEEM: a blockchain-based framework for securing electronic health records. In: *2018 IEEE Globecom Workshops (GC Workshops) 2018 Dec 9* (pp. 1–6). IEEE.

[15] Tanwar S, Parekh K, and Evans R. Blockchain-based electronic healthcare record system for Healthcare 4.0 applications. *Journal of Information Security and Applications.* 2020;50:102407.

[16] Grand View Research. Internet of Things (IoT) in Healthcare Market Size, Share and Trends Analysis Report by Component (Medical Devices, Systems and Software, Services), by Application, by End-use, by Region, and Segment Forecasts, 2021–2028, 2021. https://www.grandviewresearch.com/industry-analysis/iot-healthcare-market. Accessed on May 11, 2023.

[17] The Scope of IoT in the Healthcare Industry. https://community.nasscom.in/communities/healthtech-and-life-sciences/scope-iot-healthcare-industry. Accessed in May 11, 2023.

[18] Pang Z, Yang G, Khedri R, and Zhang YT. Introduction to the special section: convergence of automation technology, biomedical engineering, and health informatics toward the Healthcare 4.0. *IEEE Reviews in Biomedical Engineering.* 2018;11:249–259.

[19] Gandomi A and Haider M. Beyond the hype: big data concepts, methods, and analytics. *International Journal of Information Management.* 2015;35 (2):137–144. https://doi.org/10.1016/j.ijinfomgt.2014.10.007.

[20] Jiang F, Jiang Y, Zhi H, *et al.* Artificial intelligence in healthcare: past, present and future. *Stroke and Vascular Neurology.* 2017;2(4):230–243. https://doi.org/10.1136/svn-2017-000101.

[21] Kishor A and Chakraborty C. Artificial intelligence and Internet of Things based Healthcare 4.0 monitoring system. In: *Wireless Personal Communications* (vol. 127, issue 2, pp. 1615–1631), 2021. Springer Science and Business Media LLC. https://doi.org/10.1007/s11277-021-08708-5.

[22] "What Is the Scope of the Hospital and Health Care Management Course?" D Y Patil Online, www.dypatilonline.com/Blogs/what-is-the-scope-of-the-hospital-and-health-care-management-course. Accessed May 11, 2023.

[23] Omni Academy Consulting & Technologies. "Industry 4.0: The Fourth Industrial Revolution – Guide to Industrie 4.0." https://www.omni-academy.com/industry-4-0-the-fourth-industrial-revolution-guide-to-industrie-4-0/. Accessed May 11, 2023.

[24]  Kagermann H, Wahlster W, and Helbig J. Securing the future of German manufacturing industry: recommendations for implementing the strategic initiative INDUSTRIE 4.0. *Final Report of the Industrie 4.0 Working Group (April), 2013*, pp. 1–84.

[25]  Yang F and Gu S. Industry 4.0, a revolution that requires technology and national strategies. *Complex & Intelligent Systems*. 2021;7(3):1311–1325. https://doi.org/10.1007/s40747-020-00267-9.

[26]  European Commission: The Netherlands: Smart Industry. Digital Trans-tnqh_9; formation Monitor (January), 8 (2017). https://ec.europa.eu/growth/tools-databases/dem/monitor/content/netherlands-smart-industry.

[27]  Li L. China's manufacturing locus in 2025: with a comparison of "Made-in-China 2025" and "Industry 4.0." *Technological Forecasting and Social Change*. 2018;135:66–74. https://doi.org/10.1016/j.techfore.2017.05.028.

[28]  Moon H-C, Chung J-E, and Choi S-B. Korea's manufacturing innovation 3.0 initiative. *Journal of Information Management*. 2018;38(1):26–34.

[29]  Shang J. Global healthcare spend to remain stable. https://ihsmarkit.com/research-analysis/global-healthcare-spend-to-remain-stable.html (2020). Accessed February 16, 2021.

[30]  Casey JD, Courtright KR, Rice TW, *et al.* What can a learning health care system teach us about improving outcomes? *Current Opinion in Critical Care*. 2021;27(5):527–536.

[31]  da Silveira F, Rodeghiero Neto I, Molinar Machado F, *et al.* Analysis of industry 4.0 technologies applied to the health sector: a systematic literature review. *Studies in Systems, Decision and Control*. 2019;202:701–709. https://doi.org/10.1007/978-3-030-14730-3_73.

[32]  Rehamm MU, Andargolie AE, and Pousti H. Healthcare 4.0: trends, challenges and benefits. In: *Australasian Conference on Information Systems*, 2019, pp. 556–564.

[33]  Karatas M, Eriskin L, Deveci M, Pamucar M, and Garg H. Big data for healthcare industry 4.0: applications, challenges and future perspectives. *Expert Systems with Applications*. 2022;200:116912. https://doi.org/10.1016/j.eswa.2022.116912.

[34]  Popov VV, Kudryavtseva EV, Kumar Katiyar N, *et al.* Industry 4.0 and digitalization in healthcare. *Materials*. 2022;15(6):2140. https://doi.org/10.3390/ma15062140.

[35]  Valamede LS and Santos Akkari AC. Health 4.0: a conceptual approach to evaluate the application of digital technologies in the healthcare field. In: *Brazilian Technology Symposium*, 2020, pp. 17–24.

*Chapter 2*

# Deep learning-based convolutional neural networks for healthcare systems

*Wazir Muhammad[1], Zuhaibuddin Bhutto[2], Ayaz Hussain[1] and Salman Masroor[3]*

## Abstract

Everyday chronic diseases appears in different variants and have affected the whole world community as well as disturbed the worldwide economy and human health system. However, the earlier healthcare system was monitored by conventional techniques, which is not suitable to alert the community to control the unpredictable pandemic. Furthermore, previously developed algorithms depend on manually collected information from the different locations of countries and have chances of errors. Our proposed book's chapters discuss the recent algorithms and applications used in several deep learning-based human healthcare systems including medical image classifying, image enhancement, and medical brain tumor detection. Furthermore, we also discuss different medical image datasets used during the training as well as testing for designing the novel human healthcare monitoring model to evaluate the patient status response timely. Finally, explain the latest medical imaging software packages as well as medical imaging training and test datasets to assess the performance of different diseases of a patient.

**Keywords:** MRI images; Convolutional neural networks; Healthcare

## 2.1 Introduction

Recently, the healthcare system introduced a new way in the field of artificial intelligence (AI) and computer vision tasks, where a huge amount of biomedical data is available to obtain a remarkable performance to decide the patient's disease

[1]Department of Electrical Engineering, Balochistan University of Engineering and Technology, Khuzdar, Pakistan
[2]Department of Computer System Engineering, Balochistan University of Engineering and Technology, Khuzdar, Pakistan
[3]Department of Mechanical Engineering, National Taiwan University of Science and Technology, New Taipei, Taiwan ROC

properly. By taking into account several aspects of the patient's data, including molecular feature variation, environmental influences, electronic health records (EHRs), and the patient's way of life. Precision medicine is an innovative approach, which supports the decision to take proper treatment of each patient. In this situation, doctors are allowed to decide on a treatment based on the patient's genetic information at the right time [1–3]. For research in the field of medical science, the quality of data still is a challenging task. One of the most challenging obstacles is the security of biomedical data (patient personal data), visualization, and privacy. Multiple data sources have been linked earlier in an attempt to establish mutually beneficial information, which can be involved in predictive research [4–6]. Notwithstanding the reality that machine learning-based predictive tools offer tremendous commitment, but still they have not widely used in the medical field. Biological data still face significant obstacles to effective use because of their high dimensionality, variety, time dependency, sparsity, and irregularity. Asking a subject–matter expert to arbitrarily determine the phenotypes to utilize is a tactic that is widely employed in scientific studies. The proper definition of feature space is a collection of the same class of features that are very correlated to each other. The representations required for prediction and automatically found from the raw data using representation learning techniques. Deep learning techniques are used to extract the low, medium and high-level features from the medical images to classify the different stages of diseases. Furthermore, deep learning algorithm involved in different computer vision tasks, such as speech recognition, language processing and medical image enhancement to shows the incredible potential.

## 2.2    Literature survey

This section offers a thorough evaluation of medical imaging algorithms that include current cutting-edge techniques. Brain tumors are a difficult problem in today's medical field, which is an abnormal mass of tissues. In the brain, tumor cells multiply and divide quickly and appear unrestrained by normal cell regulatory mechanisms. A deep CNN technique was advised by Gurunathan *et al.* [7] for the detection and diagnosis of brain tumors. Authors of [7] divided the whole process into three stages, such as preprocessing, classification, and segmentation stages. Hospital hygiene is a way to understand the infection pathways and implement an efficient infection control policy. One application of hospital hygiene named a hand hygiene tracking system is discussed by Abubeker *et al.* [8]. The hand hygiene tracking system approach uses an Internet of Things (IoT) technique to monitor and track hygiene as well as to reduce healthcare-related infections. Medical image processing using deep convolutional neural network (CNN) further improves disease detection and recognition performance. The initial stage of cancer detection is still a challenging task for doctors because it is one of the deadliest medical conditions. Gangurde *et al.* [9] suggested a different approach to identify the type of cancer. In this approach authors [9] select a 5,000-person of sample and is tested on the gene profile. The ability to make decisions quickly is one of the most crucial skills in healthcare. Clinicians and other healthcare professionals can reduce the risks by making treatment-related decisions in advance if they have more information beforehand. Healthcare and bioinformatics machine learning can process vast amounts of data and provide insightful information that can aid healthcare practitioners in making timely decisions. Additionally, it enables them to examine a patient's medical background and forecast results based on their course of treatment and lifestyle. On the other hand, they can also plan ahead and recommend a thorough course of therapy to the patient, which will cut costs and improve the patient's experience overall. In their comprehensive evaluation of explainable deep learning in healthcare, Jin *et al.* [10] placed a strong emphasis on the models' interpretability. Additionally, the author of [10] provides an algorithm-based reference to open the window for future work in the field of medical science. Abdel-Jaber *et al.* [11] reviewed a number of commonly employed deep CNN-based deep learning techniques, as well as their network architectures, real-world applications, and its challenging tasks.

Cloud and IoT-based health-preserving deep learning-based algorithms were introduced by Munirathinam *et al.* [12]. In [12], authors mainly focus on developing a novel technique for e-healthcare systems to track the level of decreased diseases through IoT and cloud technologies, as well as a deep learning technique and also employed the sets of fuzzy for temporal characteristics. The proposed system [12] collects medical information from a variety of patients who are using e-healthcare helping gadgets and are spread across different locations. Additionally, to increase the diagnosis research quality of disease, more medical-related areas will adopt deep learning algorithms in the future, as shown by Faust *et al.* in their study [13]. Electronic-based healthcare medical data and their observations are typically irregular and periodic in nature. To keep accurate medical records, store information about previous illnesses, extrapolate present ailment states, and forecast upcoming healthcare results, DeepCare approach is one neural network-based approach that was suggested by Pham *et al.* [14]. Initially, features of the DeepCare network model have used the historical records of patient health and portray care episodes as a vector. DeepCare algorithm is used to maintain the periodic interval of time events because it uses the concept of long short-term memory (LSTM). Additionally, DeepCare directly simulates medical procedures that alter the development of sickness and influence potential medical risks that appear in the future. In their discussion of the construction and operation of deep neural networks, Kaul *et al.* [15] put particular emphasis on how these networks might be used to diagnose and treat conditions, such as cancer disease detection, Alzheimer's, diabetes, and Parkinson type disease. A thorough analysis of [16] compares deep learning models' diagnosis performance to that of medical practitioners. A key conclusion of the review is that a few publications offered data that were superficially validated or contrasted to show the effectiveness of deep learning architectures and medical experts apply a similar type of samples.

Another problem during the training of redundant features and the unnecessary class imbalance was proposed by Sreejith *et al.* [17] known as a clinical decision support system (CDSS). This method balances the dataset at the present level of data and employs a wrapper technique for feature selection. The review study by Kashani *et al.* [18] discuss 146 studies published between 2015 and 2020. The authors of that review study list, contrast, and taxonomically categorize current investigations in the Healthcare IoT (HIoT) systems. A computer-aided diagnosis (CAD) method is presented by Sweetlin *et al.* [19] to increase the diagnostic consistency and accuracy of image understanding of pulmonary tuberculosis. To choose the best feature subset, the authors of this approach [19] combined approaches like cuckoo search optimization and a one-against-all support vector machine (SVM) classifier. The treatment for urticaria, a common allergy illness that affects people of all ages, is provided by Christopher *et al.* in their article from [20]. To classify diseases and enhance clinicians' decision-making, Leema *et al.* [21] discuss a differential evolution with global information and backpropagation (DEGI-BP) optimized ANN supported by a CAD system. This method's improved best mutation strategy as well as increase the exploration of search space. A movement-based illness that disturbs the patient's neurological system is known as Parkinson's disease (PD). In PD, a patient uses a wearable sensor, which gathers the information frequently. It becomes difficult to analyze gait abnormalities in PD because sensors produce a time-sampled sequence of data. The difficult task of creating an accurate clinical decision-making system (CDMS) helps the doctor to determine the degree of gait irregularities due to Parkinson's disease in patients as suggested by Jane *et al.* [22].

## 2.3   Deep learning algorithms

Artificial neural networks (ANNs) and representation learning include as unsupervised, semi-supervised, or supervised learning as a subclass of machine learning (ML) algorithms known as deep learning. Deep learning approaches involved in different fields include meteorology, bioinformatics, medication research, and analysis of medical images. Medical imaging-based deep learning frameworks are vision transformers, CNNs, recurrent neural networks, deep belief networks, and reinforcement learning. ANNs were modeled after the biological systems' scattered information processing and communication nodes. The differences between biological brains and ANNs are numerous. The organic brain of most living organisms is an analogue and dynamic. In contrast, ANNs are typically static and symbolic. The use of more layers in a serial fashion is what is meant by the phrase "deep learning." Boltzmann machine, autoencoder, CNN, recurrent neural network, and multilayer perceptron (MLP) are the principal algorithms. Table 2.1 gives a general overview of deep learning techniques.

### 2.3.1   Multilayer perceptron

Multilayer perceptron (ML) is a fully connected type of feedforward ANN, which is popularly read as an MLP. The word "MLP" is vague. It may be employed to describe any feedforward ANN, but particularly, those networks composed of numerous layers of perceptron (with threshold activation). Particularly when they

*Table 2.1   Summary of deep learning algorithms used in healthcare system*

| Methods | Category of disease | Type of DL algorithms | Year |
| --- | --- | --- | --- |
| Potghan *et al.* [23] | Lung tumor | MLP | 2018 |
| Ting *et al.* [24] | Breast cancer | MLP | 2017 |
| Lorencin *et al.* [25] | Bladder cancer diagnosis | MLP | 2020 |
| Sonawane *et al.* [26] | Heart disease | MLP | 2014 |
| Selwal *et al.* [27] | Thyroid disease | MLP | 2020 |
| Petrosian *et al.* [28] | Alzheimer's | RNN | 2001 |
| Liu *et al.* [29] | Influenza | RNN | 2018 |
| Krishnan *et al.* [30] | Heart disease | RNN | 2021 |
| Rejaibi *et al.* [31] | Depression | RNN | 2022 |
| Chovatiya *et al.* [32] | Dengue | RNN | 2019 |
| Abiyev *et al.* [33] | Chest diseases | CNN | 2018 |
| Muhammad *et al.* [34,35] | COVID-19 | CNN | 2022 |
| Ahmad *et al.* [36] | Alzheimer's disease | CNN | 2020 |
| Juneja *et al.* [37] | Thoracic syndrome | CNN | 2021 |
| Tariq *et al.* [38] | Lung disease | CNN | 2019 |
| Rathod *et al.* [39] | Skin diseases | CNN | 2018 |
| Muhammad *et al.* [40] | MRI | CNN | 2023 |
| de Souza *et al.* [41] | Parkinson's disease | Boltzmann Machines | 2021 |
| Pranata *et al.* [42] | Respiratory infections | Boltzmann Machines | 2022 |
| Jayashree *et al.* [43] | COVID-19 | Boltzmann Machines | 2022 |
| Wahid *et al.* [44] | Pneumonia | Boltzmann Machines | 2022 |
| Pandey *et al.* [45] | Arrhythmia | Boltzmann Machines | 2021 |
| Benyelles *et al.* [46] | COVID-19 | Autoencoder | 2021 |
| Saravanan *et al.* [47] | Glaucoma | Autoencoder | 2022 |
| Martinez-Murcia *et al.* [48] | Alzheimer's disease | Autoencoder | 2019 |
| Xiao *et al.* [49] | Thorax disease | Autoencoder | 2023 |
| Nasser *et al.* [50] | Osteoporosis disease | Autoencoder | 2017 |

comprise a single hidden layer, multilayer perceptron neural network is normally named "vanilla" neural networks [51]. A simple architecture of MLP is used: input, hidden, and out layers, which are designed as three layers of nodes. Each node, except an input node, a neuron is used followed by a nonlinear type of activation function, as depicted in Figure 2.1. MLP utilizes a chain rule [52] based supervised learning technique called backpropagation or reverse mode of automatic differentiation for training. The main difference between MLP and linear perceptron is the number of layers because MLP uses more layers with different types of nonlinear activation functions [53].

## 2.3.2   Recurrent neural network

A recurrent neural network (RNN) is a subclass member of ANN that creates feedback (cycle) between the nodes as illustrated in Figure 2.2. In Figure 2.2, the resultant output of ANN gives the back response to hidden layers. The RNN network type of architecture creates a progressive dynamic performance. RNN is an advanced and modified version of feedforward neural networks. The performance

Input layers          Hidden layers          Output layers

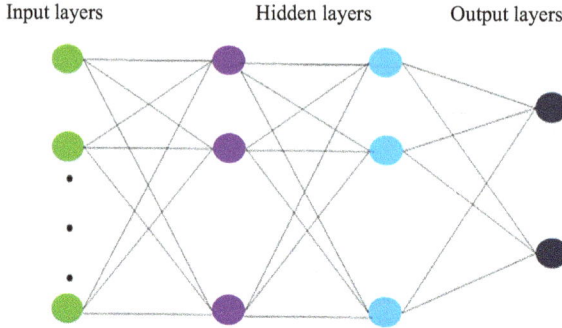

*Figure 2.1   General diagram of MLP*

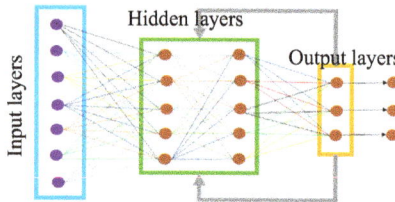

*Figure 2.2   General diagram of RNN*

process of the RNN network depends on a variable length of an input set of data samples by employing its internal memory or state [54–56]. Furthermore, it can be used in different tasks such as unsegmented handwriting recognition [23] or speech recognition [24]. Additionally, we explain RNN behavior as a network with an infinite number of responses, while CNN has a limited number of impulse types of response. Both classes of architecture exhibit dynamic response.

## 2.3.3   CNN

The gap between human and computer skills is increasingly being closed by AI. To get exceptional outcomes, both experts and lay people concentrate on a variety of aspects of the subject. The aim of this area is to give robots the ability to see the world in a way that is comparable to how humans do. To use the knowledge of a variety of tasks, such as image enhancement, video recognition, natural language processing, media reconstruction to provide the healthy and timely response to the end user (patients). A deep learning-based CNN/ConvNet method selects an input image with different components and objects in the image weights and biases that can be learned and be able to differentiate across them. A ConvNet significantly requires a fewer pre-processing compared to other classification methods as shown in Figure 2.3. Different from the basic hand-designed approach, CNN filters learn features and properties with sufficient training. The design of a CNN was based on how the visual cortex is planned and mirrors the human brain's linking network of neurons. There is just one section of the visual field where individual neurons respond to stimuli, called the receptive field.

## 2.3.4   Boltzmann machine

A Sherrington–Kirkpatrick model, also known as a stochastic spin-glass model with an external field, is a Boltzmann machine [54]. It uses a statistical physics method that is applied to cognitive science [55] due to the locality and Hebbian character of their training algorithm (being trained by Hebb's rule), parallelism, and similarity of their dynamics to straightforward physical processes, as depicted in Figure 2.4. However, if the connection is appropriately restricted, the learning can be made efficient enough to be effective for practical applications. Boltzmann machines with uncontrolled connectivity have not been demonstrated to be useful for actual problems in machine learning or inference.

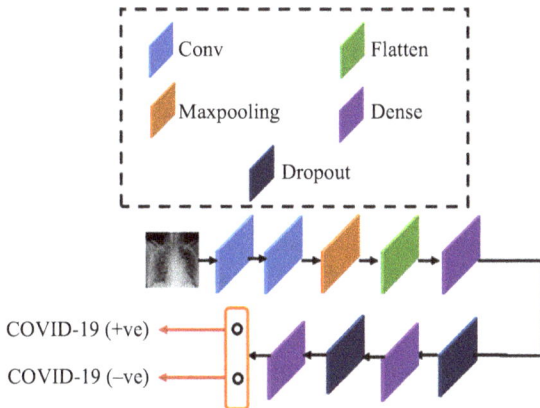

*Figure 2.3   Basic CNN architecture of chest X-ray images for classification task*

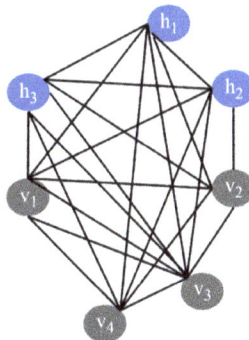

*Figure 2.4   General view of Boltzmann machine*

## 2.3.5   Autoencoder

An ANN called an autoencoder is used to learn effective coding of unlabeled data (unsupervised learning) [56] as shown in Figure 2.5. An autoencoder learns two operations: an encoding operation that modifies the input data and a decoding operation that reconstructs the input data from the encoded representation. For dimensionality reduction, typically, the autoencoder learns an effective representation (encoding) for a set of data. Autoencoders are used to solve a variety of issues, such as word meaning acquisition, feature detection, anomaly detection, and facial recognition.

## 2.3.6   Major applications of deep learning-based healthcare system

CNNs are built on deep learning and have recently obtained remarkably improved performance in the areas of computer vision and medical imaging. Advances in computational power graphics processing units (GPUs), parallelized computing, privacy-preserving Edge AI (on-device processing), and more effective frameworks for modeling training with annotated data are driving deep learning. To recognize patterns, the GPU computer first receives raw data before producing its own representations. Very complex functions that offer high accuracy in medical image identification applications can be trained using deep learning methods. The uses of deep learning in healthcare systems are covered here in the following subsections.

### 2.3.6.1   Clinical research

A branch of medical science called clinical research, which can assess the efficacy and security of medical devices, medications, diagnostic instruments, and treatment regimens, intended for human use. These can be used to treat, diagnose, or relieve the symptoms of illnesses. Clinical research is a separate discipline from clinical practice. While established treatments are used in clinical practice, gathering evidence to support treatment is the focus of clinical research.

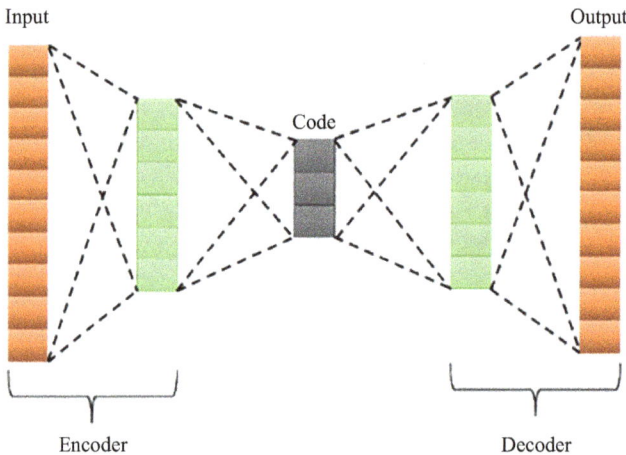

*Figure 2.5   General architecture of autoencoder*

## 2.3.6.2    Drug discovery

Drug discovery is a method in which new candidates of medications are obtained in the areas of medicine, pharmacology, and biotechnology. In the past, drugs were discovered accidentally, like penicillin, or by extracting the active ingredient from therapies that were already in use. A method referred to as conventional pharmacology was used in recent years for searching chemical archives of manufactured small molecules, natural products, or extracts in whole cells or organisms for substances that had the essential therapeutic impact. Since the comprehensive sequencing of the human genome made it feasible to perform rapid cloning and synthesis of enormous quantities of purified proteins, reverse pharmacology has evolved into an established method for high throughput screening of large compound libraries against isolated biological targets that are hypothesized to be disease-modifying. The complete drug cycle is shown in Figure 2.6.

## 2.3.6.3    Electronic health record

An electronic health record (EHR) converts a patient's paper medical record to a digital one. EHRs are patient-centered, real-time records that give authorized users easy and secure access to information. An EHR system may give a broader view of how a patient is being treated, regardless of whether it incorporates the patient's health and treatment history and is intended to go above the standard clinical data collected in a provider's office.

## 2.3.6.4    COVID-19 detection and classification

In late December 2019, a Chinese doctor in Wuhan, the provincial capital of Hubei, China's mainland, discovered the current coronavirus outbreak. This new virus is very contagious and has spread quickly throughout the entire world. As a result of the

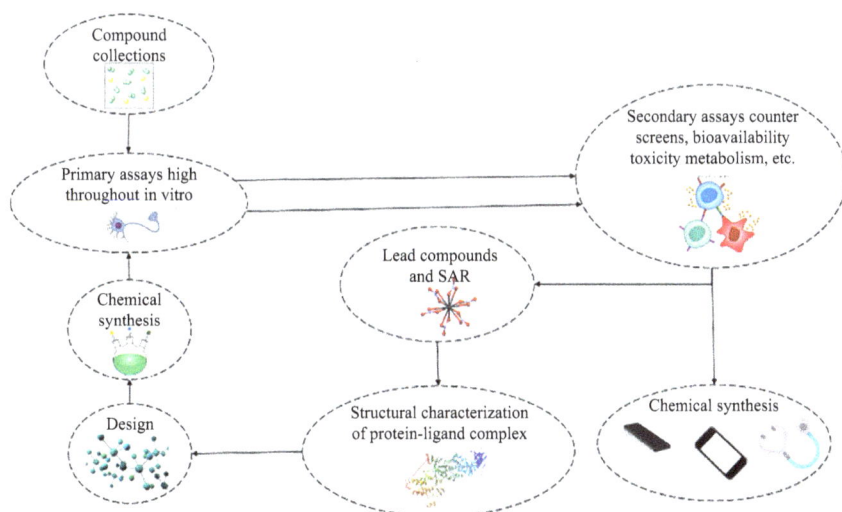

*Figure 2.6    Drug discovery cycle*

outbreak spreading to 216 nations, on January 30, 2020, the World Health Organization (WHO) designated it a worldwide health emergency with global concern. The WHO designated this new coronavirus-associated acute respiratory disorder as COVID-19 on February 11, 2020. Computer vision can greatly aid in meeting this problem as nations all over the world struggle to fight against the disease.

### 2.3.6.5    Genomics analysis

Deep learning models improve biological data's interpretability and understanding. With the aid of these models' comprehensive data analysis tools, investigators can better comprehend and interpret genetic variation to create genome-based therapies. Scientists can extract properties from fixed-size deoxyribonucleic acid (DNA) sequence windows by using CNNs, which are often employed.

### 2.3.6.6    Healthcare data analytics

Models based on deep learning have the best degree of correctness and can evaluate EHR faster than traditional methods. Medical notes, results of laboratory tests, diagnoses, and prescription information are just a few examples of organized and unorganized information that can be found in EHR. Additionally, smartphones and wearable technology offer helpful information about lifestyle.

### 2.3.6.7    Health monitoring

Medical professionals are increasingly using AI and computer vision technologies to track their patients' fitness and well-being. These evaluations allow medical professionals to make faster, better judgments, even in life-threatening situations. The amount of blood lost during operations can be measured by computer vision models to detect whether the patient has reached a critical stage or not.

### 2.3.6.8    Medical imaging

Computer vision is used in a range of healthcare applications to help medical personnel treat more effectively. Medical imaging, also known as an analysis of medical images, is one such method that makes particular tissues and organs visible to help with diagnosis. Surgeons and physicians can effortlessly inspect a patient's interior organs and spot any issues or abnormalities through medical image analysis. Medical imaging includes X-rays radiography, ultrasound, magnetic resonance imaging (MRI), endoscopy, and other specialties.

### 2.3.6.9    Remote online patient health monitoring

It has become more and more common for patients to be able to monitor some aspects of their health from their own place or home as well as manage both acute and chronic diseases thanks to remote patient health monitoring. Infection risk and travel expenses for patients are also decreased. Remote patient health monitoring and telehealth are effective together when patients need to be followed up on for certain medical issues. Additionally, it can help individuals who find it difficult to travel to avoid health problems. Remote patient monitoring can be employed to monitor a wide range of symptoms and illnesses, including diabetes, chronic obstructive, pulmonary disease, cardiac problems, high blood pressure, sleep apnea, and weight loss or gain.

## 2.4 Datasets used for deep learning algorithms in healthcare system

In this section, we are present the different algorithms that used for specific diseases with proper datasets. The main category of diseases includes such as cancer, Parkinson, heart failure, COVID, and chest X-ray images in Table 2.2. The complete information in Table 2.2 is discussed by Shamshirband *et al.* [57].

*Table 2.2   Summary of the articles that have been used in deep learning DL in healthcare system [57]*

| Disease category | Article | Year | Data | DL method |
|---|---|---|---|---|
| Breast cancer | Dhungel *et al.* [58] | 2017 | INbreast | CNN+DBN |
| | Jiao *et al.* [59] | 2018 | DDSM MIAS | CNN |
| | Samala *et al.* [60] | 2016 | DM, SFM-UMDM, SFM-USF | DCNN |
| | Wahab *et al.* [61] | 2017 | MITOS12 TUPAC16 | CNN |
| | Zhang *et al.* [62] | 2016 | 227 SWE images of 121 female patients | DBN (PGBM) |
| Gastric cancer | Sharma *et al.* [63] | 2017 | – | CNN |
| Lung cancer | Sun *et al.* [64] | 2017 | LIDC/IDRI | CNN+DBN +SDAE |
| Brain cancer | Zhao *et al.* [65] | 2018 | BRATS 2013, 2015, 2016 | FCNN+CRF-RNN |
| | Tabbar and Halici [66] | 2016 | Dataset III from BCI Competition II dataset 2b from BCI Competition IV | CNN+SAE |
| Cancer | Xiao *et al.* [67] | 2018 | RNA-seq (LUAD + STAD + BRCA) | DNN |
| Multiple sclerosis | Yoo *et al.* [68] | 2017 | Myelin and T1w images | CNN |
| | Yoo *et al.* [69] | 2018 | Myelin and T1w images | DBN |
| Parkinson | Choi *et al.* [70] | 2017 | PPMI SNUH | CNN |
| Heart failure | Choi *et al.* [71] | 2016 | Sutter Palo Alto Medical Foundation (Sutter-PAMF) | RNN adopted by GRU |
| | Al Rahhal *et al.* [72] | 2016 | MIT-BIH INCART SVDB | DNN + DAE |
| Epilepsy and seizure | Acharya *et al.* [73] | 2017 | EEG signals from the Bonn University database | CNN |
| Mental workload | Yin and Zhang [74] | 2017 | – | SDAE |
| Multiple diseases | Miotto *et al.* [75] | 2016 | – | SDN |
| | Nie *et al.* [76] | 2015 | EveryoneHealthy WebMD MedlinePlus | SCDP |

## 2.5    Medical imaging software

Both medical professionals and patients as end users tremendously benefit from the implementation of medical image analysis tools. Recently, hospitals, diagnostic centers, ambulatory surgical centers, academic institutions, and research centers have all adopted the practice of using medical image processing. However, the market for medical imaging analysis software is projected to grow as a result of the rising demand for medical imaging, particularly in light of the fact that some of the market's major competitors are enormous leading brands that are taking an innovative approach to medicine. The main software packages to analyze the medical imaging are the following:

- Nova RIS.
- NovaPACS.
- UltraLinQ.
- Ambra Health.
- Dicom Systems Unifier Platform.
- ProtonPACS.
- Intelligent Medical Software (IMS).
- ARANZ MEDICAL.

## 2.6    Common medical imaging datasets

There are many datasets available for medical image enhancement using deep learning-based CNNs. In this section, we can discuss some important medical imaging datasets.

### 2.6.1    Alzheimer's disease neuroimaging initiative

The Alzheimer's disease neuroimaging initiative (ADNI) image datasets are a collection of brain scans and related data from people with Alzheimer's disease, healthy older people, and younger people. The datasets are used by researchers to study the progression of Alzheimer's disease and to develop and test new treatments.

### 2.6.2    The Cancer Imaging Archive

The Cancer Imaging Archive (TCIA) is a sizable repository of cancer-related medical images that are open to download by anyone. The National Cancer Institute (NCI) is head of maintaining the archive, which features images from various cancer types.

### 2.6.3    CheXlocalize

A segmentation dataset on chest X-rays called CheXlocalize has been annotated by radiologists [77]. The dataset consists of pixel-level segmentations and most-representative points, which are two different forms of radiologist annotations for the localization of 10 diseases. Images from the CheXpert validation and test sets were annotated. The dataset also includes two different sets of radiologist annotations: (1) benchmark pixel-level segmentations and most representative points on the test set, drawn by a separate team of three board-certified radiologists; and (2) ground-truth pixel-level segmentations on the validation and test sets, drawn by two board-certified radiologists. About 234 chest X-rays from 200 patients make up the validation set, whereas 668 chest X-rays from 500 patients make up the test set.

### 2.6.4    CheXphoto

As a part of the validation and test sets for CheXpert, all 234 X-rays from 200 patients and 668 X-rays from 500 patients, respectively, underwent both natural and artificial modifications. Randomly chosen from the CheXpert training set, 10,507 X-rays from 3,000 distinct patients were then exposed to a training set comprising genuine images and fake modifications.

### 2.6.5    CheXplanation

Radiologists' annotations and competition for automated pathological segmentation are included in the chest X-ray segmentation dataset. The dataset can be used to evaluate the model assumptions for X-ray interpretation.

### 2.6.6    CheXpert

CheXpert is a competition for automated chest X-ray interpretation that includes radiologist-labeled reference standard assessment sets, uncertainty labels, and a sizable chest X-ray dataset [78]. When it comes to clinical decision support and workflow prioritization, large-scale screening and global population health programs perform better in a variety of medical situations. It may be very helpful to have an automated interpretation of chest radiographs on par with expert radiologists.

### 2.6.7    Diverse dermatology images

Triage of skin diseases may be facilitated by AI. The majority of AI models, however, have not been thoroughly tested on photos of people with different skin tones or rare disorders [79]. To identify potential biases in algorithm performance, we created the diverse dermatology images (DDI) dataset, the first meticulously curated, pathologically verified picture collection with a diversity of skin tones.

### 2.6.8    EchoNet-dynamic

A baseline for analyzing heart motion and chamber sizes is provided by this dataset, which includes 10,030 tagged echocardiography films and human expert annotations (measurements, tracings, and computations) [80].

### 2.6.9    EchoNet-LVH

The 12,000 tagged echocardiography films in the EchoNet-LVH dataset, along with the measurements, tracings, and calculations made by human experts, serve as a baseline for the investigation of heart chamber size and wall thickness [81].

## 2.6.10    ImageNet

ImageNet is a large-scale medical image dataset that contains more than 1 million images of various diseases and conditions. The dataset is divided into several categories, such as cancer, diabetes, and Alzheimer's disease.

## 2.6.11    Kaggle

Kaggle medical image datasets are collections of medical images that have been organized and annotated for use in machine learning and deep learning applications. The datasets typically contain a large number of images, often in the tens of thousands, and are organized into categories or classes. The images in the datasets can be of any type, including X-rays, MRI scans, and computerized tomography (CT) scans.

## 2.6.12    LERA—lower extremity radiographs

A total of 182 patients who had radiographic tests at Stanford between 2003 and 2014 have been incorporated into this dataset. There are additional pictures of each patient's foot, knee, ankle, and hip.

## 2.6.13    The Lung Image Database Consortium

Thoracic CT images from diagnostic and screening lung cancer CT scans are included in the Lung Imaging Database Consortium image collection (LIDC-IDRI). These images have been labeled with identified lesions. There is a global resource available online for the creation, instruction, and assessment of computer-assisted diagnostic (CAD) approaches for the early identification and diagnosis of lung cancer. This public–private partnership, which was started by the NCI and promoted by the Foundation for the National Institutes of Health (FNIH) with active engagement from the Food and Drug Administration (FDA), highlights the effectiveness of a consortium built utilizing a consensus-based technique.

## 2.6.14    MRNet dataset

The 1,370 knee MRI tests conducted at Stanford University Medical Center make up the MRNet dataset. The dataset has 1,104 abnormal examinations (80.6%), including 508 meniscal tears and 319 anterior cruciate ligament (ACL) tears (33.3%). Labels were manually extracted from clinical records.

## 2.6.15    Multimodal pulmonary embolism dataset

In this dataset, 1,794 Stanford patients are used who are at risk for pulmonary embolism. Chest CT images, patient demographics, and medical background make up the dataset.

## 2.6.16    Musculoskeletal radiographs

A sizable dataset of bone X-rays is known as musculoskeletal radiographs (MURA). The task of classifying an X-ray scan as normal or abnormal is left to algorithms [82]. More than 1.7 billion individuals worldwide are affected by musculoskeletal problems, which account for 30 million visits to emergency rooms each year and are steadily rising.

## 2.6.17    National Institutes of Health Image Gallery

The NIH medical image datasets are a collection of medical images that have been collected and made available by the National Institutes of Health (NIH) [83]. The images in the dataset can be used to train and test algorithms for various medical image analysis tasks.

## 2.6.18    National Library of Medicine MedPix

In MedPix, there are roughly 9,000 participants, 12,000 patient case scenarios, and 59,000 photos. The National Library of Medicine makes available this website as a free, open-access online repository of clinical themes, teaching cases, and medical imagery. Our primary target audience is made up of physicians, nurses, allied health professionals, nursing and medical students, as well as those who are interested in medicine. The information is arranged according to the organ system in which the disease occurs, the pathology category, the patient profiles, the image classification, and the image captions. Patients' symptoms and indicators, diagnoses, organ systems, picture modalities, and image descriptions can all be used to search the collection.

## 2.6.19    Open Images Dataset

The Open Images Dataset is an extensive, open-source dataset that contains over 9 million images. The dataset is organized into over 15,000 categories, and each image is labeled with one or more of these categories.

## 2.6.20    Public lung database to address drug response

The Prevent Cancer Foundation (PCF), which works with the National Cancer Institute (NCI) to speed the development of computer-aided quantitative disease monitoring techniques, provided gracious financing that made this database possible [84]. NCI research funds have helped to fund a portion of Cornell Medical Center's imaging research projects. This tool is an inspiring example of a public–private partnership working together to advance the treatment of lung cancer, the deadliest of all malignancies. There are currently a few annotated CT imaging scans in the database that demonstrate many of the important issues with evaluating massive lung lesions. On the website, you may download each image for free. Upon establishing an acceptable file format, the annotations will also be made accessible. Both the CT images and their annotations can be seen using a variety of interactive image viewing tools on the website. Lesion measurements and growth analysis presentations are also included.

## 2.6.21    RadFusion

RadFusion Multimodal Pulmonary Embolism Dataset collected the data from 1,794 patients susceptible to pulmonary embolism at the Stanford University Medical Center [85]. Chest computed tomography (CT), patient characteristics, and medical history make up the dataset.

## 2.6.22    RadGraph

The RadGraph dataset, which contains radiological reports from various entities, is built on an original approach to information extraction. There are 221K papers with 10.5M automatically generated annotations and 600 reports with 30K radiologist annotations. Two sets of board-certified radiologist annotations for 100 radiology reports from the MIMIC-CXR and CheXpert databases make up the test dataset. A development dataset includes radiologist annotations for 500 radiological reports from the MIMIC-CXR dataset. Together with mappings to related chest radiographs, the inference dataset includes automatically produced annotations for 500 CheXpert reports (13,783 people and 9,908 relations) and 220,763 MIMIC-CXR reports (6 million entities and 4 million relations).

## 2.6.23    Re3Data

Re3 is an open-access scientific service to provide research funding, access to libraries and a list of all publishers with repositories of international data. It includes research data repositories from several academic disciplines. For its 2012 debut, money was granted by the German Research Foundation. Re3Data contains information from more than 2,000 research subjects that have been divided into numerous key categories.

## 2.6.24    The Reference Image Database to Evaluate Response

The Reference Image Database to Evaluate Response (RIDER) dataset to come up with a unanimous agreement technique to optimize the tumor reaction with the help of software tools. Furthermore, a comparative analysis of software tools for evaluating the efficacy of tumor reaction to therapy. Additionally, we create a freely available collection of serial images obtained during lung cancer drug and radiation therapy clinical trials. In RIDER, a photograph of real people and phantoms is also available which were shot in settings where the biology or size of the tumors were known to be unaffected. Thanks to the RIDER studies, crucial clinical assessments, like figuring out whether a certain tumor is responding to treatment, will be less ambiguous.

## 2.6.25    Stanford knee MRI with multi-task evaluation

Stanford knee MRI with multi-task evaluation (SKM-TEA) provides a 155 quantitative double echo steady-state MRI knee images. In SKM-TEA, dataset having complete annotations and imaging information was collected. The information comprises bounding boxes for 16 diseases, segmentations of six tissues, and the raw k-space and digital imaging and communications in medicine (DICOM).

## 2.6.26    Stanford Medical ImageNet

The Stanford Medical ImageNet medical image datasets are a set of image datasets that were created by Stanford University for use in research on medical image analysis. The databases include X-rays, MRI scans, and CT scans among other types of imaging.

## 2.6.27    *Thyroid Ultrasound Cine-clip*

Thyroid Ultrasound Cine-clip used 167 Stanford participants ($n$=192) with thyroid nodules verified by biopsy. The dataset includes histological diagnoses, lesion size and location, patient demographics, radiologist-annotated segmentations, and ultrasound cine-clip pictures.

## 2.6.28    *UCI Machine Learning Repository*

The UCI Machine Learning Repository [86] currently available 622 datasets provide a facility to AI research community. UCI serves as a repository for datasets, domain theories, and data generators used by the machine learning community to develop and evaluate machine learning algorithms. The repository provides a source for research-related medical imaging collections.

## 2.6.29    *COVID-19 dataset*

COVID-19 dataset is a novel data repository maintained by Johns Hopkins University Center for Systems Science and Engineering (JHU CSSE) [87]. This dataset is continuously updated with the guidance of medical experts. COVID-19 dataset collected the best information about data to facilitate the policymaker, public, and doctors to a proper vaccine for patients.

## 2.7    Conclusion

CNN applications on DL performed a crucial part in the area of healthcare because deep learning is a promising field of AI. In the AI, CNN-based medical image processing has attained special attention for disease diagnosis purposes. In addition to its use in the image processing area, CNN has also had extraordinary success with other notable deep learning applications like object recognition, image segmentation, and recommendation systems. This chapter discussed the main applications of deep learning-based medical health system, its related training as well as testing datasets and medical imaging software to identify the disease efficiently.

## References

[1]    Miotto, R., Wang, F., Wang, S., Jiang, X. and Dudley, J.T., Deep learning for healthcare: review, opportunities and challenges. *Briefings in Bioinformatics*, 2018. **19**(6): p. 1236–1246.

[2]    Collins, F.S. and H. Varmus, A new initiative on precision medicine. *New England Journal of Medicine*, 2015. **372**(9): p. 793–795.

[3]    Lyman, G.H. and H.L. Moses, Biomarker tests for molecularly targeted therapies – the key to unlocking precision medicine. *The New England Journal of Medicine*, 2016. **375**(1): p. 4–6.

[4]    Wang, B., Mezlini, A.M., Demir, F., *et al.*, Similarity network fusion for aggregating data types on a genomic scale. *Nature Methods*, 2014. **11**(3): p. 333–337.

[5]   Chen, Y., Li, L., Zhang, G.Q. and Xu, R., Phenome-driven disease genetics prediction toward drug discovery. *Bioinformatics*, 2015. **31**(12): p. i276–i283.

[6]   Xu, R., L. Li, and Q. Wang, dRiskKB: a large-scale disease-disease risk relationship knowledge base constructed from biomedical text. *BMC Bioinformatics*, 2014. **15**(1): p. 1–13.

[7]   Gurunathan, A. and B. Krishnan, Detection and diagnosis of brain tumors using deep learning convolutional neural networks. *International Journal of Imaging Systems and Technology*, 2021. **31**(3): p. 1174–1184.

[8]   Abubeker, K. and S. Baskar, A hand hygiene tracking system with LoRaWAN network for the abolition of hospital-acquired infections. *IEEE Sensors Journal*, 2023. **23**(7): p. 7608–7615.

[9]   Gangurde, R., Jagota, V., Khan, M.S., *et al.*, Developing an efficient cancer detection and prediction tool using convolution neural network integrated with neural pattern recognition. *BioMed Research International*, 2023.

[10]  Jin, D., Sergeeva, E., Weng, W.H., Chauhan, G. and Szolovits, P., Explainable deep learning in healthcare: A methodological survey from an attribution view. *WIREs Mechanisms of Disease*, 2022. **14**(3), p. e1548.

[11]  Abdel-Jaber, H., Devassy, D., Al Salam, A., Hidaytallah, L. and El-Amir, M., A review of deep learning algorithms and their applications in health-care. *Algorithms*, 2022. **15**(2), p. 71.

[12]  Munirathinam, T., S. Ganapathy, and A. Kannan, Cloud and IoT based privacy preserved e-Healthcare system using secured storage algorithm and deep learning. *Journal of Intelligent & Fuzzy Systems*, 2020. **39**(3): p. 3011–3023.

[13]  Faust, O., Hagiwara, Y., Hong, T.J., Lih, O.S. and Acharya, U.R., Deep learning for healthcare applications based on physiological signals: A review. *Computer Methods and Programs in Biomedicine*, 2018. **161**: p. 1–13.

[14]  Pham, T., Tran, T., Phung, D. and Venkatesh, S., Predicting healthcare trajectories from medical records: A deep learning approach. *Journal of Biomedical Informatics*, 2017. **69**: p. 218–229.

[15]  Kaul, D., H. Raju, and B. Tripathy, Deep learning in healthcare. *Deep Learning in Data Analytics: Recent Techniques, Practices and Applications*, 2022: p. 97–115.

[16]  Liu, X., Faes, L., Kale, A.U., *et al.*, A comparison of deep learning performance against health-care professionals in detecting diseases from medical imaging: a systematic review and meta-analysis. *The Lancet Digital Health*, 2019. **1**(6): p. e271–e297.

[17]  Sreejith, S., H.K. Nehemiah, and A. Kannan, Clinical data classification using an enhanced SMOTE and chaotic evolutionary feature selection. *Computers in Biology and Medicine*, 2020. **126**: p. 103991.

[18]  Kashani, M.H., Madanipour, M., Nikravan, M., Asghari, P. and Mahdipour, E., A systematic review of IoT in healthcare: Applications, techniques, and trends. *Journal of Network and Computer Applications*, 2021. **192**, p.103164.

[19]  Sweetlin, J.D., H.K. Nehemiah, and A. Kannan, Computer aided diagnosis of drug sensitive pulmonary tuberculosis with cavities, consolidations and nodular manifestations on lung CT images. *International Journal of Bio-Inspired Computation*, 2019. **13**(2): p. 71–85.

[20]  Christopher, J.J., Nehemiah, H.K., Arputharaj, K. and Moses, G.L., Computer-assisted medical decision-making system for diagnosis of Urticaria. *MDM Policy & Practice*, 2016. **1**(1), p. 2381468316677752.

[21]  Leema, N., H.K. Nehemiah, and A. Kannan, Neural network classifier optimization using differential evolution with global information and back propagation algorithm for clinical datasets. *Applied Soft Computing*, 2016. **49**: p. 834–844.

[22]  Jane, Y.N., H.K. Nehemiah, and K. Arputharaj, A Q-backpropagated time delay neural network for diagnosing severity of gait disturbances in Parkinson's disease. *Journal of Biomedical Informatics*, 2016. **60**: p. 169–176.

[23]  Potghan, S., R. Rajamenakshi, and A. Bhise. Multi-layer perceptron based lung tumor classification. In *2018 Second International Conference on Electronics, Communication and Aerospace Technology (ICECA)*, 2018.

[24]  Ting, F. and K. Sim. Self-regulated multilayer perceptron neural network for breast cancer classification. In *2017 International Conference on Robotics, Automation and Sciences (ICORAS)*, 2017. IEEE.

[25]  Lorencin, I., Anelić, N., Španjol, J. and Car, Z., Using multi-layer perceptron with Laplacian edge detector for bladder cancer diagnosis. *Artificial Intelligence in Medicine*, 2020. **102**, p.101746.

[26]  Sonawane, J.S. and D.R. Patil. Prediction of heart disease using multilayer perceptron neural network. In *International Conference on Information Communication and Embedded Systems (ICICES2014)*, 2014. IEEE.

[27]  Selwal, A. and I. Raoof, A Multi-layer perceptron based intelligent thyroid disease prediction system. *Indonesian Journal of Electrical Engineering and Computer Science*, 2020. **17**(1): p. 524–533.

[28]  Petrosian, A.A., Prokhorov, D.V., Lajara-Nanson, W. and Schiffer, R.B., Recurrent neural network-based approach for early recognition of Alzheimer's disease in EEG. *Clinical Neurophysiology*, 2001. **112**(8): p. 1378–1387.

[29]  Liu, L., Han, M., Zhou, Y. and Wang, Y., LSTM recurrent neural networks for influenza trends prediction. In *Bioinformatics Research and Applications: 14th International Symposium, ISBRA 2018, Beijing, China, June 8-11, 2018, Proceedings 14*, 2018 (pp. 259–264). Springer International Publishing.

[30]  Krishnan, S., P. Magalingam, and R. Ibrahim, Hybrid deep learning model using recurrent neural network and gated recurrent unit for heart disease prediction. *International Journal of Electrical & Computer Engineering (2088–8708)*, 2021. **11**(6).

[31]  Rejaibi, E., Komaty, A., Meriaudeau, F., Agrebi, S. and Othmani, A., MFCC-based recurrent neural network for automatic clinical depression

recognition and assessment from speech. *Biomedical Signal Processing and Control*, 2022. **71**, p.103107.

[32]  Chovatiya, M., Dhameliya, A., Deokar, J., Gonsalves, J. and Mathur, A., Prediction of dengue using recurrent neural network. In *2019 3rd International Conference on Trends in Electronics and Informatics (ICOEI)*, 2019 (pp. 926–929). IEEE.

[33]  Abiyev, R.H. and M.K.S. Ma'aitah, Deep convolutional neural networks for chest diseases detection. Journal of Healthcare Engineering, 2018. 2018: 11 pages.

[34]  Muhammad, W., Gupta, M. and Bhutto, Z., Role of deep learning in medical image super-resolution. In *Principles and Methods of Explainable Artificial Intelligence in Healthcare*, 2022 (pp. 55–93). IGI Global.

[35]  Muhammad, W., Bhutto, Z., Shah, S.A.R., *et al.*, Deep transfer learning CNN based approach for COVID-19 detection. *International Journal of Advanced and Applied Sciences*, 2022. **9**: p. 44–52.

[36]  Ahmad, I. and K. Pothuganti, Analysis of different convolution neural network models to diagnose Alzheimer's disease. In *Materials Today: Proceedings*, 2020.

[37]  Juneja, S., Juneja, A., Dhiman, G., Behl, S. and Kautish, S., An approach for thoracic syndrome classification with convolutional neural networks. *Computational and Mathematical Methods in Medicine*, 2021.

[38]  Tariq, Z., S.K. Shah, and Y. Lee. Lung disease classification using deep convolutional neural network. In *2019 IEEE International Conference on Bioinformatics and Biomedicine (BIBM)*. 2019. IEEE.

[39]  Rathod, J., Waghmode, V., Sodha, A. and Bhavathankar, P., Diagnosis of skin diseases using Convolutional Neural Networks. In *2018 Second International Conference on Electronics, Communication and Aerospace Technology (ICECA)*, 2018 (pp. 1048–1051). IEEE.

[40]  Muhammad, W., Bhutto, Z., Masroor, S., Shaikh, M.H., Shah, J. and Hussain, A., IRMIRS: Inception-ResNet-based network for MRI image super-resolution. *CMES-Computer Modeling in Engineering & Sciences*, 2023. **136**(2).

[41]  de Souza, R.W., Silva, D.S., Passos, L.A., *et al.*, Computer-assisted Parkinson's disease diagnosis using fuzzy optimum-path forest and Restricted Boltzmann Machines. *Computers in Biology and Medicine*, 2021. **131**, p. 104260.

[42]  Pranata, A.R., Alamsyah, A., Prasetiyo, B. and Vember, H., Restricted Boltzmann machine and softmax regression for acute respiratory infections disease identification. *Journal of Soft Computing Exploration*, 2022. **3**(2): p. 77–84.

[43]  Jayashree, R., Enhanced classification using restricted Boltzmann machine method in deep learning for COVID-19. *Understanding COVID-19: The Role of Computational Intelligence*, 2022: p. 425–446.

[44]  Wahid, F., Azhar, S., Ali, S., Zia, M.S., Almisned, F.A. and Gumaei, A., Pneumonia detection in chest x-ray images using enhanced restricted Boltzmann machine. *Journal of Healthcare Engineering*, 2022.

[45]  Pandey, S.K., Janghel, R.R., Dev, A.V. and Mishra, P.K., Automated arrhythmia detection from electrocardiogram signal using stacked restricted Boltzmann machine model. *SN Applied Sciences*, 2021. **3**(6), p. 624.

[46]  Benyelles, F.Z., A. Sekkal, and N. Settouti. Content based COVID-19 chest X-Ray and CT images retrieval framework using stacked auto-encoders. In *2020 2nd International Workshop on Human-Centric Smart Environments for Health and Well-Being (IHSH)*, 2021. IEEE.

[47]  Saravanan, V., Samuel, R.D.J., Krishnamoorthy, S. and Manickam, A., Deep learning assisted convolutional auto-encoders framework for glaucoma detection and anterior visual pathway recognition from retinal fundus images. *Journal of Ambient Intelligence and Humanized Computing*, 2022: p. 1–11.

[48]  Martinez-Murcia, F.J., Ortiz, A., Gorriz, J.M., Ramirez, J. and Castillo-Barnes, D., Studying the manifold structure of Alzheimer's disease: a deep learning approach using convolutional autoencoders. *IEEE Journal of biomedical and Health Informatics*, 2019. **24**(1): p. 17–26.

[49]  Xiao, J., Bai, Y., Yuille, A. and Zhou, Z., Delving into masked autoencoders for multi-label thorax disease classification. In *Proceedings of the IEEE/ CVF Winter Conference on Applications of Computer Vision*, 2023 (pp. 3588-3600).

[50]  Nasser, Y., El Hassouni, M., Brahim, A., Toumi, H., Lespessailles, E. and Jennane, R., Diagnosis of osteoporosis disease from bone X-ray images with stacked sparse autoencoder and SVM classifier. In *2017 international conference on advanced technologies for signal and image processing (ATSIP)*, 2017 (pp. 1–5). IEEE.

[51]  Hastie, T., Tibshirani, R., Friedman, J.H. and Friedman, J.H., *The Elements of Statistical Learning: Data Mining, Inference, and Prediction*, 2009 (vol. 2: p. 1–758). New York: Springer.

[52]  Millidge, B., A. Tschantz, and C.L. Buckley, Predictive coding approximates backprop along arbitrary computation graphs. *Neural Computation*, 2022. **34**(6): p. 1329–1368.

[53]  Cybenko, G., Approximation by superpositions of a sigmoidal function. *Mathematics of Control, Signals and Systems*, 1989. **2**(4): p. 303–314.

[54]  Sherrington, D. and S. Kirkpatrick, Solvable model of a spin-glass. *Physical Review Letters*, 1975. **35**(26): p. 1792.

[55]  Ackley, D., G. Hinton, and T. Sejnowski, Boltzmann machines: constraint satisfaction networks that learn. *Cognitive Science*, 1985. **9**: p. 147.

[56]  Kramer, M.A., Nonlinear principal component analysis using auto-associative neural networks. *AIChE Journal*, 1991. **37**(2): p. 233–243.

[57]  Shamshirband, S., Fathi, M., Dehzangi, A., Chronopoulos, A.T. and Alinejad-Rokny, H., A review on deep learning approaches in healthcare systems: Taxonomies, challenges, and open issues. *Journal of Biomedical Informatics*, 2021. **113**, p. 103627.

[58]    Dhungel, N., G. Carneiro, and A.P. Bradley, A deep learning approach for the analysis of masses in mammograms with minimal user intervention. *Medical Image Analysis*, 2017. **37**: p. 114–128.

[59]    Jiao, Z., Gao, X., Wang, Y. and Li, J., A parasitic metric learning net for breast mass classification based on mammography. *Pattern Recognition*, 2018. **75**: p. 292–301.

[60]    Samala, R.K., Chan, H.P., Hadjiiski, L., Helvie, M.A., Wei, J. and Cha, K., Mass detection in digital breast tomosynthesis: Deep convolutional neural network with transfer learning from mammography. *Medical Physics*, 2016. **43**(12): p. 6654–6666.

[61]    Wahab, N., A. Khan, and Y.S. Lee, Two-phase deep convolutional neural network for reducing class skewness in histopathological images based breast cancer detection. *Computers in Biology and Medicine*, 2017. **85**: p. 86–97.

[62]    Zhang, Q., Xiao, Y., Dai, W., *et al.*, Deep learning based classification of breast tumors with shear-wave elastography. *Ultrasonics*, 2016. **72**: p. 150–157.

[63]    Sharma, H., Zerbe, N., Klempert, I., Hellwich, O. and Hufnagl, P., Deep convolutional neural networks for automatic classification of gastric carcinoma using whole slide images in digital histopathology. *Computerized Medical Imaging and Graphics*, 2017. **61**: p. 2–13.

[64]    Sun, W., B. Zheng, and W. Qian, Automatic feature learning using multi-channel ROI based on deep structured algorithms for computerized lung cancer diagnosis. *Computers in Biology and Medicine*, 2017. **89**: p. 530–539.

[65]    Zhao, X., Wu, Y., Song, G., Li, Z., Zhang, Y. and Fan, Y., A deep learning model integrating FCNNs and CRFs for brain tumor segmentation. *Medical Image Analysis*, 2018. **43**: p. 98–111.

[66]    Tabar, Y.R. and U. Halici, A novel deep learning approach for classification of EEG motor imagery signals. *Journal of Neural Engineering*, 2016. **14**(1): p. 016003.

[67]    Xiao, Y., Wu, J., Lin, Z. and Zhao, X., A deep learning-based multi-model ensemble method for cancer prediction. *Computer Methods and Programs in Biomedicine*, 2018. **153**: p. 1–9.

[68]    Yoo, Y., Tang, L.Y., Li, D.K., *et al.*, Deep learning of brain lesion patterns and user-defined clinical and MRI features for predicting conversion to multiple sclerosis from clinically isolated syndrome. *Computer Methods in Biomechanics and Biomedical Engineering: Imaging & Visualization*, 2019. **7**(3): p. 250–259.

[69]    Yoo, Y., Tang, L.Y., Brosch, T., *et al.*, Deep learning of joint myelin and T1w MRI features in normal-appearing brain tissue to distinguish between multiple sclerosis patients and healthy controls. *NeuroImage: Clinical*, 2018. **17**: p. 169–178.

[70]    Choi, H., Ha, S., Im, H.J., Paek, S.H. and Lee, D.S., Refining diagnosis of Parkinson's disease with deep learning-based interpretation of dopamine transporter imaging. *NeuroImage: Clinical*, 2017. **16**: p. 586–594.

[71]    Choi, E., Schuetz, A., Stewart, W.F. and Sun, J., Using recurrent neural network models for early detection of heart failure onset. *Journal of the American Medical Informatics Association*, 2017. **24**(2): p. 361–370.

[72] Al Rahhal, M.M., Bazi, Y., AlHichri, H., Alajlan, N., Melgani, F. and Yager, R.R., Deep learning approach for active classification of electrocardiogram signals. *Information Sciences*, 2016. **345**: p. 340–354.

[73] Acharya, U.R., Oh, S.L., Hagiwara, Y., Tan, J.H. and Adeli, H., Deep convolutional neural network for the automated detection and diagnosis of seizure using EEG signals. *Computers in Biology and Medicine*, 2018. **100**: p. 270–278.

[74] Yin, Z. and J. Zhang, Cross-session classification of mental workload levels using EEG and an adaptive deep learning model. *Biomedical Signal Processing and Control*, 2017. **33**: p. 30–47.

[75] Miotto, R., Li, L., Kidd, B.A. and Dudley, J.T., Deep patient: an unsupervised representation to predict the future of patients from the electronic health records. *Scientific Reports*, 2016. **6**(1): p. 1–10.

[76] Nie, L., Wang, M., Zhang, L., Yan, S., Zhang, B. and Chua, T.S., Disease inference from health-related questions via sparse deep learning. *IEEE Transactions on Knowledge and Data Engineering*, 2015. **27**(8): p. 2107–2119.

[77] Saporta, A., Gui, X., Agrawal, A., *et al.*, Benchmarking saliency methods for chest x-ray interpretation. medRxiv. 2021.

[78] Irvin, J., Rajpurkar, P., Ko, M., *et al.*, Chexpert: A large chest radiograph dataset with uncertainty labels and expert comparison. *In Proceedings of the AAAI Conference on Artificial Intelligence*, 2019 (vol. 33: p. 590–597).

[79] Daneshjou, R., Vodrahalli, K., Novoa, R.A., *et al.*, Disparities in dermatology AI performance on a diverse, curated clinical image set. *Science Advances*, 2022. **8**(31), p. eabq6147.

[80] Ouyang, D., He, B., Ghorbani, A., *et al.*, Video-based AI for beat-to-beat assessment of cardiac function. *Nature*, 2020. **580**(7802): p. 252–256.

[81] Duffy, G., Cheng, P.P., Yuan, N., *et al.*, High-throughput precision phenotyping of left ventricular hypertrophy with cardiovascular deep learning. *JAMA Cardiology*, 2022. **7**(4): p. 386–395.

[82] Rajpurkar, P., Irvin, J., Bagul, A., *et al.*, Mura: Large dataset for abnormality detection in musculoskeletal radiographs. *arXiv preprint arXiv:1712.06957.* 2017.

[83] Health, N.I.O., *NIH Clinical Center Provides One of the Largest Publicly Available Chest X-Ray Datasets to Scientific Community,* 2022.

[84] Reeves, A.P., Biancardi, A.M., Yankelevitz, D., *et al.*, A public image database to support research in computer aided diagnosis. In *2009 Annual International Conference of the IEEE Engineering in Medicine and Biology Society*, 2009, p. 3715–3718. IEEE.

[85] Zhou, Y., Huang, S.C., Fries, J.A., *et al.*, Radfusion: Benchmarking performance and fairness for multimodal pulmonary embolism detection from CT and EHR. *arXiv preprint arXiv:2111.11665.* 2021.

[86] Frank, A., *UCI Machine Learning Repository*, 2010. http://archive.ics.uci.edu/ml.

[87] Dong, E., H. Du, and L. Gardner, An interactive web-based dashboard to track COVID-19 in real time. *The Lancet Infectious Diseases*, 2020. **20**(5): p. 533–534.

*Chapter 3*

# Investigations on the impact of AI models in human health using nutrient analysis from food images

*E.S. Sreetha[1,2], G. Naveen Sundar[1], D. Narmadha[1], K. Martin Sagayam[1] and Ahmed A. Elngar[3,4]*

## Abstract

Humans have a basic requirement for nutrition, which is also necessary for a healthy life. Getting enough nutrients on a regular basis is essential for maintaining human well-being. Malnutrition is mostly to blame for the majority of health problems. Diseases including stunted growth, eye issues, diabetes, and heart disease are primarily brought on by inadequate nutrition consumed on a regular basis. Malnutrition is not only a result of poverty; it is also a result of people's ignorance of the nutrients in the foods they eat. In this day and age, it is crucial to recognize food correctly and to be able to identify its characteristics and nutritional value. The objective of this study is to identify the best techniques to recognize the food item and its nutrient content by using deep learning (DL) algorithms. Through this, a point-by-point analysis of malnutrition and treatment for malnutrition are reviewed. Different algorithms such as machine learning, DL, and various convolutional neural network architectures are reviewed, for recognizing the food items from food images. Inception V4 gives more accuracy when compared with other techniques. Food 101 is the selected dataset for comparing the accuracy of the food image identification. The nutrient contents of all the 101 classes of food items are also reviewed.

**Keywords:** Malnutrition; Machine learning; Deep learning; Convolutional neural network

[1]Department of Computer Science and Engineering, Karunya Institute of Technology and Sciences, Coimbatore, India
[2]Department of Computer Science and Engineering, Sahrdaya College of Engineering and Technology, Kerala, India
[3]Department of Electronics and Communication Engineering, Karunya Institute of Technology and Science, Coimbatore, India
[4]Faculty of Computers and Artificial Intelligence, Beni-Suef University, Beni-Suef City, Egypt

## 3.1    Introduction

According to a report from the World Health Organization (WHO), nutrition is a crucial factor in both health and development [1]. Better nutrition is linked to stronger immune systems, safer pregnancies and deliveries, and a lower risk of non-communicable diseases (including diabetes and cardiovascular disease), and longer life spans. People who are well nourished are more productive and can open doors to progressively end the cycles of hunger and poverty.

The State of Food Security and Nutrition in the World 2022 report finds that hunger and malnutrition are significant global issues in all of its manifestations [2]. The COVID-19 pandemic's residual impacts, together with the disruption of the food supply brought on by escalating violence and extreme weather occurrences, continue to obstruct efforts to meet the sustainable development goals (SDGs) targets. More than 3 billion people worldwide lack access to a healthy diet. Poor diets contribute to millions of deaths each year by, for instance, consuming insufficient amounts of whole grains, legumes, vegetables, and fruit as well as sodium/salt, sweets, and unhealthy fats. The report's main takeaway is that the government's existing support of the food and agricultural industries frequently does not correspond to the promotion of a healthy diet. This report demonstrates how readjusting food and agricultural policy can broaden access to wholesome foods and improve the sustainability, equity, and health of food systems. To encourage the production of more nutrient-dense foods, enhance their availability, and lower their prices so that a healthy diet is affordable, different public budgetary resources need to be allocated. These initiatives must be supported by other food system policies to maximize their impact by fostering conditions that encourage and promote a healthy diet.

### 3.1.1    *Malnutrition*

Malnutrition, according to WHO, is a cellular imbalance that results from a discrepancy between the body's supply of nutrients and energy sources and the physical need for these elements. The body's capacity to grow and sustain the appropriate performance of a number of functions of the body may be affected by this imbalance. Malnutrition can therefore result in a weakened state of health and raise a person's chance of developing a number of various illnesses. Every type of malnutrition poses serious risks to human health. Undernutrition and overweight are both major causes of malnutrition in today's globe, particularly in low- and middle-income nations. Undernutrition and malnutrition linked to micro-nutrients are two further classifications for malnutrition. Undernutrition can be further broken down into four categories: wasting, stunting, underweight, and vitamin and mineral deficiencies.

Obesity and being overweight, non-communicable diseases linked to diet, and insufficient consumption of micronutrients are a few of the various malnutrition problems that are associated with micronutrients.

### 3.1.1.1 Causes of malnutrition

Malnutrition, mainly undernutrition, is due to a deficiency in nutrients, which can be brought on by a poor diet or issues with food absorption. Malnutrition has several causes [3], including:

• Lack of food is a problem that both persons with low incomes and the homeless experience frequently.
• Decrease in appetite. Cancers, tumors, mental diseases like depression and other mental illnesses, liver or kidney disease, chronic infections, etc. are common causes of lack of appetite.
• The risk of malnutrition is increased in elderly people, particularly those residing in care institutions. These people may also have trouble feeding themselves because of chronic conditions that impede their capacity to eat and absorb nutrients from meal undernutrition, some mental conditions like depression may have an impact on appetite and food consumption.
• Those who struggle with eating disorders like anorexia nervosa find it challenging to maintain a healthy diet.
• People who struggle to assimilate the nutrients in their diet due to digestive problems such as ulcerative colitis, Crohn's disease, or malabsorption syndrome may become undernourished.
• Food consumption is outweighed by the need for energy. This covers those who have undergone major surgery or who have sustained a serious injury, burn, or burns. This also applies to youngsters and pregnant women, whose higher needs for nutrients and calories—which may be insufficient in a typical diet—are a result of their growth and those of the unborn child.

### 3.1.1.2 Treatment

Depending on the underlying cause and the severity of the malnutrition, a person may require treatment [4]. People shall receive advice from a dietitian regarding beneficial dietary adjustments. They could design a personalized food plan for you to make sure you get adequate nutrients. They might also advise:

• eating "fortified" foods that contain additional nutrients,
• leading to a healthier, more balanced diet,
• between-meal snacks,
• drinking calorically rich beverages.

Supplementing with additional nutrients may be advised if these actions are insufficient. These must only be taken when directed by a medical practitioner [5].

The artificial neural network (ANN) approach was found to dominate the group of studies on the creation of nutrients and dietary composition [6]. However, studies on the impact of nutrition on how the human body functions in health and sickness heavily utilized machine learning (ML) techniques. In a collection of studies on clinical nutritional consumption, deep learning (DL) algorithms took the lead [7]. AI-based dietary system development may result in the establishment of a global network that can actively support and keep track of the provision of nutrients that are specifically tailored to each individual.

## 3.2   Image recognition

To recognize and classify different components of images or videos, image recognition is a computer vision task. When given an image as input, image recognition models are trained to produce one or more labels that describe the image. Target classes relate to the set of potential output labels. Image recognition algorithms may also produce a confidence score that indicates how certain the model is that an image belongs to a class in addition to a predicted class. For example, the pipeline would essentially resemble the following if you wanted to create an image recognition model that could automatically assess whether or not a food item was present in a given image [8]:

- On photos that have been classified as "fruit" or "not fruit," an image recognition model has been trained.
- Model data: video or picture frame.
- Model output: class name (in this case, "fruit") together with a confidence score that shows how likely it is that the object class is present in the image.

The area of food recognition has many uses for image recognition technology, including [9]:

- Automated food monitoring: by simply taking pictures of their meals, users of automated food monitoring apps can easily keep track of how many calories they consume each day.
- Image recognition technology can be used to analyze menus at cafeterias and restaurants, giving customers nutritional information about each dish and guiding them toward healthier options.
- Food safety: image recognition technology can be used to find contaminants in foods, enhancing food security and reducing the risk of foodborne diseases.
- Inventory management: image recognition can be used to identify and monitor food items in food retail and supply chain management, which reduces waste and enhances inventory management.

### 3.2.1   ML models for image recognition

A mathematical representation of a process in the actual world is an ML model. The learning algorithm looks for patterns in the training data to translate the input parameters to the target. An ML model used for prediction is the result of the training process. A few examples of ML models are represented in Figure 3.1.

- In ML, *regression algorithms* are employed to forecast a continuous numerical value based on one or more input factors. Regression methods that are frequently used include support vector regression, decision tree regression, random forest regression, ridge regression, polynomial regression, and lasso regression. The specific issue being solved and the properties of the available data determine the algorithm to use.
- Instead of trying to learn an explicit model of the relationship between the input variables and the output, instance-based learning is a sort of ML algorithm that learns from examples in the training data. Instance-based learning

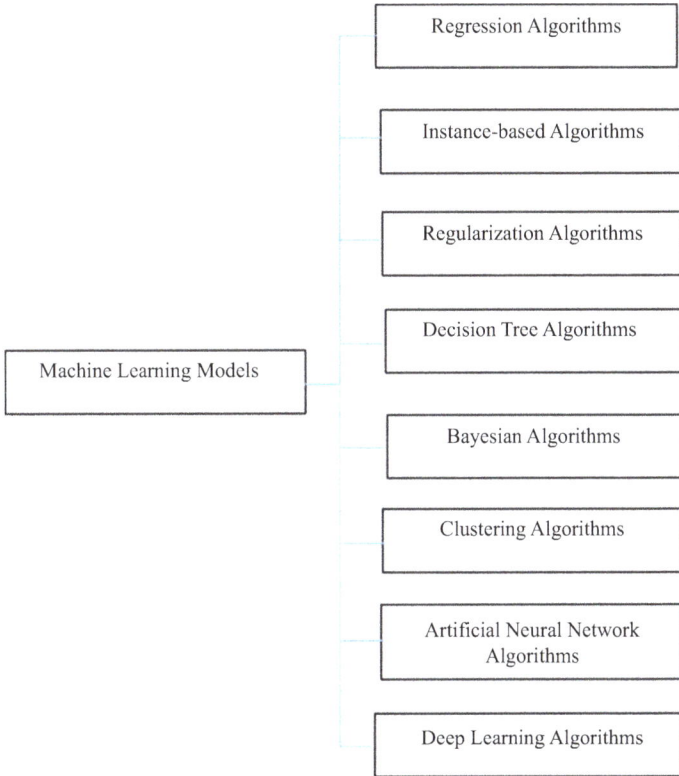

*Figure 3.1    Different ML algorithms for image recognition*

algorithms store the training examples and use them to make predictions for new input data by locating the most similar examples in the training set, as opposed to fitting a model to the complete training dataset.

- *Regularization* is an ML technique that adds a penalty term to the loss function the model is optimizing to avoid overfitting. ML algorithms that use regularization to enhance the model's generalization capabilities are known as regularization algorithms.
- A type of ML algorithm called a *decision tree* builds a model that resembles a tree to make predictions based on a collection of input features. Internal nodes in the tree represent features, and branches represent the various potential values for those features. The algorithm chooses the feature at each internal node that divides the data into distinct classes or groups according to some criteria, such as information gain or Gini defect. Until all of the tree's leaves, which correlate to the expected output values, have been reached, the process is repeated recursively.
- A family of ML algorithms known as *Bayesian algorithms* uses Bayesian inference to model and forecast the data. Observed data and prior information are combined in the statistical technique of Bayesian inference to update the likelihood of a hypothesis. The parameters of the model are modeled.

- In an unsupervised ML algorithm called *clustering*, comparable data points are grouped together into clusters according to how similar they are. Without previous knowledge of the class labels, clustering aims to find natural groups or patterns in the data. Although there are many clustering methods, they can be roughly divided into two groups: partitioning and hierarchical using prior distributions in the framework of ML, and the posterior distribution of the parameters is updated based on the observed data.
- ML algorithms called ANN algorithms are modeled after the form and operation of organic neural networks found in the human brain. ANNs are made up of interconnected nodes that analyze and transmit data using a network of interconnected layers. Multilayer perceptron, convolutional neural network (CNN), and recurrent neural network are a few popular ANN methods. ANNs have attained cutting-edge success in a variety of tasks, but they can be prone to overfitting and costly to train and test computationally.

### 3.2.1.1    Food recognition models using ML

Kawano *et al.* proposed a system in which the user begins by roughly drawing bounding boxes on the image with dragging. Each window image within the specified bounding boundaries is subjected to food recognition [10]. First, each window's picture attributes are retrieved, then feature vectors based on the pre-calculated codebook are generated, and then assessed and compared the efficiency and computational costs of several global and local image characteristics, such as color auto correlogram, color histogram, color moment, HoG, PHoG, Gabor texture feature, and Bag-of-SURF. Finally, Bag-of-SURF and color histogram combinations are used and tested using trained linear SVMs on 50 different food categories. When given ground-truth bounding boxes, the top five candidates have a classification rate of 81.55.

The following terms are defined by the Random Forest mining framework that is covered in this work proposed by Bossard *et al.* [11]: First, as compared to independently, it simultaneously mines all classes for discriminative components. This expedites the learning process and permits information transfer between classes. Second, rather than sampling random picture patches, restrict the region to search for discriminative portions to patches that are aligned by superpixels in line with successful ideas made in the field of object detection. They can therefore afford to manipulate regions with continuous color and texture in addition to extracting more effective visual clues to assist in classification. The classification difficulty on test images is also greatly decreased as a result of the common use of just a few dozen superpixels per image as opposed to tens of thousands of sliding windows. This is due to the fact that there may be a lot of component classifiers and detectors.

The Fisher Kernel framework, where patches are defined in terms of how they vary from a "universal" generative Gaussian mixture model, was proposed by Sa'nchez *et al.* as an alternative patch encoding approach [12]. This representation, known as the Fisher Vector (FV), offers a number of advantages, including exceptional performance even with effective linear classifiers and the capacity to be compressed through product quantization without sacrificing accuracy.

Aizawa *et al.* suggested an approach that underlies the Bayesian framework [13]. A Bayesian framework was utilized to extract image features such as colors, the circle feature, and BoF of local features, instead of using the deterministic method. Every time a user-corrected estimation result is used in a Bayesian framework, the model can be customized and updated. The accuracy increased to 92% for one individual user's 100 test photographs.

Anthimopoulos proposed a system in which a visual collection with approximately 5,000 photographs of home-cooked food was produced to reflect central European dietary preferences [14]. The foods depicted in the photographs have been divided into 11 high-intra variability classes. They conducted a thorough analysis of the ideal elements and parameters within the BoF design based on the aforementioned dataset. Six classifiers, fourteen local image descriptors, two clustering algorithms for building the visual dictionary, and three key point extraction techniques were examined and compared. The fusion of descriptors and feature selection were both tested. Additionally, numerous tests show the effects of several parameters including the number of key points retrieved, the size(s) of descriptors, and the number of visual words for one individual user's 100 test photographs.

## 3.2.2   DL

Artificial intelligence is achieved via DL, a subset of ML [15]. DL is a method of learning that allows us to build a machine that mimics the neuronal network seen in the human brain. It is made up of algorithms that provide computers the ability to learn to execute functions like speech recognition, natural language processing, and image recognition. This statistical method is based on deep networks and divides a task into ML algorithms. These algorithms' building blocks consist of interconnected layers. Between the input and the output layer, there will be several hidden layers. The word "Deep," which describes networks that connect neurons in more than two layers, originated as a result of these hidden layers.

The various applications of DL include healthcare, computer vision and pattern recognition, computer games, robots and self-driving cars, voice-activated intelligent assistants, advertising, predicting natural calamities, finance, etc. Food image identification is a developing area of study because it has so many applications in the medical and health fields. Future systems for tracking diets, calculating calories, and more will undoubtedly benefit from automated food recognition capabilities that employ DL techniques.

### 3.2.2.1   CNN

CNNs, also referred to as ConvNets, are a type of ANN with a feed-forward architecture whose connectivity layout is based on how the visual cortex of animals is laid out. CNNs are ANNs that analyze visual input in DL applications. Texts, movies, photographs, audio, and other sorts of media can all be handled via these networks. In the 1990s, Yann LeCunn successfully developed the first convolution networks. Figure 3.2 illustrates typical CNN architecture.

CNNs can learn complicated objects and patterns because they have different layers such as a hidden layer or layers, millions of parameters, an input layer, and

**Convolution Neural Network**

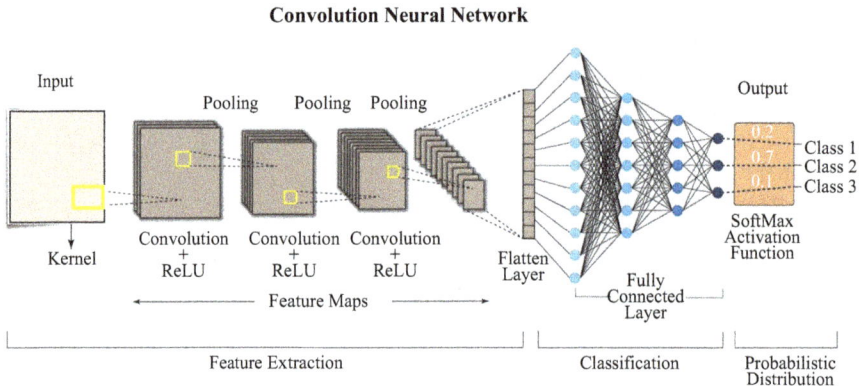

*Figure 3.2   Typical CNN architecture*

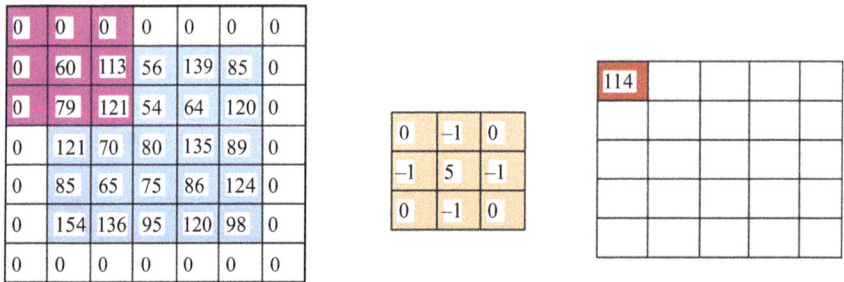

*Figure 3.3   Process of convolution*

an output layer [16]. It subsamples the input using convolution and pooling methods before utilizing an activation function. The output layer is the last fully linked layer after all of the hidden layers, which are initially only partially connected. The input image's size and the output shape are similar.

Convolution is a technique where two functions are combined to produce the output of another function. A feature map is produced after CNNs apply filters to a complex input image. Weights and biases in filters are network vectors that were produced at random. The weights and biases used by CNN are the same for all neurons as opposed to being unique for each neuron. There are many different filters that may be created, and each one extracts a certain aspect of the input image. Kernels are another name for filters.

*Convolutional layer*
Convolutional layers are the main building blocks of CNNs. Input vectors like an image, filters like a feature detector, and output vectors like a feature map are commonly included in this layer. A convolutional layer runs through the input image. The image is then transformed into a feature map, also referred to as an activation map. Figure 3.3 describes the process of convolution.

## Pooling layer

It intends to significantly decrease the spatial dimension of the representation to decrease the number of parameters and also the calculations in the network. The pooling layer treats each feature map separately. The features that are present in a specific area are summarized in the feature map produced by the feature pooling layer of a convolution layer. In place of the precisely positioned features that are produced by the convolution layer, subsequent actions are therefore performed utilizing summarized features. Since the features' locations in the input image can change, the model is consequently more adaptable. Figure 3.4 shows two types of pooling.

## Pooling layer types

**Max pooling:** From the feature map area, which the filter has covered, the "max pooling" method of pooling chooses the largest element. The outcome of the max-pooling layer would then result in a feature map that featured the salient elements from the prior feature map.

**Average pooling:** The items that are present in the feature map region that the filter is covering are averaged out using average pooling. Therefore, average pooling represents the mean of the features that are available in a portion, whereas max pooling offers the outstanding feature in a certain portion of the feature map.

## Rectified linear unit

The piecewise linear function rectified linear unit (ReLU), also referred to as the rectified linear activation function, produces zero when the input is negative and the input straight away when the input is positive. Since a model that employs it trains more rapidly and frequently outperforms other models, it has developed into the standard activation function for numerous varieties of neural networks.

## Fully connected layer

A layer of fully linked neurons makes up the last layer of the CNN. The performance of neurons in a completely linked layer is similar to that of neurons in traditional neural networks due to the fact that they are fully connected to all activations in the layer above. Utilizing the feature vector from the fully connected

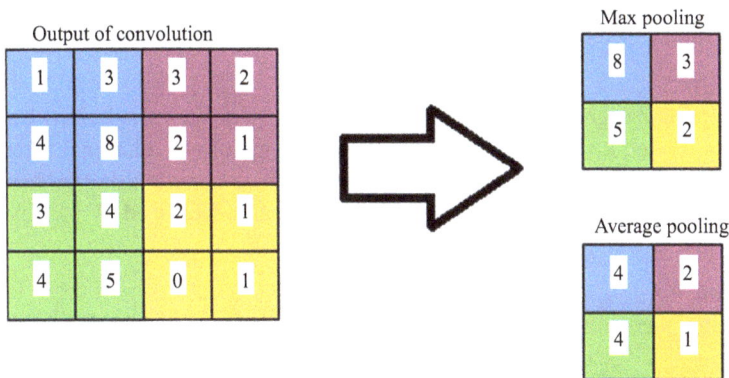

*Figure 3.4   Process of pooling*

layer, pictures are categorized after training. This layer's inputs are connected to each activation module in the layer beneath. The fully-connected layer uses all the parameters, which leads to overfitting. Several strategies, including dropout, can be used to lessen overfitting.

## Classifier

The final layer of the network, known as a classifier, is often where the activation layer known as soft-max is used. This layer is in charge of classifying the input into several kinds. The output of a network is transformed from non-normalized to a probability distribution by the SoftMax function.

### 3.2.2.2    CNN models

*AlexNet*

An eight-layer CNN architecture is called AlexNet [17]. The supplied image has a dimension of 227 by 227 by 3. It has three fully linked layers and five convolutional layers (FC). To extract numerous features, the first two convolutional layers are combined with overlapping max-pooling layers. The output layer is activated using the SoftMax algorithm. During training, a dropout layer lessens overfitting. The neurons that "dropped out" are not a part of the forward pass or the back-propagation. The first two FC layers are where the neurons that have fallen out are found.

*LeNet-5*

Yann LeCun created the LeNet-5 CNN model, which was first used to recognize handwritten digits in 1998 [18]. It was one of the first effective DL implementations, and it has since evolved into a standard architecture for image recognition tasks. LeNet-5 has seven layers, including three completely connected layers, two convolutional layers, and two subsampling layers. A collection of filters is applied to the input image by the convolutional layer's first layer to extract local features. A subsampling layer in the second layer lowers the geographic dimensionality of the features while maintaining the most important data. The characteristics are further refined in the third and fourth layers, which are again convolutional and sub-sampling layers, respectively. Fully linked layers five, six, and seven carry out the classification based on the features extracted by the earlier layers.

*GoogLeNet*

The Inception design serves as the foundation for CNNs like GoogLeNet. Utilizing Inception modules, the network has access to a range of convolutional filter sizes for each block. These modules are piled on top of one another using an Inception network, and the resolution of the grid is occasionally decreased by half by max-pooling layers with stride 2.

*Inception V3*

The image recognition model Inception V3 has been shown to be capable of exceeding 78.1% accuracy on the ImageNet dataset. The model is the outcome of several ideas that have been developed over the years by various scholars. It is based on the original research done by Szegedy *et al.* [19]. The model's symmetric and asymmetric building blocks include convolutions, average pooling, max pooling, concatenations, dropouts, and completely linked layers. Batch normalization, which is also used for the activation inputs, is heavily utilized by the model. SoftMax is employed to determine loss.

An image recognition system influenced by LeNet-5, AlexNet, and GoogleNet was proposed by Chang *et al.* [20]. This system employs a CNN with three convolutional layers, two subsampling layers, and one fully connected layer. This system made use of the UEC-100/UEC-256 and Food 101 public databases. A customized food classification system based on Inception V3 has been proposed by Burkapalli *et al.* [21]. This CNN-based model achieved a 98.7% accuracy after being trained on more than a thousand food photos.

The performance of various CNN models (CNNFood, Multitask, MultitaskCNN, FoodNet, DeepFood, Module, ResNet, InceptionV3, and WISer) [22] using datasets such as Food101, UECFood-256, and UECFood-100 is described in Table 3.1.

### 3.2.2.3   Dataset

The key to achieving the best classification accuracy is a strong dataset of images. Taking into account the number of food classes and the type of food, a dataset is constructed. Table 3.2 lists the number of food-related datasets that are currently accessible, including the number of food classes and the number of food photos. A huge number of food photos is needed to train a food classification model because

*Table 3.1   Performance of various CNN models*

| Model | Dataset | Top 1% | Top 5% |
|---|---|---|---|
| | Food101 | 70.41 | – |
| CNNFood | UECFood 256 | 67.57 | 88.97 |
| | UECFood 100 | 78.48 | 94.85 |
| Multitask | Food101 | 72.11 | – |
| MultiTaskCNN | UECFood 100 | 82.42 | 97.29 |
| FoodNet | Food101 | 72.12 | 91.61 |
| | Food101 | 77.40 | 93.70 |
| DeepFood | UECFood 256 | 54.70 | 81.50 |
| | UECFood 100 | 76.3 | 94.6 |
| | Food101 | 77.00 | 94.00 |
| InceptionModule | UECFood 256 | 63.00 | 87.00 |
| | UECFood 100 | 76.30 | 94.60 |
| | Food101 | 78.50 | 94.10 |
| ResNet | UECFood 256 | 71.20 | 91.10 |
| | UECFood 100 | 80.60 | 95.90 |
| | Food101 | 87.96 | – |
| InceptionV3 | UECFood 256 | 76.17 | 92.58 |
| | UECFood 100 | 81.45 | 97.27 |
| | Food101 | 90.27 | 98.71 |
| WISeR | UECFood 256 | 83.15 | 95.45 |
| | UECFood 100 | 89.58 | 99.23 |

*Table 3.2   Details of dataset*

| S. no. | Dataset | Authors | Number of classes | Total number of images |
|---|---|---|---|---|
| 1 | PFID | Chen *et al.* | 61 | 1,038 |
| 2 | TADA | Mariapen *et al.* | 11 | 256 |
| 3 | Food50 | Yanai *et al.* | 50 | 5,000 |
| 4 | Food85 | Haoshi *et al.* | 85 | 8,000 |
| 5 | Foodlog | Miyaski *et al.* | 2,000 | 6,512 |
| 6 | UECFood-100 | Matsuda *et al.* | 100 | 14,361 |
| 7 | Food101 | Bossard *et al.* | 101 | 101,000 |
| 8 | UECFood-256 | Kawano *et al.* | 256 | 256 |
| 9 | UNCIT-FD889 | Farinella *et al.* | 899 | 899 |
| 10 | Food-975 | Zhou *et al.* | 975 | 975 |
| 11 | Food524DB | Ciocca *et al.* | 524 | 524 |

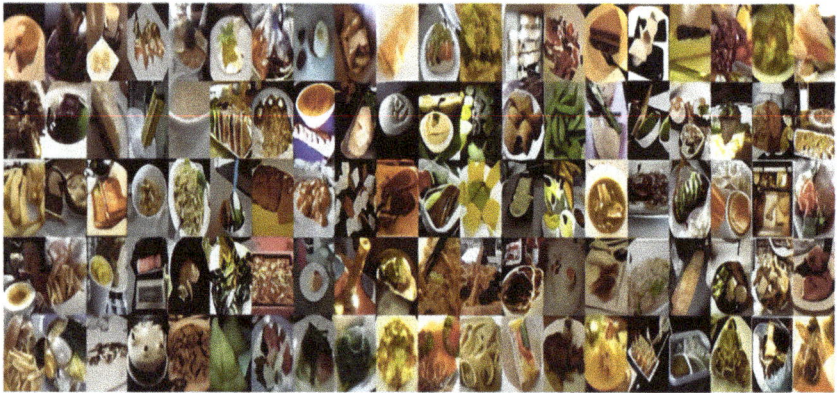

*Figure 3.5   Sample images from Food101 dataset*

DL is data-hungry. A single food image, a mixed food image, a non-mixed food image, multiple food groups, a liquid food image, the type of cuisine, and the total number of images per food class are just a few of the many differences across food image collections. Table 3.2 provides a list of the most popular datasets, together with information on the total number of classes and photos in each dataset.

### Food101 dataset

The system proposed by Bossard *et al.* uses the Food101 dataset. The huge dataset is useful for testing computer vision algorithms. The huge dataset is useful for testing computer vision algorithms. We present a difficult data set with 101 food categories and 101,000 photos. Each class receives 750 training photos and 250 test photographs that have been manually examined. The training images were not cleaned on purpose and still have some noise in them. Each image was resized to have a side length that could not exceed 512 pixels. Sample images from each class of Food101 are shown in Figure 3.5.

#### 3.2.2.4 Image preprocessing

Images need to be processed before they can be used for model training and inference [23]. This includes, but is not limited to, changes in color, size, and direction. To improve the quality of the image, preprocessing is done, so we can analyze it more successfully. Through preprocessing, we can get rid of undesired distortions and enhance certain qualities that are crucial for the application we are developing. Those qualities could alter based on the application. For software to work properly and deliver the required results, an image must be preprocessed.

Preprocessing must be done on the image data before it can be used as model input. For instance, the fully connected layers of CNNs required that all the images be in arrays of the same size. Model preprocessing may also speed up model inference and reduce the amount of time needed for model training. The amount of time required to train the model will be dramatically reduced if the input photos are reduced in size without significantly compromising model performance if the input images are quite large. Preprocessing of the image data that suppresses unintentional distortions or enhances some image features essential for subsequent processing, despite the fact that geometric transformations of images (like rotation, scaling, and translation) are classified as preprocessing techniques.

*Data augmentation*

Making little changes to already-existing data to broaden its diversity without gathering new data is known as data augmentation [24]. It is a method for increasing a dataset. Standard data augmentation methods include flipping data horizontally and vertically, rotating data, cropping data, shearing data, etc. Data augmentation can assist in stopping a neural network from picking up unrelated features. As a result, the model performs better.

Sample image from Food101 dataset and the output of image augmentation such as rotation and shearing flipping are shown in Figure 3.6.

#### 3.2.2.5 Inception V4

The Inception-V4 architecture is shown in Figure 3.7. The stem, inception, reduction, average pooling, dropout, and fully connected modules make up the Inception V4 model. The stem in this sense refers to the initial set of processes performed before inserting the Inception blocks. Images with three RGB channels and a size

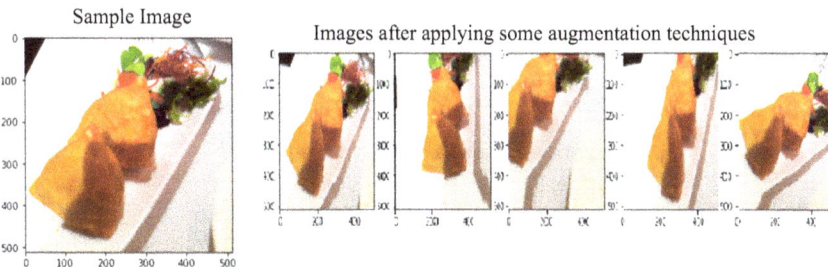

*Figure 3.6   Image augmentation*

| | |
|---|---|
| Input (299×299×3) | 299×299×3 |
| Stem | Output: 35×35×384 |
| 4×Inception-A | Output: 35×35×384 |
| Reduction-A | Output: 17×17×1024 |
| 7×Inception-B | Output: 17×17×1024 |
| Reduction-B | Output: 8×8×1536 |
| 3×Inception-C | Output: 8×8×1536 |
| Average Pooling | Output: 1536 |
| Dropout (Keep 0.8) | Output: 1536 |
| Softmax | Output: 1000 |

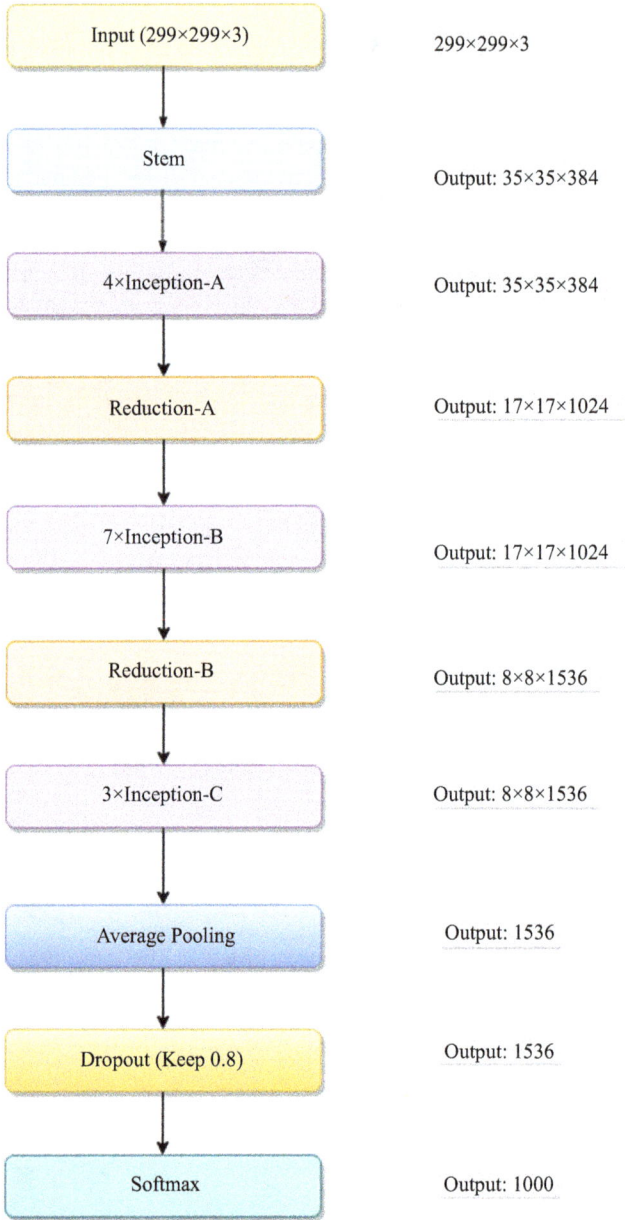

*Figure 3.7   Inception V4 architecture*

of 299 × 299 are utilized as input. The RGB image channels of the sample image are represented in Figure 3.8. Before the activation, batch normalization is conducted following each convolution. ReLU is the activation function applied to each convolution. The output layer uses an activation function called SoftMax.

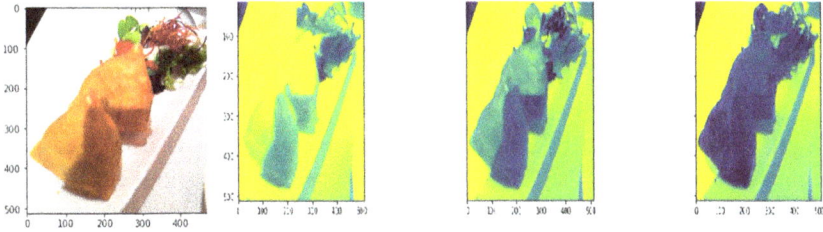

*Figure 3.8   RGB image channels*

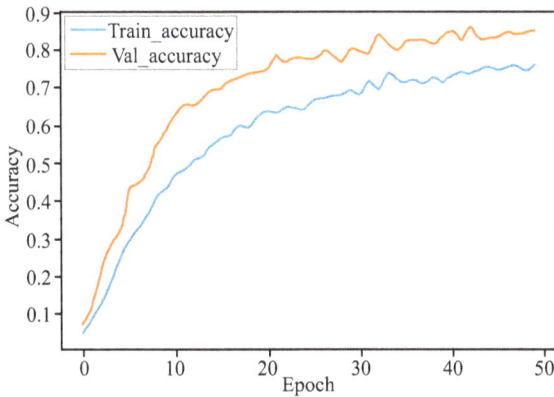

*Figure 3.9   Accuracy*

Thirty-two data samples are used in each batch for training, which is done using micro batch learning in the implementation. Additionally used as loss functions and learning functions, respectively, are cross entropy and the Adam optimizer. The training and validation accuracy of the same model with 50 epoch is shown in Figure 3.9.

## 3.3   Nutrition evaluation

Historically, techniques such as 24-hour recall or meal frequency questionnaires have been used to quantify food intake [25]. Despite being frequently employed, these techniques are acknowledged to have serious issues. Digital alternatives have emerged recently in an effort to capitalize on how simple many mobile applications are to use. However, applications that simply allow study participants to manually record their food intake via text do not significantly beat paper-based methods in terms of usability because of the difficulty of text entry on mobile devices. More promising are applications that scan the bar codes of food items and then extract the nutritional data from associated databases.

After identifying the food item and examining the nutrition of the meal, the system ought to be able to do dietary evaluation [26]. From each meal image, we basically compute the calories, lipids, carbohydrates, and proteins. In a real-world setting, the system should elicit from users basic physical data such as age, gender, weight, height, and level of exercise. Based on their profile, we can predict how much food and nutrition they should consume to maintain a healthy diet. How can one tell if a user is getting the right amount of energy and food? As the go-to resource for dietary assessment, the USDA National Nutrient Database (NNDB), which contains nutritional data on 8,618 staple foods, is employed. Create a reference table of nutrition facts using the data provided by the USDA and all of the food items in the databases. The amount of nutritional components for the food items users have captured is then determined by mapping the identified food to the reference table.

An illustration of our food nutrition reference table can be found in Tables 3.3 and 3.4. The reference table lists the food's protein, calories, fat, carbohydrates, and vitamins in each row. The Food101 dataset has 101 different food categories, hence the table will have 101 rows. We can offer a diet calculator based on the user profile details.

*Table 3.3    Food nutrition reference table of classes 0–50 in Food101 dataset*

| Class | Name | Protein | Calcium | Fat | Carbohydrates | Vitamins |
|---|---|---|---|---|---|---|
| 0 | Apple pie | 2.63 | 0.018 | 14.04 | 35.09 | 0 |
| 1 | Baby back ribs | 18.75 | 0.026 | 9.82 | 0 | 0 |
| 2 | Baklava | 6.64 | 0.04 | 29.13 | 37.53 | 0.0013 |
| 3 | Beef carpaccio | 27.1 | 0.012 | 14.93 | 0 | 0 |
| 4 | Beef tartare | 15.67 | 0.032 | 13.84 | 1.56 | 0.0052 |
| 5 | Beet salad | 1.32 | 0.018 | 5.29 | 11.01 | 0.4542 |
| 6 | Beignets | 12.5 | 0.25 | 0 | 75 | 0 |
| 7 | Bibimbap | 5.38 | 0.033 | 2.81 | 8.34 | 0.0055 |
| 8 | Bread pudding | 4.42 | 0.044 | 12.39 | 43.36 | 0.398 |
| 9 | Breakfast burrito | 5.16 | 0.052 | 5.16 | 18.06 | 0.1305 |
| 10 | Bruschetta | 4.03 | 0.039 | 7.7 | 22.18 | 0.1366 |
| 11 | Caesar salad | 5.91 | 0.157 | 15.75 | 7.48 | 4.1505 |
| 12 | Cannoli | 6.32 | 0.021 | 14.74 | 42.11 | 0 |
| 13 | Caprese salad | 3.52 | 0.106 | 11.97 | 8.45 | 1.0602 |
| 14 | Carrot cake | 3.85 | 0.046 | 29.23 | 56.15 | 1.923 |
| 15 | Ceviche | 10.34 | 0.025 | 0.75 | 3.58 | 1.939 |
| 16 | Cheese plate | 6.46 | 0.146 | 11.51 | 15.58 | 0.27 |
| 17 | Cheesecake | 5.5 | 0.051 | 22.5 | 25.5 | 0.2544 |
| 18 | Chicken curry | 5.73 | 0.032 | 3.85 | 6.67 | 0.263 |
| 19 | Chicken quesadilla | 14.16 | 0.221 | 10.62 | 22.12 | 0.2661 |
| 20 | Chicken wings | 18.58 | 0 | 18.58 | 0 | 0 |
| 21 | Chocolate cake | 3.53 | 0.024 | 12.94 | 60 | 0 |
| 22 | Chocolate mousse | 1.19 | 0.036 | 23.81 | 19.05 | 0.0007 |
| 23 | Churros | 3.02 | 0.007 | 30.58 | 49.8 | 0 |
| 24 | Clam chowder | 2.68 | 0.007 | 3.12 | 8.48 | 0 |

*(Continues)*

*Table 3.3*    (*Continued*)

| Class | Name | Protein | Calcium | Fat | Carbohydrates | Vitamins |
|---|---|---|---|---|---|---|
| 25 | Club sandwich | 14.04 | 0.171 | 12.33 | 20.21 | 0.7741 |
| 26 | Crab cakes | 11.76 | 0.024 | 5.88 | 15.29 | 0 |
| 27 | Creme brulee | 3.64 | 0.055 | 18.18 | 17.27 | 0.909 |
| 28 | Croque madame | 15 | 0 | 7.5 | 70 | 0 |
| 29 | Cup cakes | 2.22 | 0.222 | 11.11 | 60 | 0 |
| 30 | Deviled eggs | 10.71 | 0 | 25 | 0 | 0.714 |
| 31 | Donuts | 4 | 0.08 | 26 | 64 | 0 |
| 32 | Dumplings | 14.29 | 0 | 0.89 | 73.21 | 0 |
| 33 | Edamame | 10.59 | 0.059 | 4.71 | 8.24 | 0 |
| 34 | Eggs benedict | 12.65 | 0.06 | 22.55 | 8.25 | 0.0011 |
| 35 | Escargots | 16.95 | 0.169 | 0.85 | 1.69 | 0.169 |
| 36 | Falafel | 8.33 | 0.087 | 40.54 | 29.32 | 0.1767 |
| 37 | Filet mignon | 15.18 | 0 | 15.18 | 0 | 0.089 |
| 38 | Fish and chips | 13.9 | 0.028 | 10.66 | 12.63 | 0.0926 |
| 39 | Foie gras | 11.4 | 0.07 | 43.84 | 4.67 | 3.335 |
| 40 | French fries | 2.38 | 0.011 | 4.76 | 25 | 3.335 |
| 41 | French onion soup | 4.21 | 0.088 | 3.51 | 6.32 | 0.1421 |
| 42 | French toast | 6.78 | 0.068 | 3.39 | 33.05 | 0 |
| 43 | Fried calamari | 2.07 | 0.05 | 18.1 | 34.05 | 0.0068 |
| 44 | Fried rice | 7.69 | 0.013 | 3.21 | 27.24 | 0.2419 |
| 45 | Frozen yogurt | 4.41 | 0.368 | 2.21 | 32.35 | 0.441 |
| 46 | Garlic bread | 8.51 | 0.085 | 12.77 | 40.43 | 0 |
| 47 | Gnocchi | 3.33 | 0 | 0 | 33.33 | 0.001 |
| 48 | Greek salad | 2.01 | 0.034 | 4.03 | 7.38 | 3.2001 |
| 49 | Grilled cheese sandwich | 15.33 | 0.4 | 18 | 31.33 | 0.137 |
| 50 | Grilled salmon | 24.64 | 0.014 | 9.42 | 0 | 0.1467 |

*Table 3.4    Food nutrition reference table of classes 51–101 in Food101 dataset*

| Class | Name | Protein | Calcium | Fat | Carbohydrates | Vitamins |
|---|---|---|---|---|---|---|
| 51 | Guacamole | 3.57 | 0 | 7.14 | 10.71 | 0.3741 |
| 52 | Gyoza | 3.33 | 0 | 7.14 | 33.33 | 0.3741 |
| 53 | Hamburger | 9.3 | 0.093 | 2.33 | 44.19 | 0 |
| 54 | Hot and sour soup | 2.58 | 0.019 | 1.21 | 4.35 | 0 |
| 55 | Hot dog | 19.3 | 0.035 | 14.04 | 1.75 | 0.2651 |
| 56 | Huevos rancheros | 6.87 | 0.049 | 6.48 | 8.72 | 0.264 |
| 57 | Hummus | 10.71 | 0.071 | 8.93 | 28.57 | 0 |
| 58 | Ice cream | 4.29 | 0.086 | 8.57 | 37.14 | 0 |
| 59 | Lasagna | 12.5 | 0.018 | 1.79 | 75 | 0 |
| 60 | Lobster bisque | 5.22 | 0.052 | 2.6 | 1.7 | 0.0013 |
| 61 | Lobster roll sandwich | 21.64 | 0.052 | 8.12 | 16.5 | 0.0004 |
| 62 | Macaroni and cheese | 6.09 | 0.085 | 4.78 | 18.7 | 0.0004 |
| 63 | Macarons | 10 | 0.083 | 23.33 | 53.33 | 0.0004 |
| 64 | Miso soup | 1.92 | 0.027 | 0.8 | 2.08 | 0.0004 |

*(Continues)*

*Table 3.4    (Continued)*

| Class | Name | Protein | Calcium | Fat | Carbohydrates | Vitamins |
|-------|------|---------|---------|-----|---------------|----------|
| 65 | Mussels | 23.89 | 0.033 | 4.42 | 7.08 | 0.0004 |
| 66 | Nachos | 4.32 | 0.063 | 21.5 | 34.91 | 0.0011 |
| 67 | Omelet | 7.93 | 0.066 | 3.96 | 4.85 | 0.1386 |
| 68 | Onion rings | 0 | 0.071 | 21.43 | 71.43 | 0 |
| 69 | Oysters | 4.77 | 0.075 | 10.78 | 18.41 | 0.0018 |
| 70 | Pad thai | 8.12 | 0.021 | 7.39 | 14.32 | 0.0047 |
| 71 | Paella | 13.33 | 0.067 | 3.33 | 82.22 | 1.341 |
| 72 | Pancakes | 6.45 | 0.097 | 2.42 | 53.23 | 0.161 |
| 73 | Panna cotta | 3 | 0.15 | 10 | 30 | 0.161 |
| 74 | Peking duck | 0.36 | 0.011 | 0.13 | 60.61 | 0.1619 |
| 75 | Pho | 6.14 | 0.011 | 2.24 | 10.39 | 0.1625 |
| 76 | Pizza | 10.59 | 0.294 | 9.41 | 23.53 | 0.2378 |
| 77 | Pork chop | 27.69 | 0.008 | 10.5 | 0 | 0.235 |
| 78 | Poutine | 11.25 | 0.188 | 18.75 | 20 | 0.375 |
| 79 | Prime rib | 16.15 | 0.009 | 31.66 | 0 | 0 |
| 80 | Pulled pork sandwich | 10.33 | 0.033 | 7.07 | 31.52 | 0.109 |
| 81 | Ramen | 12.73 | 0.036 | 2.73 | 63.64 | 0.7281 |
| 82 | Ravioli | 13 | 0.25 | 10 | 29 | 1.75 |
| 83 | Red velvet cake | 4.67 | 0.037 | 22.43 | 57.01 | 0.374 |
| 84 | Risotto | 8.11 | 0 | 2.7 | 75.68 | 0.8207 |
| 85 | Samosa | 4.66 | 0.027 | 17.87 | 32.21 | 0.8154 |
| 86 | Sashimi | 14.73 | 0.016 | 9.3 | 3.1 | 0.0037 |
| 87 | Scallops | 15.04 | 0 | 0.88 | 0.88 | 0 |
| 88 | Seaweed salad | 0 | 0.111 | 2.78 | 11.11 | 0.222 |
| 89 | Shrimp and grits | 8.82 | 0.074 | 8.33 | 9.8 | 0.3798 |
| 90 | Spaghetti bolognese | 1.39 | 0.026 | 1.61 | 7.43 | 0.37 |
| 91 | Spaghetti carbonara | 1.39 | 0.026 | 1.61 | 7.43 | 0.37 |
| 92 | Spring rolls | 11.9 | 0.048 | 7.14 | 19.05 | 0.595 |
| 93 | Steak | 0 | 0 | 0 | 111.11 | 0 |
| 94 | Strawberry shortcake | 5.26 | 0 | 21.05 | 57.89 | 0 |
| 95 | Sushi | 0 | 0 | 0 | 3.57 | 0 |
| 96 | Tacos | 10.94 | 0.016 | 4.69 | 23.44 | 0.1607 |
| 97 | Octopus balls | 12.3 | 0.035 | 0.8 | 0 | 0 |
| 98 | Tiramisu | 5.91 | 0.066 | 24.26 | 29.61 | 0.0011 |
| 99 | Tuna tartare | 15.67 | 0.032 | 13.84 | 1.56 | 0.0052 |
| 100 | Waffles | 4.69 | 0.031 | 17.19 | 51.56 | 0 |

## 3.4   Application

Systems that automatically monitor nutrients are useful in daily living. That implies that those who are concerned about their daily intake can monitor the components of their meals and the nutrients they contain. This system may also be used in health care. Based on the patient's condition, it is possible to determine their nutritional needs and create a suitable diet plan. With potential applications in personalized nutrition, clinical nutrition, public health, the food industry, agriculture, and research, AI models can analyze food photos for nutrient analysis. AI models can be used to measure nutrient consumption, monitor population nutrition, aid healthcare professionals in determining a patient's nutritional state, optimize food products, increase agricultural yields and nutritional value, and facilitate large-scale research. The use of AI models in the analysis of food photographs has the potential to enhance public health outcomes and deepen our knowledge of the connection between diet and health.

## 3.5    Conclusion

Malnutrition-related health problems of various kinds were explored. Additionally, several nutrition classes and their suppliers were noted. Proper processes for maintaining the nutrient level are also determined by determining the nutritional content from food photos. People of all ages are using smartphones more and more, and also care about their health. Currently, there are numerous techniques for creating a customized diet. Using the ideas presented here, a smartphone can handle the complete system automatically. The development of more precise and thorough AI models that can examine food photos for a larger variety of nutrients and dietary components can be the subject of future research. This will make nutrient analysis and nutrition advice more accurate and individualized. Also future studies can evaluate the effectiveness of AI nutrient analysis models across various ethnicities and cultures to make sure they deliver appropriate recommendations for a larger range of people.

## References

[1]  https://www.who.int/health-topics/nutrition#tab=tab 1.

[2]  FAO, IFAD, UNICEF, WFP and WHO. 2022. The State of Food Security and Nutrition in the World 2022. Repurposing Food and Agricultural Policies to Make Healthy Diets More Affordable. Rome, FAO. https://doi.org/10.4060/cc0639en.

[3]  J. Saunders and T. Smith. Malnutrition: causes and consequences. *Clin Med (Lond)*. 2010;10(6):624–627. doi:10.7861/clinmedicine.10-6-624. PMID: 21413492; PMCID: PMC4951875.

[4]  A.L. Cawood, M. Elia, and R.J. Stratton. Treatment of malnutrition in chronic nonmalignant disease. *Am. J. Clin. Nutr.* 2011;93(2):247–254. doi:10.3945/ajcn.110.003485.

[5]  S.E. Sreetha, G.N. Sundar, and D. Narmadha. An investigation on impact of malnutrition in human health and technique to evaluate the nutrient intake from the food image. In: *2022 IEEE International Power and Renewable Energy Conference (IPRECON)*, Kollam, India, 2022, pp. 1–5. doi: 10.1109/IPRECON55716.2022.10059560.

[6]  J. Sak and M. Suchodolska. Artificial intelligence in nutrients science research: a review. *Nutrients* 2021;13:322. https://doi.org/10.3390/nu13020322.

[7]    E.S. Sreetha, G. Naveen Sundar, and D. Narmadha. Comparative study on recognition of food item from images for analyzing the nutritional contents. In: Peter, J.D., Fernandes, S.L., and Alavi, A.H. (eds.), *Disruptive Technologies for Big Data and Cloud Applications. Lecture Notes in Electrical Engineering*, vol. 905, 2022. Singapore: Springer. https://doi.org/10.1007/978-981-19-2177-3_27.

[8]    https://www.fritz.ai/image-recognition.

[9]    https://nanonets.com/image-recognition.

[10]   Y. Kawano and K. Yanai. Real-time mobile food recognition system. In: *2013 IEEE Conference on Computer Vision and Pattern Recognition Workshops*, 2013, pp. 1–7.

[11]   L. Bossard, M. Guillaumin, and L. Van Gool. Food-101 – mining discriminative components with random forests. In: *European Conference on Computer Vision*, 2014.

[12]   J. Sánchez, F. Perronnin, T. Mensink, *et al.* Image classification with the Fisher vector: theory and practice. *Int. J. Comput. Vis.* 2013;105:222–245. https://doi.org/10.1007/s11263-013-0636-x.

[13]   K. Aizawa, Y. Maruyama, H. Li, and C. Morikawa, Food balance estimation by using personal dietary tendencies in a multimedia food log. *IEEE Trans. Multimed.* 2013;15(8):2176–2185.

[14]   J.M.M. Anthimopoulos, L. Gianola, L. Scarnato, P. Diem, and S.G. Mougiakakou. A food recognition system for diabetic patients based on an optimized bag-of-features model. *IEEE J. Biomed. Health Inform.* 2014;18 (4):1261.

[15]   https://intellipaat.com/blog/tutorial/machine-learning-tutorial/introduction-deep learning.

[16]   https://www.analyticsvidhya.com/blog/2022/03/basics-of-cnn-in-deep-learning.

[17]   C. Szegedy, W. Liu, Y. Jia, *et al.* Going deeper with convolutions. In: *2015 IEEE Conference on Computer Vision and Pattern Recognition (CVPR)*, 2015, pp. 1–9, doi: 10.1109/CVPR.2015.7298594.

[18]   Y. LeCun, L. Bottou, Y. Bengio, and P. Haffner. Gradient based learning applied to document recognition. In: *Proceedings of the IEEE*, November 1998.

[19]   C. Szegedy, V. Vanhoucke, S. Ioffe, J. Shlens, and W. Zbigniew. Rethinking the inception architecture for computer vision, arXiv:1512.00567, doi.org/10.48550/arXiv.1512.00567.

[20]   C.K. Chang, L. Chiari, Y. Cao, *et al.* Inclusive smart cities and digital health – deep-food: deep learning-based food image recognition for computer-aided dietary assessment, vol. 9677. In: *Lecture Notes in Computer Science*, 2016 (Chapter 4), pp. 37–48, doi:10.1007/978-3-319-39601-9.

[21]   V.C. Burkapalli and P.C. Patil. Transfer learning: Inception-V3 based custom classification approach for food images. *IC-TACT J. Image Video Process.* 2020;11(1):2261–2267. doi:10.21917/ijivp.2020.0321.

[22]   L. Zhou, C. Zhang, F. Liu, Z. Qiu, and Y. He. Application of deep learning in food: a review. *Comprehen. Rev. Food Science Food Safety*, 2019;18:1541–4337.12492. doi:10.1111/1541-4337.12492.

[23] https://www.isahit.com/blog/what-is-the-purpose-of-image-preprocessing-in-deep-learning.

[24] https://www.section.io/engineering-education/image-preprocessing-in-python/.

[25] S.P. Mohanty, G. Singhal, E.A. Scuccimarra, *et al.* The food recognition benchmark: using deep learning to recognize food in images. *Front. Nutr.* 2022;9:875143. doi: 10.3389/fnut.2022.875143.

[26] Md Riyazudin, M.A. Chaurasia, S. Ibaad, A. Lalani, and S. Fathima. Estimation of quantity and nutritional information of food using image processing. In: *Contactless Healthcare Facilitation and Commodity Delivery Management during COVID-19 Pandemic,* 2022. 10.1007/978-981-16-5411-4 11.

*Chapter 4*

# Medical diagnosis of human heart diseases using supervised learning techniques

*S. Muthurajkumar[1], R. Praveen, A.A. Abd El-Aziz[2], R. Shangeeth[1], S. Anika Lakshmi[1] and R. Gaythrisri[1]*

## Abstract

All around the world, machine learning (ML) is employed in a variety of domains. The healthcare sector is no different. In recent years, predictive analytics has become a potential tool for decision-making and problem-solving in the healthcare industry. The data processing is automated, increasing the medical system's durability and efficiency. To deliver higher quality healthcare at a lower cost, it demonstrates critical and evaluates healthcare data. The likelihood of developing cardiac disease can be predicted with the aid of ML. If foreseen, such information can offer physicians vital intuitions, enabling them to customize each patient's diagnosis and therapy. A range of diagnostic tests are advised for patients to take part in. Foreseeing potential cardiac problems in patients is done using ML techniques. The primary aim of the research work is to use fewer indicators to predict the prevalence of heart disease (HD). Thirteen characteristics were first employed to forecast cardiac disease. A simplified genetic algorithm is employed to determine the characteristics that are most important for the diagnosis of cardiac issues, hence minimizing the amount of testing that a patient must undergo. Thirteen features are whittled down to five via genetic search. The system takes into consideration a fuzzy logic in one of those five features. Making the best judgment feasible given the data requires taking into account all available information. The system compares various classifiers, including the naive Bayes classifier, the random forest classifier, the decision tree classifier, and the logistic regression classifier. These four classifiers have been employed in the system to predict HDs using potential risk data extracted from health records. The cardiac data set has been put through a number of tests, and results indicate that decision trees surpass cross-validation and train-test split techniques, with accuracy rates of 88.52% and 82.51%, respectively. The second finding is that all algorithms' accuracy has been reduced when cross-validation is used. Finally, the system applies

[1]Department of Computer Technology, Madras Institute of Technology (MIT) Campus, Anna University, Chennai, India
[2]Department of Information Systems and Technology, Faculty of Graduate Studies for Statistical Research, Cairo University, Cairo, Egypt

several validation procedures with evidence that was gathered prospectively to confirm the validity of the suggested approach.

**Keywords:** Machine learning; Decision tree classifier; Fuzzy logic; Logistic regression; Heart disease prediction; e-Healthcare

## 4.1  Introduction

Healthcare is one of humanity's primary concerns. According to World Health Organization (WHO) recommendations, everyone has the fundamental right to good health. It is believed that suitable medical services should be made available for regular health examinations. Over 31% of fatalities worldwide are attributable to heart disease (HD). Due to a shortage of diagnostic facilities, qualified physicians, and other factors that affect the accuracy of HD prediction, the early diagnosis and treatment of several heart disorders are extremely difficult, especially in poor nations [1,2]. In light of this, medical aid software that supports the early detection of cardiac disease has been developed recently using the approaches of computer technology and machine learning (ML). Any heart condition that is detected early can reduce mortality. To understand the data pattern and derive predictions from it, a variety of ML techniques are applied to health data. Healthcare data is frequently massive in size and expertly organized [3,4]. Large-scale data management and information mining are capabilities of ML algorithms. ML algorithms learn from and forecast real-time events using historical data [5]. The ML architecture for early HD prediction enables unskilled practitioners to detect angina type more quickly, potentially saving a significant number of lives. Heat disease was diagnosed utilizing ML, which employed the flow of several modules from data analysis to classification while employing the best possible search technique. Each module's output is evaluated and provided. The system attempts to more precisely and economically forecast a patient's heart condition. The system provides the performance, analysis, multi-validation methodologies, and effects of each module in a well-documented manner. Designing a suitable dataset with a fuzzy logic feature that can be utilized to predict the kind of angina is the major goal of this study. The cross-validation technique will be employed to solve the overfitting issue. To increase accuracy, the differences between the cross-validation and split data approaches will be examined. The most accurate model will be determined by comparing the classifier models logistic regression, decision tree, naive Bayes, and random forest taking into account two validation approaches. Additionally, the user may choose to have a report with the generated results mailed to the physician.

## 4.2  Literature survey

In the field of HD detection and prediction, researchers have explored various ML and deep learning techniques to improve accuracy. Ibomoiye Domor Mienye *et al.* [6]

proposed the accuracy-based weighted aging classifier ensemble (AB-WAE), which used an average-based splitting technique to divide the dataset into minor portions and merge Classification and Regression Tree (CART) models into a homogeneous ensemble. The AB-WAE achieved an accuracy of 93% and 91% for the Cleveland and Framingham datasets, respectively. Rohit Bharti *et al.* [7] used the isolation forest for feature selection and handling outliers and employed a sequential model deep learning approach to overcome overfitting. The deep learning approach had an accuracy rate of 94.2%, outperforming ML models, with KNeighbors achieving a maximum accuracy of 3.29%. Finally, Hamdaoui *et al.* [8] focused on developing a clinical support system for forecasting cardiac disease using risk factor information collected from medical files. They found naive Bayes to be the algorithm of choice, achieving an accuracy of 82.16% for cross-validation and 84.21% for train-test split approaches. However, the study noted that the cross-validation technique caused a drop in accuracy for all algorithms, highlighting the importance of careful evaluation of ML models in the medical field.

Several ML models have been compared in studies aimed at predicting HD, including decision trees, naive Bayes, random forests, support vector machines, k-nearest neighbors, and logistic regression. The performance of these models was assessed using metrics such as precision, accuracy, area under the ROC curve (AUC), and F1-score. Random forest was found to be particularly effective at identifying heart disorders, with an accuracy rate of 83.57% and AUC and accuracy scores of 87.24% and 88.89%, respectively, according to Sujatha *et al.* [9]. Saw *et al.* [10] used a random search method to find the best model solution with random combinations of hyperparameters and achieved an accuracy of 87% in the prediction of the logistic regression model. Fitriyani *et al.* [11] balanced the uneven training dataset using the synthetic minority over-sampling technique and edited nearest neighbor (SMOTE-ENN) and utilized density-based spatial clustering of applications along with noise (DBSCAN) to find and remove anomalous data. They compared several ML models, including naive Bayes, logistic regression, multi-player perceptron, support vector machine, decision tree, and random forest.

To diagnose heart illness, a number of ML models have been developed. Umarani Nagavelli *et al.* [12] proposed a hybrid approach using the Waikato Environment for Knowledge Analysis (WEKA) and Knowledge Extraction based on Evolutionary Learning (KEEL) tools to evaluate the performance of these algorithms. Principal component analysis (PCA) is the widely used dimensionality reduction technique for feature extraction under WEKA tool, while the wrapper method is used for feature selection under KEEL tool. Swain *et al.* [13] aimed to discover the best forecasting algorithm and employed a variety of ML methods, including logistic regression, support vector machines, k-nearest neighbors, Gaussian naive Bayes, decision trees, and random forests. Logistic regression was shown to have the best prediction accuracy of 88.29%. Dengqing Zhang *et al.* [14] aimed to enhance accuracy by examining ML algorithms using several performance criteria. The study required using the mean value to replace missing data in the pre-processing step and achieved a scoring accuracy of 86.8% using SVM with a linear kernel.

Sajja *et al.* [15] use the WEKA tool to pre-process the raw dataset and apply different ML techniques. Support vector machine (SVM) is found to be the most dependable procedure for categorizing and predicting cardiac disease. Amen *et al.* [16] aim to predict the five stages of HD using hyperparameters to optimize the performance of classifiers. Logistic regression (LR) outperforms the other five algorithms, with an accuracy of 82%. Anna Karen Garate-Escamila *et al.* [17] propose a feature selection strategy with a dimensionality reduction method to achieve higher accuracy rates. The best outcomes come from CHI-PCA with RF, which had accuracy rates of 98.7%, 99.0%, and 99.4% for Cleveland, Hungarian, and CH, respectively. The studies use various performance criteria such as f-measure, precision, recall, and accuracy to assess the performance of the algorithms.

A hybrid strategy has been suggested by Ashri *et al.* [18] to increase prediction accuracy for identifying cardiac disease. The authors applied an ensemble model and recommended pre-processing and feature selection based on a genetic algorithm to enhance performance and reduce time complexity. The proposed ensemble classifier model achieved a classification accuracy of 98.18%. In a similar vein, Hager Ahmed *et al.* [19] suggested the most effective ML strategy for forecasting cardiac disease by using univariate feature selection and Relief methods for feature selection. They optimized four different types of ML algorithms using cross-validation and hyperparameter optimization. The random forest classifier was found to perform better than the other models with a high accuracy of 94.9%. The proposed architecture can be employed with Apache Kafka and Apache Spark to effectively manage Twitter data streams containing patient data [20–22].

## 4.3    Proposed work

HD has been responsible for a large number of deaths during the past ten years, and this trend is still present today. Depending on a person's gender, color, and ethnicity, different numbers of people pass away from HD. As a result, earlier detection of cardiac disease has become increasingly challenging. Naive Bayes, logistic regression, support vector machine, decision tree, and random forest models have been proposed for predicting HD based on the references of research publications from the last 4–5 years. The above-mentioned standard models have yielded superior outcomes in the diagnosis of HD and have achieved notable results. These standard models in research publications influenced the idea behind the model of classification and pre-processing phases in HD prediction among patients.

Accompanying Figure 4.1 depicts the entire architecture of the implemented model. Feature extraction, validation, and classification are used to build the model. Furthermore, the dataset being used here had been newly created, and its crucial variable Exang (Exercise-induced Angina) was acquired in decimals using fuzzy logic. Fuzzy logic has been applied to consider the Exang to various degrees to better effectively forecast stable and unstable angina. Using the patient's medical records, the model can predict the patient's outcome once it has been trained. To select the best model, the accuracy of each model is compared, and the model with

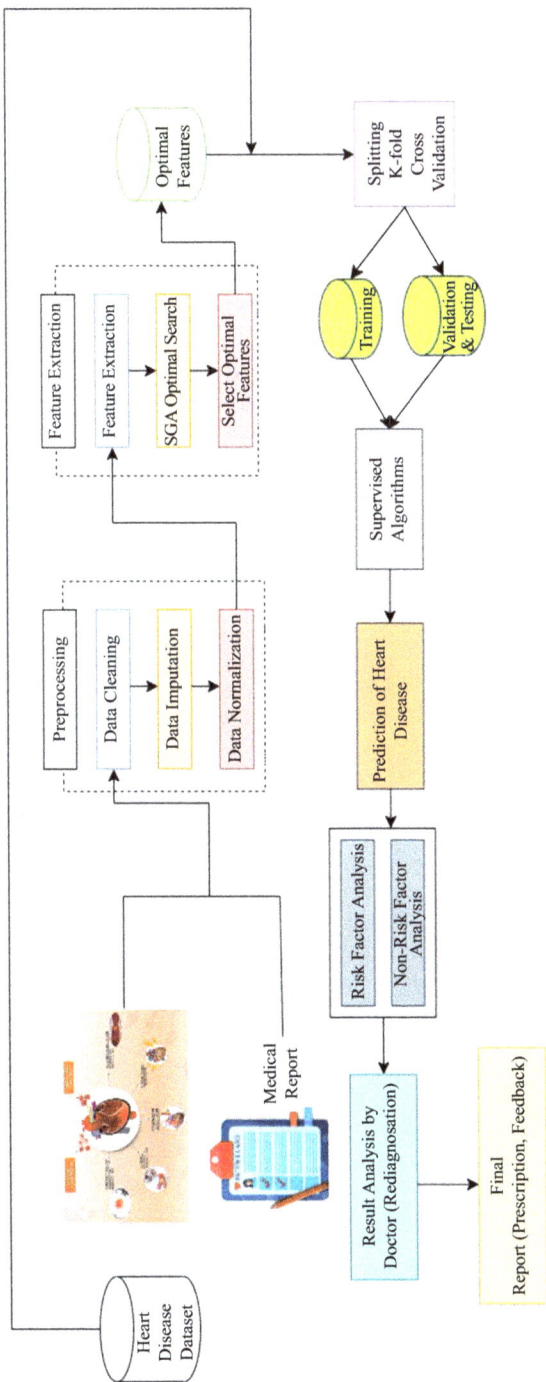

*Figure 4.1   Architecture diagram*

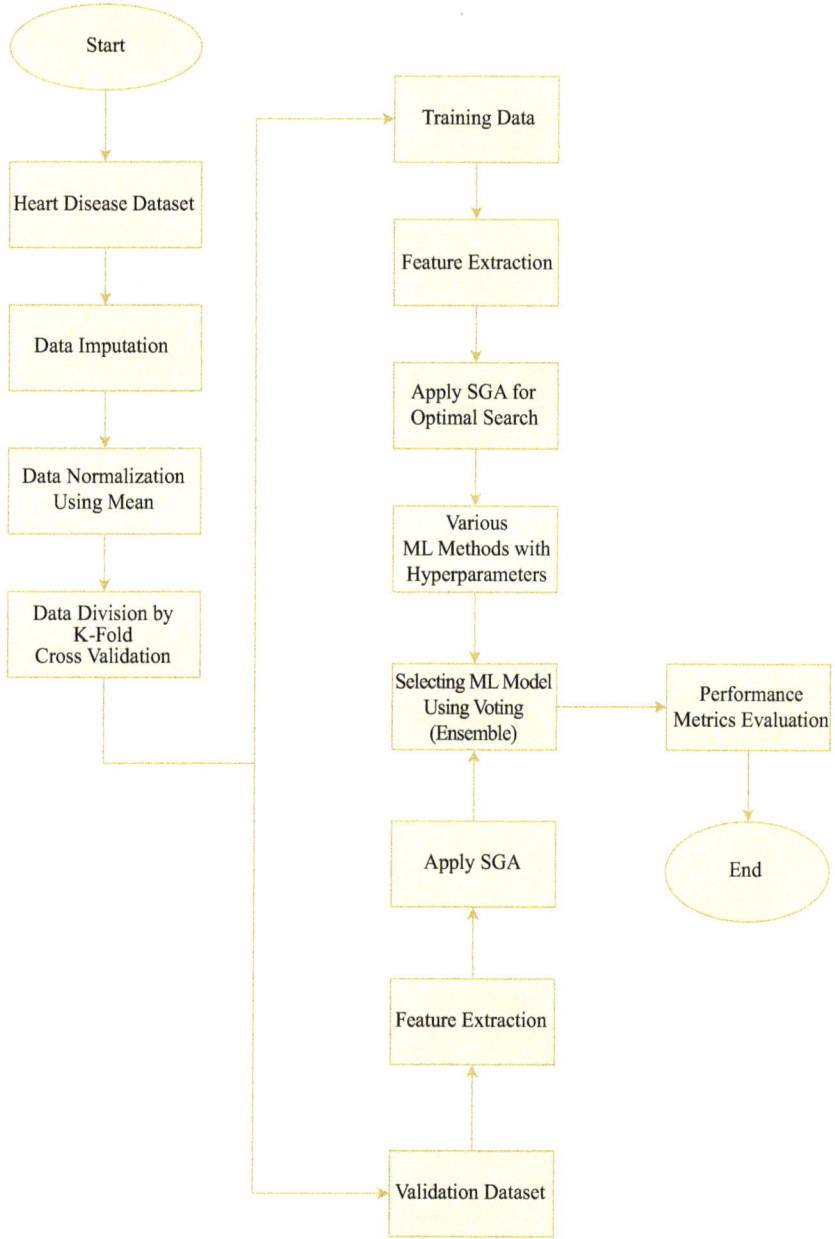

*Figure 4.2   System workflow*

the highest accuracy is chosen to represent the result. Additionally, a report containing the model's output and the user's entered values will be forwarded to the registered user and the doctor.

The pre-processing phase receives the provided medical data. Then, using the simple genetic approach (SGA), the best features are retrieved. The dataset is validated purely on the basis of the optimal features. The dataset is separated into train and test sets in an 80:20 ratio. Following that, features retrieved from the train data are employed to classify the output. The performance of the classifiers is investigated and compared. The system can forecast the patient's outcome after examining the model's output.

### 4.3.1    Workflow

The workflow of HD diagnosis is the dataset that has been provided with the patient's medical details as shown in Figure 4.2. A new dataset is considered by using an attribute with fuzzy logic. In the proposed work and conclusion, the importance of interpreting Exang feature as fuzzy logic is covered. After pre-processing, the data K-fold cross-validation is applied. The feature extraction is done by SGA. The optimal features are extracted from the entire dataset. Then, the classification model is fed with these features as input and trained. The ML models are compared and performance is analyzed.

## 4.4    Implementation

Figure 4.3 depicts the processes involved in developing the Heart Disease Prediction (HDP) system. The dataset is initially acquired with 14 attributes. It was pre-processed to improve the data quality by converting the raw dataset into a cleaned data to enhance prediction results more accurately. Utilizing feature extraction improves prediction's ideal speed. The best features are derived from the other attributes through feature extraction. The various ML models are evaluated with hyperparameters. By doing a comparison research on split data and the cross-validation technique, the validity is also improved. The accuracy results indicate the presence or absence of a cardiac disease.

### 4.4.1    Data accumulation

The Cleveland-Hungarian dataset has been gathered from the University of California, Irvine ML Repository. The dataset has around 1,300 instances and 14 attributes including age, sex, chest pain type, blood pressure, serum cholesterol levels, and others. Two among the 14 attributes are demographic while the other 11 are clinical measurements of cardiovascular state and performance. The target variable in this dataset is a binary variable indicating the presence or absence of HD. Exang which stands for exercise-induced angina is 1 of the 11 clinical attributes that are listed after data imputation. Angina is a type of chest pain that occurs when the heart is not receiving enough oxygen. Exercise can cause a specific type of angina called exercise-induced angina. A mathematical framework called fuzzy logic enables the depiction of ambiguity and imprecision. Instead of just being true or false, values in fuzzy logic might range from entirely false to completely true, with the middle values signifying different levels of truth. Fuzzy logic representation of the Exang feature will aid in capturing the uncertainty and imprecision contained in

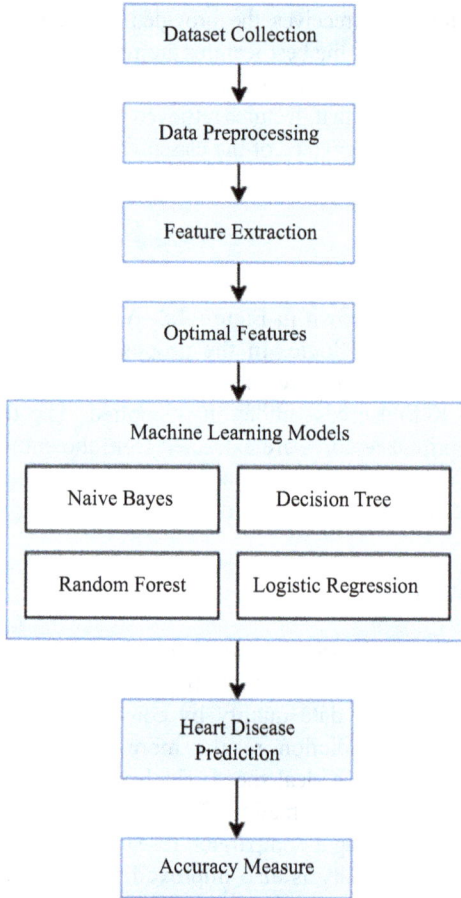

*Figure 4.3   System model*

clinical data, improving clinical decision-making and prediction accuracy. As a result, a new attribute called Exang (Fuzzy-based) is introduced for more precise prediction, especially for angina, and a newly modified dataset is obtained.

## 4.4.2   Description of features used

Taking into account the 14 characteristics provided in the "Feature name" column. Target field one of those 14 characteristics refers to the patient's presence of HD. Its values are 0 for no disease, 1 for disease, and 1 for male and 2 for female in the sex field. An integer number of 1 indicates stable angina, while an integer value of 2 indicates unstable angina. The ST phase of the peak exercise was graded as follows: 1 = Unsloping, 2 = Flat, and 3 = Unsloping. Based on the specified domain range, an integer input is required for age, maximum heart rate, old peak, Exang, and major vessels colored by fluoroscopy (Table 4.1).

*Table 4.1  Feature description*

| ID | Representation | Feature name | Datatype | Measurement | Domain range | Missing values |
|---|---|---|---|---|---|---|
| 1 | Age | AGE | Continuous-Real | Age in years | 29–79 | NO |
| 2 | Sex | SEX | Discrete Binary | Gender of patient | 0, 1 | NO |
| 3 | CD | CPT | Discrete Categorical | 1 = Stable Angina<br>2 = Unstable Angina | 12 | YES |
| 4 | trestbps | RBP | Continuous-Real | mm Hg | 94–200 | NO |
| 5 | chol | CHOL | Continuous-Real | mg/dl | 126–564 | NO |
| 6 | fbs | FBS | Discrete Binary | mg/dl | 0, 1 | YES |
| 7 | restecg | EGR | Discrete Categorical | 0 = Normal<br>1 = ST-T Waveabnormal<br>2 = Left ventricular | 0, 1, 2 | NO |
| 8 | thalach | MHR | Continuous-Real | Numeric | 71–202 | NO |
| 9 | Exang | EIG | Decimal | Numeric | 0–1 | NO |
| 10 | old peak | ST | Continuous-Real | Numeric | 0–61 | NO |
| 11 | slope | The Slope of the Peak Exercise | Discrete Categorical | 1 = Unsloping<br>2 = Flat<br>3 = Down slopping | •1,2,3 | NO |
| 12 | ca | NMV | Discrete Real | Colored by fluoroscopy | 0–3 | YES |
| 13 | thalach | Exercise Thallium Scintigraphy | Discrete Categorical | 3 = Normal<br>6 = Fixed Defect<br>7 = Reversible Effect | 3, 6, 7 | YES |
| 14 | class | Target | Discrete Binary | 0 = Absence<br>1 = Presence | 0 or 1 | NO |

Table 4.2 Statistical analysis of the dataset

| | Age | Sex | Cp | trestbps | Chol | fbs | restecg | thalach | oldpeak | slope | ca | thal | target |
|---|---|---|---|---|---|---|---|---|---|---|---|---|---|
| count | 1025.0000 | 1025.00000 | 1025.00000 | 1025.00000 | 1025.00000 | 1025.00000 | 1025.00000 | 1025.00000 | 1025.00000 | 1025.00000 | 1025.00000 | 1025.00000 | 1025.00000 |
| mean | 54.434146 | 0.695610 | 0.942439 | 131.611707 | 246.00000 | 0.149268 | 0.529756 | 149.114146 | 1.071512 | 1.385366 | 0.754146 | 2.323902 | 0.513171 |
| std | 9.072290 | 0.460373 | 1.029641 | 17.516718 | 51.59251 | 0.356527 | 0.527878 | 23.005724 | 1.175053 | 0.617755 | 1.030798 | 0.620660 | 0.500070 |
| min | 29.000000 | 0.000000 | 0.000000 | 94.000000 | 126.00000 | 0.000000 | 0.000000 | 71.000000 | 0.000000 | 0.000000 | 0.000000 | 0.000000 | 0.000000 |
| 25% | 48.000000 | 0.000000 | 0.000000 | 120.000000 | 211.00000 | 0.000000 | 0.000000 | 132.000000 | 0.000000 | 1.000000 | 0.000000 | 2.000000 | 0.000000 |
| 50% | 56.000000 | 1.000000 | 1.000000 | 130.000000 | 240.00000 | 0.000000 | 1.000000 | 152.000000 | 0.800000 | 1.000000 | 0.000000 | 2.000000 | 1.000000 |
| 75% | 61.000000 | 1.000000 | 2.000000 | 140.000000 | 275.00000 | 0.000000 | 1.000000 | 166.000000 | 1.800000 | 2.000000 | 1.000000 | 3.000000 | 1.000000 |
| max | 77.000000 | 1.000000 | 3.000000 | 200.000000 | 564.00000 | 1.000000 | 2.000000 | 202.000000 | 6.200000 | 2.000000 | 4.000000 | 3.000000 | 1.000000 |

### 4.4.3  Data descriptive analysis

Several descriptive statistics using the Pandas library's "describe ()" function have been retrieved. The descriptive statistics retrieved include the average, total, standard deviation, max–min values, and data quantiles. The majority of values are categorized as indicated in Table 4.2. The average value of a character is represented by its mean value. The distribution of the target feature vs the age feature distribution is shown in Figure 4.4.

The "target" feature vs. the "sex" feature distribution is shown in Figure 4.5. Visualizes the association between the dataset's attributes using the Python Matplotlib library function and seaborn routines as demonstrated in the heat map in Figure 4.6. Between the variable "goal" and the other data variable the degree of correlation is low. Using visualization to uncover the relationships between the data's attributes can help us infer the key characteristics. Considering the below-mentioned heatmap, there is a positive link between the

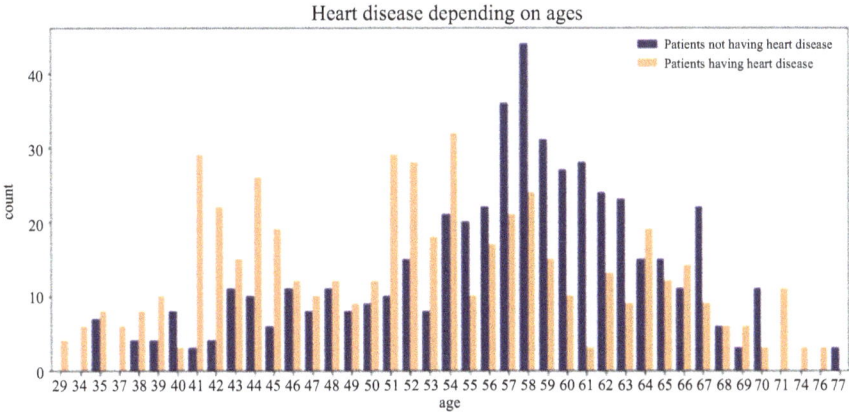

*Figure 4.4   Distribution of "target" with "age" attribute*

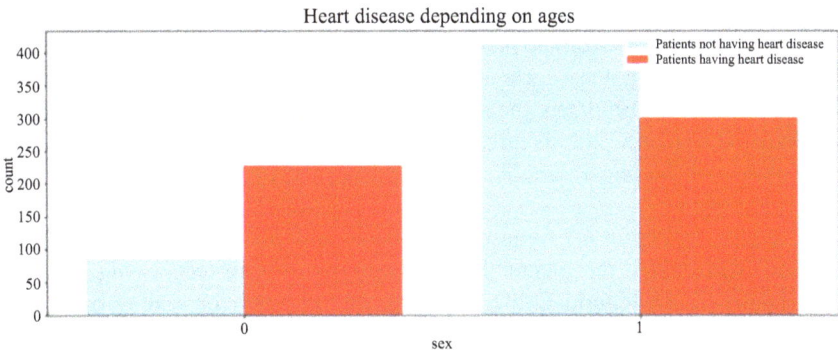

*Figure 4.5   Distribution of "sex" with "age" attribute*

|        | age   | sex    | θ      | trestbps | chol   | fbs     | restecg | thalach | oldpeak | slope   | ca     | thal   | target |
|--------|-------|--------|--------|----------|--------|---------|---------|---------|---------|---------|--------|--------|--------|
| age    | 1     | -0.1   | -0.072 | 0.27     | 0.22   | 0.12    | -0.13   | -0.39   | 0.21    | -0.17   | 0.27   | 0.072  | -0.23  |
| sex    | -0.1  | 1      | -0.041 | -0.079   | -0.2   | 0.027   | -0.055  | -0.049  | 0.085   | -0.027  | 0.11   | 0.2    | -0.28  |
| θ      | -0.072| -0.041 | 1      | 0.038    | -0.082 | 0.079   | 0.044   | 0.31    | -0.17   | 0.13    | -0.18  | -0.16  | 0.43   |
| trestbps| 0.27 | -0.079 | 0.038  | 1        | 0.13   | 0.18    | -0.12   | -0.039  | 0.19    | -0.12   | 0.1    | 0.059  | -0.14  |
| chol   | 0.22  | -0.2   | -0.082 | 0.13     | 1      | 0.027   | -0.15   | -0.022  | 0.065   | -0.014  | 0.074  | 0.1    | -0.1   |
| fbs    | 0.12  | 0.027  | 0.079  | 0.18     | 0.027  | 1       | -0.1    | -0.0089 | 0.011   | -0.062  | 0.14   | -0.042 | -0.041 |
| restecg| -0.13 | -0.055 | 0.044  | -0.12    | -0.15  | -0.1    | 1       | 0.048   | -0.05   | 0.086   | -0.078 | -0.021 | 0.13   |
| thalach| -0.39 | -0.049 | 0.31   | -0.039   | -0.022 | -0.0089 | 0.048   | 1       | -0.35   | 0.4     | -0.21  | -0.098 | 0.42   |
| oldpeak| 0.21  | 0.085  | -0.17  | 0.19     | 0.065  | 0.011   | -0.05   | -0.35   | 1       | -0.58   | 0.22   | 0.2    | -0.44  |
| slope  | -0.17 | -0.027 | 0.13   | -0.12    | -0.014 | -0.062  | 0.086   | 0.4     | -0.58   | 1       | -0.073 | -0.094 | 0.35   |
| ca     | 0.27  | 0.11   | -0.18  | 0.1      | 0.074  | 0.14    | -0.078  | -0.21   | 0.22    | -0.073  | 1      | 0.15   | -0.38  |
| thal   | 0.072 | 0.2    | -0.16  | 0.059    | 0.1    | -0.042  | -0.021  | -0.098  | 0.2     | -0.094  | 0.15   | 1      | -0.34  |
| target | -0.23 | -0.28  | 0.43   | -0.14    | -0.1   | -0.041  | 0.13    | 0.42    | -0.44   | 0.35    | -0.38  | -0.34  | 1      |

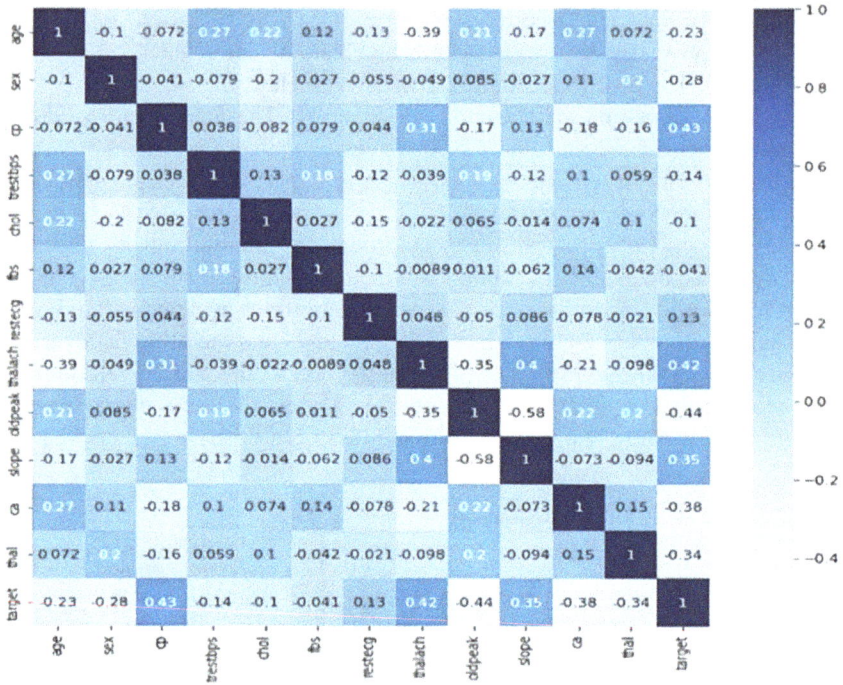

*Figure 4.6   Correlation heat-map for the dataset*

target and chest pain (cp). It implies that those who have frequent chest pain have a higher chance of getting HD. The target has a positive link with thalach, slope, and resting in addition to chest discomfort. As a result, there is a negative link between the target and exercise-induced angina (exang), which indicates that while exercising the heart needs more blood, and the blood flow is slowed down by narrower arteries. Old peak and thalach exhibit a negative connection with the objective in addition to ca.

The simultaneous correlation coefficients between variables are represented by a correlation matrix. A heatmap is then created using this correlation matrix and the specified color coding. On a scale of −1 to 1, with 1 being positively correlated and −1 being inversely correlated, the correlation matrix displays how each attribute is correlated. Considering the features that have at least a 2% (positive or negative) correlation with the target variable anything less would have a minimal impact on the target variable.

The plots in Figure 4.7 represent the presence or absence of the HD for each attribute. Histogram is represented for sex, chest pain, fbs, restecg, exang, slope, ca, thal, and target. Histogram further supports the necessity for scaling by demonstrating how each feature and label is dispersed across several ranges. The discrete bar represents the categorical variables for each attribute indicating the presence or absence of the HD.

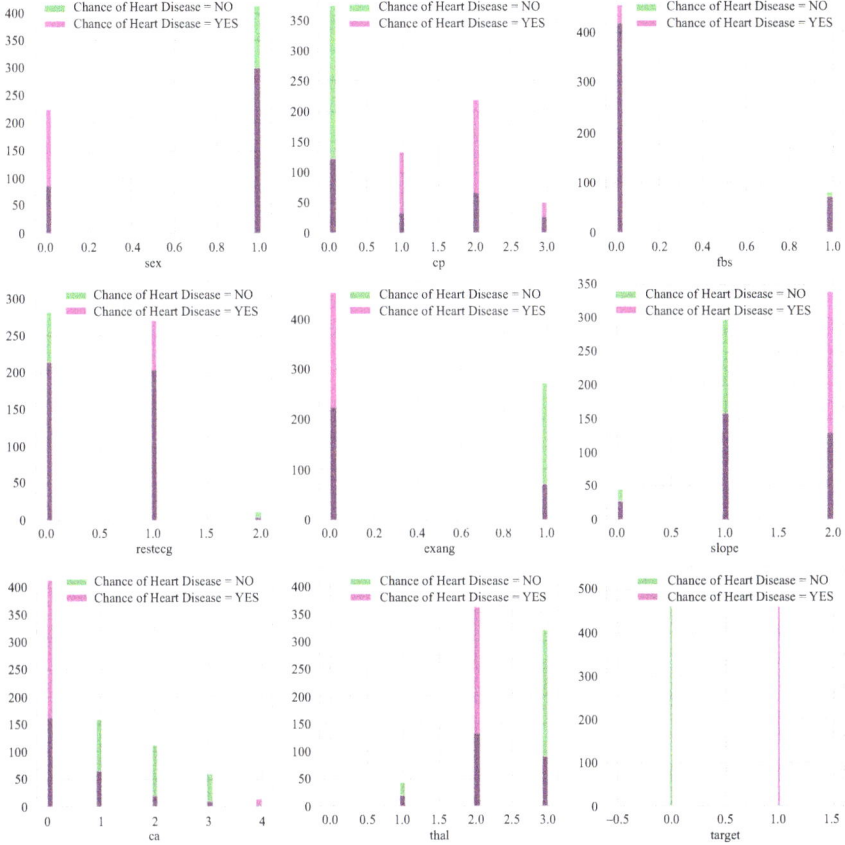

*Figure 4.7   Histogram derived through heat-map for categorical values*

## 4.4.4   Heart disorder identification framework algorithm

---

**Algorithm 4.1 Heart disorder identification framework algorithm** (HDIFA)

---

Input: Heart Disorder Dataset (DS)
Output: Performance Indicators (PI)
Start
  DS' ← Pre_prcoessing(DS)
  PV ← Performance Vector {ACC, PD}DS'
  FE ← Extract Features (DS')
  Optimal features ← Select prominent Features (Fe)
  For each method: {RF, DTC, LR, NBC}
  Technique ← Algorithm (method)
  For k==1: length (Optimal features)
  (wACC, wACUC, wF1S, wSens) ← Method

```
Performance Measure ← wACC* AC C+ wACUC* ACUC + wSens + sens)
End For
End For each
Ensemble_Algorithm ← best three Methods
For each Optimal features and Algorithm_ Ensemble
Perform Indicators (PI) ← Algorithm_ Ensemble(Optimal_features)
End For each
Return PI
Stop
```

There are multiple steps in Algorithm 4.1. First, the performance vector is established using well-known performance indicators such as precision, accuracy, ACUC, F1-score, and recall, The HDIFA then includes several processes including SGA, data imputation, feature extraction, ML techniques, and performance indicators evaluation as illustrated in Figure 4.2. In the end, the dataset is made machine-friendly by using methods of imputation to fill out the blank values with new values.

## 4.4.5   Disease diagnosing techniques

The set of key techniques involved in HD diagnosis is the following:

1.   Pre-processing
2.   Feature extraction
3.   Validation techniques
4.   Classification of models
5.   Predict disease

### 4.4.5.1   Pre-processing

Data pre-processing, the initial step, purges data by eliminating duplicates, imputes missing data, and normalizes the data. Data imputing is the process of using stand-in values for missing data. To enhance the data's quality, the records from the downloaded dataset can be normalized. The most important first step in any pre-dictive model is data preparation; it helps to turn data into a comprehensible format to increase model effectiveness. The data is pre-processed by removing duplicate entries, adding any information that is missing, and normalizing the data. Therefore, pre-processing data is crucial to increasing the model's accuracy.

### 4.4.5.2   Feature extraction

Identifying and eliminating unnecessary, tangentially related or redundant aspects or dimensions from a data source is done using feature extraction. The objective of feature extraction is to identify the lowest set of characteristics that produce a probabilistic distribution of value categories that is equivalent to the initial setup produced with all attributes. A data collection D with $n$ attributes can have $2n$ subsets. Finding the appropriate subset takes time, especially as $n$ and the variety of data categories increase. On occasions, it might become impossible. As a result, heuristic algorithms make up the majority of feature extraction techniques. By their very nature, these heuristic algorithms are greedy and seek the lowest practicable search space. Figure 4.8 represents the flowchart for feature selection using SGA. From Figure 4.8, until a population P arises with all rules meeting the fitness requirement, the generation process is repeated. With a beginning population of one hundred cases, the generation continues until the 50th generation, with a cross-over probability of 0.51 and a mutation probability of 0.21. The genetic search yielded 5 traits out of a total of 13.

## 4.4.6   Genetic algorithm for feature selection

Figure 4.9 depicts the flow of SGA. To evaluate the fitness likelihood of a single gene type, a fitness value was developed. The sum of the cumulative fitness values

```
#FEature Extraction
models = GeneticSelectionCV(
    estimator, cv=5, verbose=0,
    scoring="accuracy", max_features=5,
    n_population=100, crossover_proba=0.5,
    mutation_proba=0.2, n_generations=50,
    crossover_independent_proba=0.5,
    mutation_independent_proba=0.04,
    tournament_size=3, n_gen_no_change=10,
    caching=True, n_jobs=-1)
models = models.fit(X, y)
print('Feature Selection:', X.columns[models.support_])

Feature Selection: Index(['cp', 'exang', 'slope', 'ca', 'thal'], dtype='obje
ct')
```

*Figure 4.8   Feature selection.*

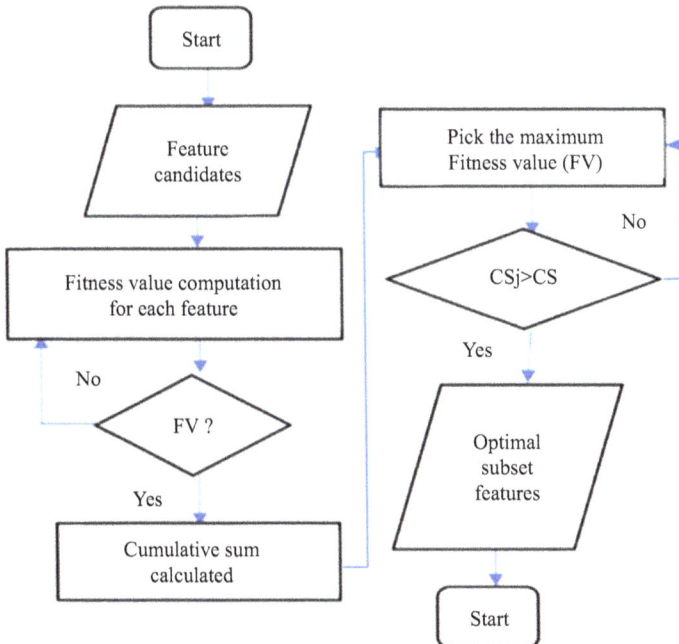

*Figure 4.9   Flow chart for SGA*

should be one. Select the greatest value for fitness *j* and determine whether the requirements are satisfied. csj csk, in which csk is a freshly created subsequence set and csj is the cumulative sum.

## 4.4.7    Validation techniques

The evaluation could largely depend on which information is employed in the training dataset and which is utilized in the test dataset. The train-test splitting validation method usually leads to overfitting. As a result, based on how the split is implemented, the evaluation may differ significantly.

Therefore, the cross-validation method as a fix for this problem is suggested. Using the original training data, cross-validation is utilized to create several micro-train-test splits to fine-tune the model. In the next experiment, ten-fold cross-validation is applied, which divides the initial dataset into ten equal-sized sub-samples and calculates the model's overall performance by averaging the accuracy over all ten trials. Each data point appears $k1$ times in the training set and $k$ times in the test set, respectively. Since majority of data is used for fitting and in the testing dataset, bias and variance have been greatly reduced. Accuracy declines after using the cross-validation method.

## 4.4.8    Classification of models

The models use Python libraries for categorization. Based on the performance metrics, four distinct classification models are compared and examined. Classification is a supervised learning technique for obtaining models that characterize pertinent data classes or forecast future trends. Classification algorithms play a key role in artificial intelligence, ML, and pattern identification. Four classifier models have been employed: logistic regression, decision tree, random forest, and naive Bayes.

The first model is a well-liked classifier, decision tree that is simple to use. It does not require any domain expertise or parameter settings and it can handle data with a lot of dimensions. As a result, it is more suited to exploratory knowledge discovery. It continues to be plagued with repetition and reproduction. As a result, suitable precautions must be taken to deal with repetition and replication.

The second model naive Bayes is a statistical classifier that assumes no attribute reliance. In determining the class, it tries to maximize the posterior probability. Despite the fact that this classifier has a theoretically low error rate, this may not always be the case. A lack of pertinent probability data and assumptions brought on by class conditional independence, however, results in errors. The findings demonstrate that naive Bayes performs well in both before and after a minimization in the number of attributes.

The logistic regression method is the third one. Logistic regression is a technique used for estimating the likelihood of a discrete outcome given an input variable. It is a powerful supervised ML technique for binary classification problems with two possible values, including true/false, yes/no, and so on. The main difference between logistic regression and linear regression is

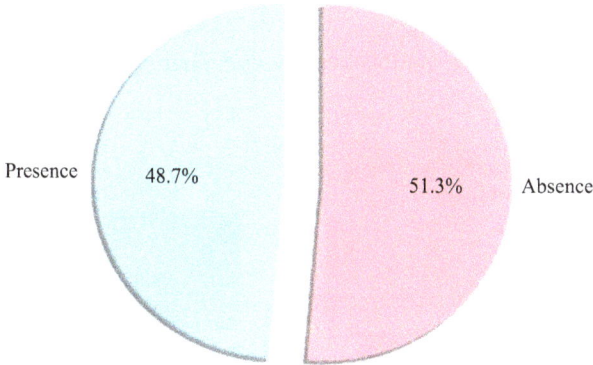

*Figure 4.10    Presence and absence of HD in the dataset*

that the range of logistic regression is restricted to values between zero and one.

The final model, called random forest, increases the expected accuracy of the dataset by averaging the results of several decision trees used on various subsets of the dataset. Instead of relying just on one decision tree, the random forest gathers predictions from each tree and predicts the final result based on the projections with the most votes.

### 4.4.9    Disease prediction

Numerous ML techniques, including decision trees, naive Bayes, random trees, and logistic regression, are used for classification. The algorithm with the highest accuracy is used after a comparative study of various techniques for the identification of HD models employing Python libraries for categorization. From the accumulated dataset, the existence of the HD is about 48.7% and the absence of HD is about 51.3% which is visualized in Figure 4.10.

## 4.5    Results and analysis

When compared to logistic regression, Gaussian naive Bayes, and random forest, decision tree did quite well according to the results of the trial. The accuracy of the decision tree-based model is 88.52% and 82.51% when split data and cross-validation procedures are used, respectively. This is around 5% more accurate than naive Bayes. Similar to this, a model created using random forest and logistic regression provides a better prediction result with an accuracy rate of 86.59%. The ML model prediction summaries in the form of matrices are depicted in Figure 4.11. The threshold for the classifier that minimizes false positives and maximizes true positives is determined using an ROC curve which is visualized in Figure 4.12.

### 4.5.1    Confusion matrix

Figure 4.11 represents the confusion matrix comparison for all the comparable methods.

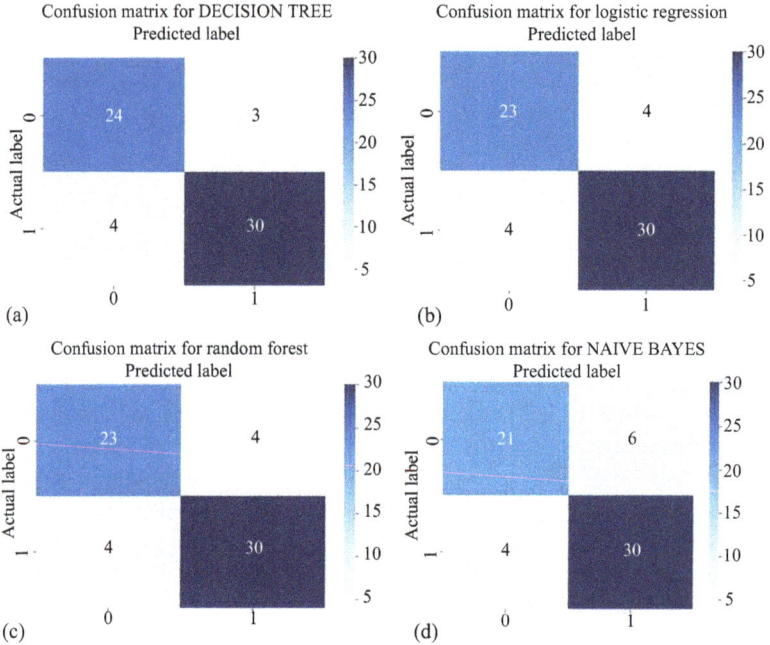

*Figure 4.11    Confusion matrices for (a) decision tree, (b) logistic regression, (c) random forest, and (d) naive Bayes*

### 4.5.2    ROC curve

Figure 4.12 represents the ROC curve results for the comparing methods.

### 4.5.3    Split data comparison

After examining the performance metrics for various ML methods, the model's performance cannot be evaluated just based on correctness. As a result, logistic regression, decision tree, naive Bayes, random forest, and others have been contrasted. Decision tree has the highest accuracy of roughly 88.52%, F1-score of approximately 89.55%, precision of approximately 90.91%, and recall of about 88.24% in comparison to the other four ML techniques. Table 4.3 shows the comparison of various models and their corresponding performance metrics.

The detailed test results can be examined more easily when using split data validation. According to the graph in Figure 4.13, the decision tree model performs better is faster and more productive and has a longer lifespan than the other model. Naive Bayes had lower accuracy than the other models.

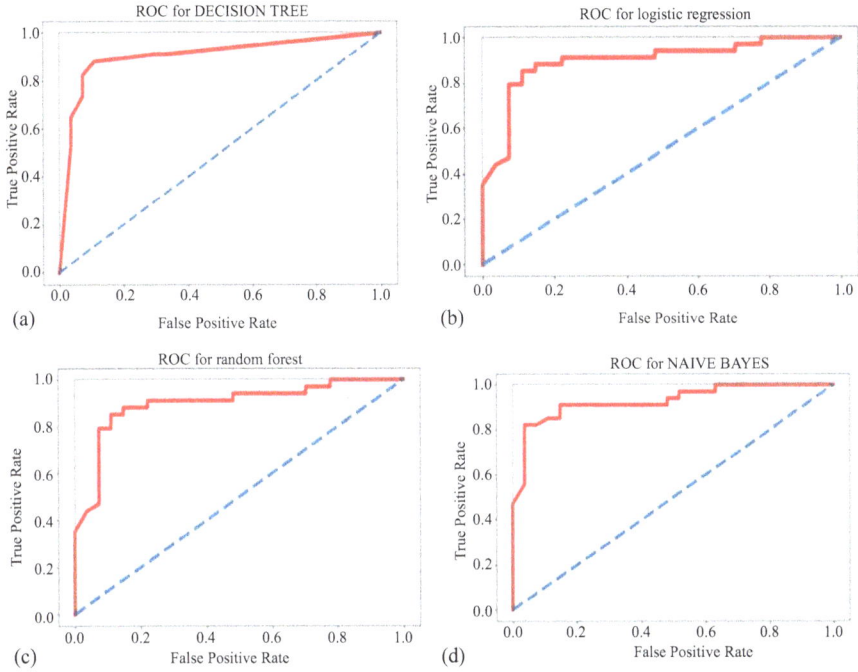

*Figure 4.12    ROC curve for (a) decision tree, (b) logistic regression, (c) random forest, and (d) naive Bayes*

*Table 4.3    Performance metrics comparison for split data*

| Models | Accuracy | F1-score | Precision | Recall |
|---|---|---|---|---|
| Decision tree | 88.52 | 89.55 | 90.91 | 88.24 |
| Naive Bayes | 83.61 | 85.71 | 83.33 | 88.24 |
| Random forest | 86.89 | 88.57 | 86.11 | 31.18 |
| Logistic regression | 86.89 | 88.24 | 88.24 | 88.24 |

## 4.5.4    Cross-validation and split data comparison

The cross-validation technique is used for solving the under-fitting problem. Table 4.4 shows the comparison examination of various ML models based on their accuracy as determined by split data and cross-validation.

To preserve consistency in testing, the statistical test on k-fold cross-validation examines the performance of each algorithm on various datasets that have been constructed with the same random seed. It also solves the issue of underfitting and among other models, decision tree stands the best. Comparatively speaking, the accuracy of naive Bayes was lower which is visualized in Figure 4.14.

|   | Algorithms | Percentage |
|---|---|---|
| 0 | Decision Tree | 88.52 |
| 1 | Logistic Regression | 86.89 |
| 2 | Random Forest | 86.89 |
| 3 | Naive Bayes | 83.61 |

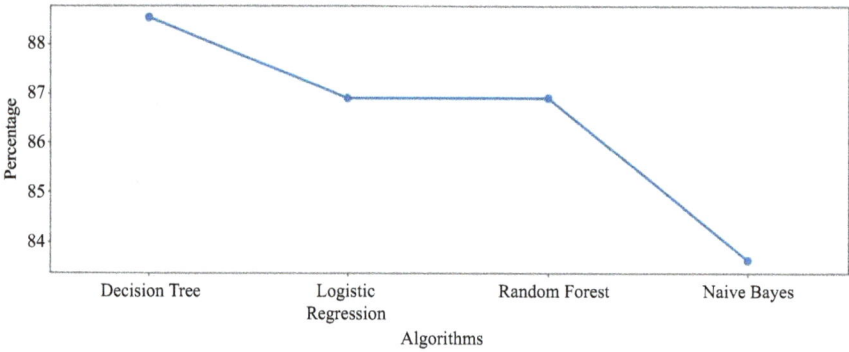

*Figure 4.13   Accuracy comparison for split data*

*Table 4.4   Accuracy comparison for split data and cross-validation*

| ML models | Accuracy (split data), % | Accuracy (cross-validation), % |
|---|---|---|
| Decision tree | 88.52 | 82.51 |
| Naive Bayes | 83.61 | 80.18 |
| Random forest | 86.89 | 81.85 |
| Logistic regression | 86.89 | 81.85 |

|   | Algorithms | Percentage |
|---|---|---|
| 0 | Decision Tree | 82.51 |
| 1 | Logistic Regression | 81.85 |
| 2 | Random Forest Classifier | 81.85 |
| 3 | Naive Bayes | 80.18 |

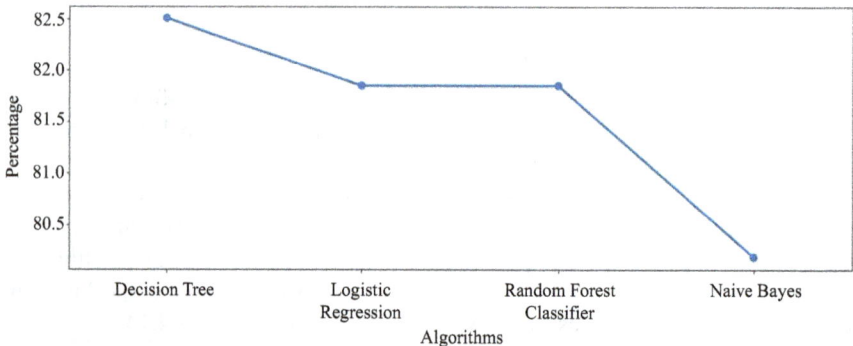

*Figure 4.14   Accuracy comparison for cross-validation*

## 4.6    Conclusion and future work

HD is a major concern in today's highly competitive environment. In a nutshell, the system recommends a model that can accurately forecast HD. The cardiac disease dataset that has 14,350 instances has been examined. For feature extraction, the system implements SGA to optimize the search. The system uses logistic regression, decision tree, naive Bayes, and random forest ML models to predict cardiac disorders in the human body based on specific medical criteria. With an accuracy rate of approximately 88.52% using split data and 82.5% using cross-validation, the decision tree classifier surpasses the other models. By comparing the performance of these existing models, you can get a better understanding of which techniques are most effective for predicting HD. Each model makes different assumptions about the data, which can impact its performance. Considering, naive Bayes assumes that all features are independent, while logistic regression assumes a linear relationship between the features and the outcome. Random forest combines multiple models to improve accuracy. By comparing these models, you can see how different assumptions impact the accuracy of the predictions.

Taking Fuzzy logic into account the different degrees of exercise-induced angina that a patient may have, rather than simply categorizing patients as either having or not having angina. This can help to improve the accuracy of predictive models based on the Cleveland-Hungarian dataset. The reason for choosing these models is to gain a comprehensive understanding of which techniques work best for predicting HD. By comparing the performance of multiple models with different assumptions and techniques, you can identify the most effective approach for this specific problem.

Future work on the automation of HD analysis could use the addition or improvement of other ML techniques. If cardiac disease is found, patients can be given regular access to medical professionals who can help them. Including a practitioner page in software simulation after the forecast can be expanded will undoubtedly assist users in obtaining a doctor consultation. The machine can provide the free-of-charge doctors' contact information as well as their areas of expertise. As a result, the user can choose the doctors of their choice. The user can upload their report to the attachment section after choosing the doctor. So that the practitioner might re-diagnose the patient's report and provide assistance to the patient based on the test outcomes regularly. An application by merging those web pages and a user interface design format can be created. And to be able to forecast the outcomes with greater accuracy.

## References

[1]    Mienye ID, Sun Y, and Wang Z. 'An improved ensemble learning approach for the prediction of heart disease risk'. *Informatics in Medicine Unlocked.* 2020;20:100402.

[2]    Bharti R, Khamparia A, Shabaz M, Dhiman G, Pande S, and Singh P. 'Prediction of heart disease using a combination of machine learning and

deep learning'. *Computational Intelligence and Neuroscience.* 2021;2021: 8387680.

[3]    El Hamdaoui H, Boujraf S, Chaoui NE, and Maaroufi M. 'A clinical support system for prediction of heart disease using machine learning techniques'. In *5th International Conference on Advanced Technologies for Signal and Image Processing (ATSIP), Sfax, Tunisia,* September 2020 (IEEE), pp. 1–5.

[4]    Sujatha P and Mahalakshmi K. 'Performance evaluation of supervised machine learning algorithms in prediction of heart disease'. In *International Conference for Innovation in Technology (INOCON),* Bangalore, India, November 2020 (IEEE), pp. 1–7.

[5]    Saw M, Saxena T, Kaithwas S, Yadav R, and Lal N. 'Estimation of prediction for getting heart disease using logistic regression model of machine learning'. In *International Conference on Computer Communication and Informatics (ICCCI),* Coimbatore, India, January 2020 (IEEE), pp. 1–6.

[6]    Fitriyani NL, Syafrudin M, Alfian G, and Rhee J. 'HDPM: an effective heart disease prediction model for a clinical decision support system'. *IEEE Access.* 2020;8:133034–50.

[7]    Nagavelli U, Samanta D, and Chakraborty P. 'Machine learning technology-based heart disease detection models'. *Journal of Healthcare Engineering.* 2022;27(2):2040–95.

[8]    Swain D, Ballal P, Dolase V, Dash B, and Santhappan J. 'An efficient heart disease prediction system using machine learning'. In *Machine Learning and Information Processing,* 2020 (Singapore, Springer, 2020), pp. 39–50.

[9]    Zhang D, Chen Y, Chen Y, *et al.* 'Heart disease prediction based on the embedded feature selection method and deep neural network'. *Journal of Healthcare Engineering.* 2021;29(9):Article ID: 6260022.

[10]   Sajja GS, Mustafa M, Phasinam K, Kaliyaperumal K, Ventayen RJ, and Kassanuk T. 'Towards application of machine learning in classification and prediction of heart disease'. In *Second International Conference on Electronics and Sustainable Communication Systems (ICESC),* Coimbatore, India, August 2021 (IEEE), pp. 1664–69.

[11]   Amen K, Zohdy M, and Mahmoud M. 'Machine learning for multiple stage heart disease prediction'. In *7th International Conference on Computer Science, Engineering and Information Technology,* Copenhagen, Denmark, September 2020 (IEEE), pp. 205–223.

[12]   Gárate-Escamila AK, El Hassani AH, and Andrès E. 'Classification models for heart disease prediction using feature selection and PCA'. *Informatics in Medicine Unlocked.* 2020;19:100330.

[13]   Ashri SE, El-Gayar MM, and El-Daydamony EM. 'HDPF: heart disease prediction framework based on hybrid classifiers and genetic algorithm'. *IEEE Access.* 2021;9:146797–809.

[14]   Ahmed H, Younis EM, Hendawi A, and Ali AA. 'Heart disease identification from patients' social posts, machine learning solution on Spark'. *Future Generation Computer Systems.* 2020;111:714–22.

[15] Surya VJ, Muthurajkumar S, Jitiendran K, Ajithkumar K, and Ibrahim SM. 'A web based application for optimization of less than truckload problem'. In *IEEE World Conference on Applied Intelligence and Computing (AIC)*, Sonbhadra, India, June 2022 (IEEE), pp. 813–817.

[16] Muthurajkumar S, Karthikeyan CA, Pradeep K, and Hariharan A. 'Privacy-preserving dynamic task scheduling for autonomous vehicles'. In *2nd International Conference on Artificial Intelligence: Advances and Applications*, Jaipur, India, February 2022 (Singapore, Springer, 2022), pp. 669–684.

[17] Priya PI, Muthurajkumar S, and Daisy SS. 'Data fault detection in wireless sensor networks using machine learning techniques'. *Wireless Personal Communications*. 2022;122(3):2441–62.

[18] Muthurajkumar S, Ganapathy S, Vijayalakshmi M, and Kannan A. 'An intelligent secured and energy efficient routing algorithm for MANETs'. *Wireless Personal Communications*. 2017;96(2):1753–69.

[19] Muthurajkumar S, Vijayalakshmi M, and Kannan A. 'Secured data storage and retrieval algorithm using map reduce techniques and chaining encryption in cloud databases'. *Wireless Personal Communications*. 2017;96 (4):5621–33.

[20] Muthurajkumar S, Vijayalakshmi M, Kannan A, and Ganapathy S. 'Optimal and energy efficient scheduling techniques for resource management in public cloud networks'. *National Academy Science Letters*. 2018;41(4):219–23.

[21] Kaladevi P, Sengathir J, Praveen R, and Muthusankar D. 'An improved ensemble classification-based secure two stage bagging pruning technique for guaranteeing privacy preservation of DNA sequences in electronic health records'. *Journal of Intelligent & Fuzzy Systems*. 2023;44(1):149–166.

[22] Deepika P, Suresh RM, and Pabitha P. 'Defending Against Child Death: Deep learning-based diagnosis method for abnormal identification of fetus ultrasound images'. *Computational Intelligence*. 2021;37(1):128–54.

*Chapter 5*

# Artificial intelligence to predict heart disease and model constructed using TabPy

*S. Senith[1], A. Alfred Kirubaraj[2], S.R. Jino Ramson[3] and M. Jegadeeswari[4]*

## Abstract

The heart is one of the most important organs in the human body. It supports metabolic processes and circulates oxygen and other vital nutrients throughout the body. Because of this, even minor heart conditions can have a significant effect on the entire body. Researchers are heavily utilising data analysis to assist doctors in foretelling heart issues. In order to anticipate who will develop coronary heart disease in the near future, this paper can explore the many machine learning techniques used in predictive analytics with an emphasis on heart disease prediction. Using Tableau, a predictive model with the highest degree of accuracy is created, allowing users to enter values and obtain predictions about the likelihood of the existence or absence of heart disease. Quick treatment will result, in saving the lives of the sufferers. The prognosis and aetiology of heart illness, as well as the classification of infections in patients who have just undergone surgery, are among the findings of this study.

**Keywords:** Prediction algorithms; Machine learning; big data analytics; Automation; Deep learning; Coronary heart disease; Sepsis; Heart attack

## 5.1 Introduction

One of the body's most important organs is the heart. By pumping blood throughout the body and supplying various organs and tissues with oxygen and other vital nutrients, it plays an important part in the circulatory system. The heart

[1]School of Management, Karunya Institute of Technology and Sciences, Coimbatore, India
[2]Department of Electronics and Communication Engineering, Karunya Institute of Technology and Sciences, Coimbatore, India
[3]Principal Engineer, Global Foundries, Santa Clara, CA, USA
[4]Department of Commerce, The Standard Fireworks Rajaratnam College for Women, Madurai Kamaraj University, Sivakasi, India

also helps in removing metabolic wastes, making it a key component of the body's metabolic functions. Thus, even minor heart problems can have a significant impact on the overall health of an individual.

To help doctors predict heart problems, researchers are turning to data analysis. Predictive analytics is an emerging field that involves using historical data to make predictions about future events or trends. Predictive analytics in the context of heart disease can assist medical professionals in identifying those who are very likely to soon develop coronary heart disease (CHD). Researchers can create predictive models that can help doctors make precise diagnoses and create treatment plans by using machine learning algorithms to analyse data from wearables, electronic health records, and other sources.

One of the primary goals of predictive analytics in the context of heart disease is to develop models that can accurately predict the likelihood of an individual developing CHD in the future. Researchers employ a range of machine learning techniques to accomplish this, including logistic regression, decision trees, random forests, and neural networks. These algorithms operate by examining data patterns and creating models that have a high degree of accuracy for forecasting future events.

Once the predictive models have been developed, they can be integrated into clinical decision support systems that can help doctors make more accurate diagnoses and treatment plans. For example, a doctor could input a patient's medical history, lifestyle factors, and other relevant information into a predictive model and receive a probability score indicating the likelihood of the patient developing CHD in the future. Based on this score, the doctor could recommend lifestyle changes or prescribe medication to reduce the patient's risk of developing CHD.

To create predictive models for heart disease, one tool that can be used is Tableau. Users of this data visualisation software can enter data and produce visualisations that can be used to spot patterns and trends in the data. Researchers may develop interactive applications that let clinicians input patient data and get real-time estimates of the likelihood of heart illness using Tableau's predictive modelling software.

In conclusion, the discipline of predictive analytics is a young one, but it has the potential to transform how medical professionals identify and treat cardiac disease. Researchers can create predictive models that can aid clinicians in developing more accurate diagnoses and treatment plans by utilising machine learning algorithms to analyse data from various sources. With the help of tools like Tableau, these predictive models can be made more accessible to doctors and other healthcare professionals, allowing for prompt treatment and potentially saving lives. The findings of this research include improved cardiac disease prognosis and aetiology, as well as better classification of infection in post-surgery patients.

To help doctors forecast heart problems, researchers are looking into the use of data analytics. To forecast future occurrences or trends, predictive analytics analyses both current and historical data using statistical techniques, machine learning algorithms, and data mining. Doctors can identify people who are at risk of developing heart disease and offer suitable preventative therapies by examining multiple risk factors and patient data.

A key element of predictive analytics is machine learning algorithms. Large volumes of data may be analysed by these algorithms, which can also spot patterns that the human eye would miss. The support vector machine (SVM) is one of the machine learning techniques utilised for heart disease prediction. A supervised learning system called SVM can divide data into two or more groups based on features and patterns.

Another machine learning algorithm used in heart disease prediction is artificial neural networks (ANN). ANN is a type of deep learning algorithm that can analyse complex data and identify patterns. It can be used to analyse medical data, including images, to identify potential heart disease risk factors.

Who will experience CHD in the near future has been the focus of research. A common form of heart disease called CHD can cause heart attacks and other severe health problems. The chance of getting CHD can be determined by examining a number of risk factors, such as age, gender, family history, blood pressure, cholesterol levels, and smoking history.

By using predictive analytics and machine learning algorithms, doctors can make more accurate predictions about future heart problems. These predictions can help patients take preventive measures, such as making lifestyle changes or starting medication, to reduce their risk of developing heart disease. The use of predictive analytics in healthcare is a promising development that could improve the prevention and treatment of heart disease and other health conditions.

Due mostly to record keeping, compliance, administrative needs, and patient care, the healthcare sector produces enormous amounts of data. With so many advantages, including better healthcare service and lower costs, this data is being digitised more and more. It is referred to as 'big data', and it has the potential to be used for a variety of medical and healthcare applications, such as clinical decision support, disease surveillance, and population health management.

However, big data in healthcare is overwhelming due to its volume as well as the variety of data types and the speed at which it must be processed. Despite these difficulties, big data analytics can glean insights from large amounts of data, allowing for more informed choices that could save lives and cut costs. Medical management, planning, measurement, and learning are all impacted by healthcare analytics, which is the methodical application of health information and business insights to decision-making.

Big data analytics has the potential to do more than just increase profits and save waste – it has the ability to predict epidemics, cure diseases, enhance life quality, and decrease avoidable deaths. To produce predictions and evaluate their predictive value, predictive analytics uses statistical and other methodologies. It is thought of as the next revolution in both statistics and medicine.

A paper by Timsina and colleagues provides an advanced analytics solution for automating medical systematic reviews. While systematic reviews are critical for evidence-based practice, they are resource-intensive to create and update. For systematic reviews, the authors automatically categorised articles for inclusion and exclusion using advanced analytics approaches.

The digitisation of healthcare has resulted in the creation of large data sets, such as electronic medical records, health claims information, radiology images, and patient-generated data from wearables and health apps. However, many healthcare providers are not effectively utilising this data to improve patient care and population health analytics. Additionally, healthcare providers are under pressure to meet the Fourfold Aims, which include improving access to care, reducing costs, improving treatment outcomes, and optimising provider satisfaction. Prescriptive analytics can be used to make data-driven recommendations for improving healthcare workflows and patient outcomes, using techniques such as machine learning and cognitive systems.

According to the World Health Organisation [1], cardiovascular disease is the main cause of mortality worldwide, taking 17.9 million lives annually. CHD, cerebrovascular disease, rheumatic heart disease, and other issues involving the heart and blood vessels are only a few of the conditions it covers. One-third of cardiovascular disease-related deaths occur before the age of 70, and heart attacks and strokes account for four out of every five of these deaths [1]. Acquired comorbidities contribute to morbidity and mortality at a higher rate as the number of patients with congenital heart disease rises.

According to Sreeniwas Kumar and Nakul Sinha [2], cardiovascular disease is one of the most prevalent diseases in India. According to them, there would be 4.77 million fatalities in India owing to cardiovascular disease by 2050, up from 2.26 million in 1990. According to Huffman *et al.* [3], the prevalence of CHD has increased in India from 1.6% to 7.4% in rural areas and from 1% to 13.2% in urban areas in recent years.

Studies suggest that risk factors such as abdominal obesity, hypertension, and diabetes have an impact on the onset of heart disease. Predictive analysis is widely used in the healthcare industry as predicting the onset of disease reduces the likelihood of people falling ill. Cardiovascular diseases have been shown to increase the mortality rate. Machine learning, which is used to create predictive models for various domains, is currently being employed in the field of medical diagnostics.

Age, gender, blood pressure, heart rate, diabetes, and other risk variables are all taken into account in this analysis of heart disease. Predictive analysis using artificial intelligence can help predict the risk of heart disease and provide healthcare professionals with valuable insights into the risk factors associated with this condition. Such insights can enable the development of effective treatment plans to prevent the onset of heart disease and reduce mortality rates.

## 5.2    Related studies

In research for the prediction of heart disease using data mining approaches, the authors of [4] explore the various information abstraction mechanisms currently being used. Algorithms are used to examine the effectiveness of the data mining techniques naive Bayes, neural network, and decision tree algorithm on medical data sets. According to the study, further research can be done on neural networks, decision trees, and naive Bayes to create an algorithm that will be useful for healthcare institutions. The K closest neighbour technique, neural network, naive Bayes, and decision tree were employed in the study by [5] to predict heart disease. With an accuracy of 80.4%, they employed data mining algorithms to properly diagnose the risk of heart disease. Prediction tries to find hidden trends in a dataset using machine learning techniques and to forecast or know the present value on a scale, according to [6] heart disease research report. Heart disease prediction requires tremendous quantities of data that are too complex and large for current methods to process and comprehend. The goal was to develop a system that was both effective and dependable for predicting heart disease. The decision tree technique was 77.58% accurate compared to the KNN method's 86.30% accuracy. In 2016, Chen *et al.* proposed the Heart Disease Prediction System, which is based on a data mining technique for heart disease prediction with a list of crucial characteristics and an artificial neural network for categorising heart illness based on crucial features. The J48 algorithm yielded a predicted accuracy percentage of about 80%. Using data mining, Sheikh [7] proposed a method for identifying CHD and predicting the numerous events connected to each patient record in 2012. Through the use of feature selection, this model lowers the number of attributes. With an accuracy rating of 60.74%, this model chose nine attributes. According to Purushottam *et al.* (2016), 'An automated method in medical diagnostics would increase medical treatment while also reducing costs'. In this study, we created a system that can quickly identify the criteria for predicting a patient's risk level based on a specific health parameter. Single models such as decision tree, artificial neural network, and naive Bayes performance 85%, 76%, and 69%, respectively. Researchers (Shanta Kumar, B. Patil, and Y. Kumaraswamy, 2011) found that recognising the risk factors for heart disease can aid medical professionals in identifying people who are at high risk for developing the disease. Healthcare professionals may employ statistical analysis and data processing methods to assist in the identification of heart illness. According to statistical study, the following conditions are prevalent: CHD (heart attacks), cerebrovascular disease (stroke), hypertension (high blood pressure), coronary artery disease, rheumatic heart disease, congenital heart disease, and heart failure. Smoking, inactivity, a poor diet, and problematic alcohol use are the main contributors to cardiovascular disease. Several classification methods have been studied by Baharami *et al.* (2018), including J48 decision tree, k-nearest neighbours (k-NN), naive Bayes (NB), and sequential minimal optimisation algorithm (SMO) (SMO is widely used for training SVM). J48 is the most accurate, with an accuracy of 83.732%. Palaniyappan *et al.* built Intelligent Heart Disease Prediction Systems (IHDPS) using naive Bayes, decision trees, and artificial neural networks. To facilitate visualisation and analysis, it offers the findings in both tabular and graphical representations. The naive Bayes model outperforms the other two, with 86.12% of accurate predictions, followed by 85.68% for neural networks and 85.68% for decision trees. The authors of [8] employed decision trees, support vector machines, deep learning, and K nearest neighbour algorithms. They aimed to reduce noise in the datasets by cleaning and pre-processing the data, as well as reducing the dataset's dimensionality. They found that neural networks can produce incredibly accurate results. Cardiovascular disease and the many symptoms of a heart attack were covered in great detail by the authors of [9]. The classification and clustering processes used a variety of methods and technologies. To obtain 89% accuracy using the dataset's 13 attributes, Banu and Gomathy used the C4.5 algorithm, MAFIA, and K-means clustering. The heart disease data contains redundant and unnecessary information, according to [10]. Arrangements must be made in advance for this. Additionally, they contend that choosing specific dataset features is necessary for improved performance. An 89% accuracy was achieved by K-means, MAFIA, and C4.5. The accuracy of KNN is 89.2%, whereas the accuracy of SVM is 85%. Data mining algorithms have been proposed by Vikas Chaurasia and Saurabh Pal to detect cardiac disease. We use the machine learning data mining programme WEKA, which has a number of machine learning methods. There are just 11 attributes used for prediction. Naive Bayes is 82.31% accurate. Chen *et al.* presented a method for forecasting the status of heart disease that leverages clinical data from patients. The 13 clinical criteria included age, sex, and the type of chest discomfort. Heart disease was categorised using an artificial neural network technique. About 80% of the time, the suggested prediction method is accurate. A classification technique based on supervised machine learning was utilised by Asha Rajkumar *et al.* [11] to identify heart disease. The data is categorised with the use of the Tanagra tool, assessed with 10-fold cross-validation, and the results are compared. For academic and research needs, Tanagra is a free data mining programme. Naive Bayes accuracy was 52.33% compared to 45.27% for k-NN. The research by Polaraju and Durga Prasad intends to apply the statistical model multiple linear regression analysis to construct a model that precisely forecasts the risk of heart disease and helps in the diagnosis of patients in time to save their lives. To create a model that can be applied to test data, multiple linear regression analysis is employed on trained data. According to a study by [12], J48 yields an accuracy of 56.76%, which is better than the Logistic Model Tree algorithm's accuracy of 55.75%. The work by [13] is broken down into two phases: the pre-processing phase, in which we chose the most crucial attributes, and the second phase, in which we utilised machine learning algorithms to identify the optimal algorithm. As a result, the accuracy increased to 90%, 85.50%, and 93%, respectively. In this study, Apurv Garg *et al.* [14] use the K-nearest neighbour (K-NN) and random forest machine learning algorithms. The prediction accuracy of the K-NN algorithm is 86.885%, compared to 81.967% for the random forest approach.

In the papers under discussion, the use of data mining and machine learning techniques for the prediction of cardiac disease is the main topic. The accuracy of the predictions has been examined using a variety of techniques, including naive Bayes, neural networks, decision trees, k-NN, and support vector machines (SVMs). The accuracy of the algorithms varies from 60.74% to 89.2%, and the results show that these techniques can be effective in predicting heart disease risk. The papers also emphasise the importance of feature selection and data pre-processing to increase the accuracy of the models. The ultimate goal is to develop effective and reliable systems to assist healthcare providers in diagnosing and treating heart disease.

## 5.3    Objective

To evaluate the efficacy of several supervised machine learning algorithms and to pinpoint the numerous risk factors that lead to heart disease and using the algorithm with the highest prediction accuracy to build a predictive model.

## 5.4    Methodology

### 5.4.1    Algorithm used

Logistic algorithm: The parameters of a logistic prototypical with a reliant on mutable with two probable principles, such as pass/fail, are estimated using logistic regression. The two values are labelled '0' and '1', respectively [15]. The following mathematical formula can be used to define the linear relationship: where $b$ is the base of the logarithm, is the log-odds, and are the model's parameters.

$$l = \log_b P/1/P = \beta 0 + \beta 1 \chi 1 + \beta 2 \chi 2$$

The naive Bayes classifiers are a group of simple probabilistic classifiers that are based on the Bayes theorem and a strong obligation on structural individuality. They are among the most fundamental representations of a Bayesian network [4]. The model must therefore be revised to make it more manageable. The Bayes theorem $(x)$ can be used to deconstruct the conditional probability as $(Ck\ x) = P(Ck)$ $p(x)\ Ck)/p(x)$. An enormous quantity of decision trees is built by a random forest during training. The random forest's productivity in sorting tasks is determined by the session that the most well-liked trees choose. The relapse tasks pay back the mean or standard estimate of the discrete trees [12]. The joint technique of bootstrap combination, or bagging, is used by the random forest training algorithm to train tree learners. Snaring repeatedly ($B$ times) creates a random sample with extra data from the training set given a training set $X = x1,..., xn$ and responses $Y = y1,..., yn$. The closest neighbour chain method loops through a series of collections A, B, C..., each of which is the collection that came before it in the chain and is next to it, until it reaches a pair of clusters that are communal nearest neighbours [16]. A decision tree and its intricately interwoven stimulus illustration are used in decision analysis as visual and investigative decision-backing aids.

### 5.4.2    Confusion matrix

An effective tool for assessing a classification algorithm's output is a confusion matrix. The criterion of accuracy alone might not be adequate when working with datasets that have more than two classes or an uneven distribution of classes. A confusion matrix summarises the classification results, breaking down the number of accurate and inaccurate predictions by class.

The main purpose of a confusion matrix is to help identify where a classification model is making correct predictions and where it is making mistakes. By breaking down the results of the model into a matrix, we can see not only the overall accuracy but also the types of errors that are being made. This information is invaluable in refining the model and improving its accuracy.

A confusion matrix's important feature is that it demonstrates how the classification model gets confused when making predictions. It provides a thorough description of the various errors being made, not just a tally of how many were made by the classifier. To understand the model's performance and potential areas for improvement, this degree of detail is essential.

In conclusion, a confusion matrix is a critical tool for assessing the effectiveness of a classification system. It offers a split of the number of precise and unreliable predictions, enabling a more in-depth analysis of the model's performance. We can recognise the kinds of errors being produced and enhance the model's accuracy over time by using a confusion matrix.

### 5.4.3  Accuracy score

Accuracy is one parameter to evaluate classification models. The percentage of accurate predictions made by our model is referred to as accuracy informally. The definition of accuracy in formal terms is as follows:

Accuracy=number of correct predictions/total number of predictions

To measure accuracy in terms of positives and negatives for binary classification, use the formula below:

$$\text{Accuracy} = \frac{\text{TP} + \text{TN}}{\text{TP} + \text{TN} + \text{FP} + \text{FN}}$$

TP denotes true positives, TN denotes true negatives, FP denotes false positives, and FN denotes false negatives. A real positive occurs when the model accurately predicts the positive class. Contrarily, a real negative is an outcome for which the model accurately predicted the negative class. When the model accurately predicts the positive class, a false positive result. When the model predicts the negative class erroneously, the consequence is a false negative.

### 5.4.4  Train-test-split procedure

The dataset is divided into the training dataset and the testing dataset using the train-test split method. The training dataset serves as the initial subset for fitting the machine learning model. The model is not trained on the second subset; rather, it is fed the dataset's input elements, which it then uses to generate predictions and compare to the expected values. The name provided for the second subset is the test dataset.

The ratio of training to testing is commonly 70:30 or 80:20, with 70–80% of the dataset going towards training and 30–80% going towards testing. To prevent bias, the dataset should be divided at random.

The train-test split approach is used to measure the output of a machine learning model using fresh data that was not used to train it. Using this strategy, it is possible to assess how well the model works when presented with data that is somewhat analogous to the training set but not exactly the same.

It is important to note that the train-test split method has some limitations. One of the limitations is that it may not work well for small datasets. In such cases, cross-validation techniques may be more appropriate. Another limitation is that it may not work well for classification problems where the dataset is unbalanced. In such cases, stratified sampling techniques may be more appropriate.

In conclusion, the train-test split method offers a straightforward and practical method for assessing the performance of machine learning models on fresh data. It is useful to predict how well the model will perform when applied to fresh data that was not utilised in model training. It should be utilised cautiously, though, especially for classification issues involving unbalanced datasets and tiny datasets, as it has certain drawbacks.

## 5.5   Dataset description

The Kaggle and UCI Machine Learning Repository are where the datasets were obtained. Following are the attributes taken into account for analysis: the datasets, which serve as the foundation for the predictive model created with Tableau, are made up of 304 samples and 462 samples, respectively. (1) Age: the person's age, expressed in years, ranging from 29 to 77; (2) sex: male or female, with 1 male and 0 female; (3) chest pain type: four levels of chest pain; (5) resting BP: at the time of hospital admission, the patient's resting blood pressure To analyse blood pressure, two facts must be excluded: systolic blood pressure, the first number, describes the amount of weight in the veins while the heart beats. The additional figure, diastolic blood pressure, actions the weight in the arteries between heartbeats; (6) serum cholesterol in mg/dl: cholesterol is often linked to heart disease; (7) fasting blood sugar: after a period of not eating, a blood sugar test is performed. A blood sample will be held after a brief interval. Less than 100 mg/dL (5.6 mmol/L) of rapid blood sugar is necessary. Blood sugar levels between 100 and 125 mg/dL (5.6–6.9 mmol/L) are considered prediabetes. If the blood sugar levels are 126 mg/dL (7 mmol/L) or higher on two different tests, diabetes is present; (8) resting ECG results: The resting ECG is a straightforward, simple, and painless procedure. The resting ECG can detect heart hypertrophy, ischemia, myocardial infarction, myocardial infarction sequelae, cardiac arrhythmias, and other heart disorders. The test takes about 5 min and there is no need to prepare; (9) maximum heart rate: To get the average heart rate associated with age, subtract age from 220. For instance, a 50-year-old male's maximum predicted age-related heart rate would be 220 – 50 years = 170 beats per minute (bpm); (10) maximum heart rate achieves – maximum heart rate during strenuous activities (71–202); exercise-induced angina: 1 – Yes, 0 – No; physical activity is commonly the cause of angina. While climbing stairs, exercising, or trekking, the heart needs more bodily fluid, but blood flow is constrained by tapering veins. In addition to physical exercise, several factors can contribute to angina, including smoking, cold weather, large meals, and emotional stress; (11) systolic blood pressure (SBP). The top number in 120/80 is systolic blood pressure, which calculates the force the heart exerts on the walls of arteries each time it beats; low-density lipoprotein cholesterol and tobacco (collective tobacco, kg): low-density lipoproteins, also known as LDL, are a type of lipoprotein. It is usually referred to as 'poor' lipid because high levels of LDL cause a build-up of fat in the veins. (13) Adiposity – an individual's BMI. The BMI is a preliminary calculation based on a person's height and weight. BMI is calculated as $kg/m^2$, where kg is a person's weight in kilograms and $m^2$ is a measurement of their height in metres squared. While the strong range is 18.5–24.9, heavy is defined as a BMI of 25.0 or higher. A BMI is present in most persons between the ages of 18 and 65; (14) Famhist – family history of heart disease, regardless of whether a family member has recovered from the condition. A variable that has the states '0 – Absent' and '1 – Present'; (15) Typea: type-A behaviour that permeates rivalry, readily aroused displeasure, haste, suddenness of gesture and speech (explosive voice), hypervigilance, and overcommitment to career or profession; (16) alcohol – present alcohol intake; (17) CHD, 0 – absent, 1 – present.

## 5.6    Tableau for predictive dashboard

Business intelligence, or BI, is a term that describes the application of technology and data analytics to the process of gathering information and making business decisions. Utilising BI software, businesses may better their operations and decision-making by analysing and transforming raw data into useful information.

With Tableau, users can quickly and simply build engaging data visualisations. Tableau is a strong and popular BI application. Spreadsheets, databases, and cloud services are just a few of the many data sources that users of Tableau may simply connect to and visualise. Structured, semi-structured, and unstructured data are just a few of the data kinds that the platform can handle.

One of Tableau's primary advantages is its capacity to transform complex data into an understandable format. Charts, graphs, maps, and tables are just a few of the visualisation possibilities that Tableau provides, enabling users to build engaging and dynamic visualisations. These visualisations can be simply shared with other employees of the company and can be altered to the user's particular needs.

With Tableau's drag-and-drop interface, non-technical users can easily construct customised dashboards that offer real-time insights into important business KPIs. Users can quickly and easily drill down into their data with Tableau to acquire deeper insights and make wiser decisions.

In addition to its visualisation capabilities, Tableau also provides powerful data analysis tools. These tools allow users to perform complex calculations, create data models, and generate forecasts. Tableau's machine learning capabilities allow users to analyse data and identify patterns and trends in their data.

Being able to interact with other BI tools and data sources is one of Tableau's key advantages. This enables customers to quickly access and examine data from numerous sources and acquire a greater understanding of their business operations.

Overall, Tableau is a strong and adaptable BI solution that can assist companies of all sizes in the analysis and visualisation of their data, as well as in gaining deeper insights and making better decisions. For anyone trying to harness the power of data and analytics to propel company success, Tableau is a crucial tool thanks to its user-friendly design and robust capabilities [17–19].

## 5.7 TabPy server

TabPy, or the Tableau Python server, is a tool that enables the use of Python code within the Tableau platform. With TabPy, Tableau users can execute Python scripts and saved functions to enhance their data analysis and visualisations. This allows for more complex data manipulation and advanced analytics within Tableau.

Python is a well-liked programming language for data analysis because of its simplicity, robust modules for data manipulation and machine learning, and a sizable user and developer community. By integrating Python into Tableau, users can leverage the strengths of both tools for their data analysis projects [20–22].

TabPy works by creating a connection between Tableau and a Python server. The Python server is a separate process that runs independently of Tableau and is responsible for executing Python scripts and functions. When a user creates a calculated field in Tableau that requires a Python script, the calculation is sent to the Python server for execution. The result is returned to Tableau and can be used for data analysis and visualisation.

One of the benefits of using TabPy is the ability to use Tableau's table calculations in Python scripts. Table calculations are powerful tools for data analysis in Tableau, allowing users to create complex calculations based on the values in a table. By using Python scripts within Tableau, users can take advantage of Python's libraries for data manipulation and machine learning to create more advanced and sophisticated calculations that may not be possible with Tableau's built-in functionality alone [22–24].

TabPy also allows users to save their Python scripts and functions as reusable modules, which can be shared and used by others within the organisation. This makes it easier to collaborate on data analysis projects and maintain consistency across multiple users and teams.

In conclusion, TabPy is a strong solution that allows Tableau users to make advantage of Python's data manipulation and machine learning libraries to improve their data analysis and visualisation abilities. Users can use Tableau to run Python scripts and stored functions and benefit from the best features of both programmes by connecting Tableau and a Python server.

## 5.8 Analysis and interpretation

When analysing data, it is essential to gather statistical information to gain insights into the dataset. Statistical details provide us with numerical information about the data set, allowing us to understand the central tendency, range, and variability of the data as shown in Figure 5.1.

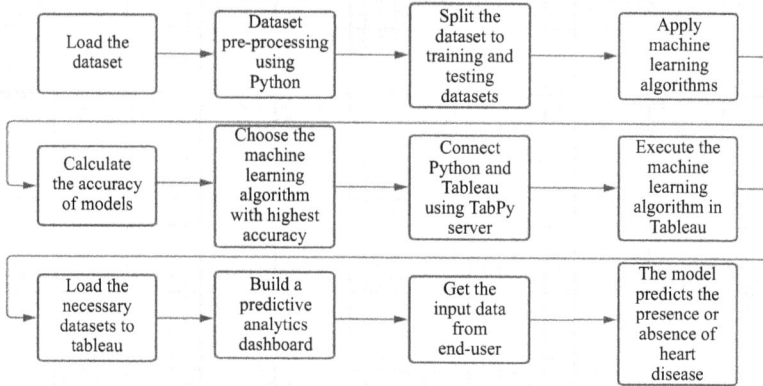

*Figure 5.1    Process of analysis*

In this data collection, the AGE column has values from 29 to 77 years old, with a mean age of 54 years. The mean is a measure of the central tendency of the data, indicating the average value of the data points. The quartile details, given in the form of 25%, 50%, and 75%, divide the data into three quartiles or four equal parts, with 25% of the values lying in each group. This provides us with an idea of how the data is distributed and how much of the data falls into each quartile.

The standard deviation is another statistical measure that provides insights into the variability of the data set. It measures how much the data deviates from the mean, indicating how spread out the data is. While a low standard deviation suggests that the data points are relatively close to the mean, a high standard deviation suggests that the data points are dispersed across a wide range.

In addition to understanding the central tendency and variability of the data set, it is also important to check for missing or null values. In this research, the data set used did not have any missing or null values. Ensuring that there are no missing or null values is critical as it ensures that the data set is complete, accurate, and reliable, providing valuable insights for analysis.

## 5.9    Data correlation analysis

Figure 5.2 illustrates how correlation quantifies how much two variables change in relation to one another. A positive correlation is indicated by values closer to +1, and a negative correlation is shown by numbers closer to −1. The following can be seen in the correlation diagram: people are more susceptible to high blood pressure as they get older. A person is more likely to get heart disease if they experience chest pain. The development of a cardiac disease is not greatly influenced by a person's sex.

| | age | sex | cp | trestbps | chol | fbs | restecg | thalach | exang | oldpeak | slope | ca | thal | target |
|---|---|---|---|---|---|---|---|---|---|---|---|---|---|---|
| age | 1 | -0.098 | -0.069 | 0.28 | 0.21 | 0.12 | -0.12 | -0.4 | 0.097 | 0.21 | -0.17 | 0.28 | 0.068 | -0.23 |
| sex | -0.098 | 1 | -0.049 | -0.057 | -0.2 | 0.045 | -0.058 | -0.044 | 0.14 | 0.096 | -0.031 | 0.12 | 0.21 | -0.28 |
| cp | -0.069 | -0.049 | 1 | 0.048 | -0.077 | 0.094 | 0.044 | 0.3 | -0.39 | -0.15 | 0.12 | -0.18 | -0.16 | 0.43 |
| trestbps | 0.28 | -0.057 | 0.048 | 1 | 0.12 | 0.18 | -0.11 | -0.047 | 0.068 | 0.19 | -0.12 | 0.1 | 0.062 | -0.14 |
| chol | 0.21 | -0.2 | -0.077 | 0.12 | 1 | 0.013 | -0.15 | -0.0099 | 0.067 | 0.054 | -0.004 | 0.071 | 0.099 | -0.085 |
| fbs | 0.12 | 0.045 | 0.094 | 0.18 | 0.013 | 1 | -0.084 | -0.0086 | 0.026 | 0.0057 | -0.06 | 0.14 | -0.032 | -0.028 |
| restecg | -0.12 | -0.058 | 0.044 | -0.11 | -0.15 | -0.084 | 1 | 0.044 | -0.071 | -0.059 | 0.093 | -0.072 | -0.012 | 0.14 |
| thalach | -0.4 | -0.044 | 0.3 | -0.047 | -0.0099 | -0.0086 | 0.044 | 1 | -0.38 | -0.34 | 0.39 | -0.21 | -0.096 | -0.42 |
| exang | 0.097 | 0.14 | -0.39 | 0.068 | 0.067 | 0.026 | -0.071 | -0.38 | 1 | 0.29 | -0.26 | 0.12 | 0.21 | -0.44 |
| oldpeak | 0.21 | 0.096 | -0.15 | 0.19 | 0.054 | 0.0057 | -0.059 | -0.34 | 0.29 | 1 | -0.58 | 0.22 | 0.21 | -0.43 |
| slope | -0.17 | -0.031 | 0.12 | -0.12 | -0.004 | -0.06 | 0.093 | 0.39 | -0.26 | -0.58 | 1 | -0.08 | -0.1 | 0.35 |
| ca | 0.28 | 0.12 | -0.18 | 0.1 | 0.071 | 0.14 | -0.072 | -0.21 | 0.12 | 0.22 | -0.08 | 1 | 0.15 | -0.39 |
| thal | 0.068 | 0.21 | -0.16 | 0.062 | 0.099 | -0.032 | -0.012 | -0.096 | 0.21 | 0.21 | -0.1 | 0.15 | 1 | -0.34 |
| target | -0.23 | -0.28 | 0.43 | -0.14 | -0.085 | -0.028 | 0.14 | -0.42 | -0.44 | -0.43 | 0.35 | -0.39 | -0.34 | 1 |

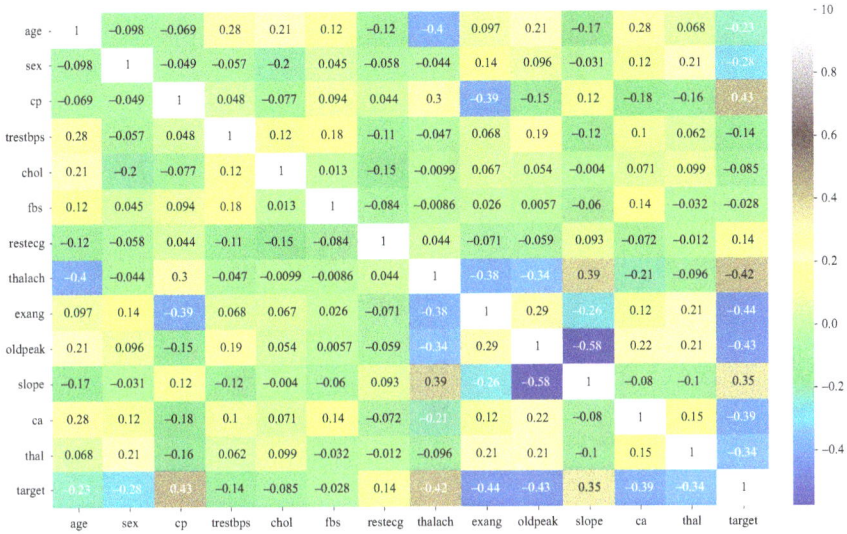

*Figure 5.2    Correlation analysis*

*Table 5.1    Algorithm accuracy*

| Algorithm | Accuracy (%) |
|---|---|
| Logistic regression | 92 |
| Naive Bayes | 89 |
| Random forest | 86 |
| KNN | 86 |
| Decision tree | 76 |

## 5.10    Algorithm accuracy results

There are several sets of data for testing and training. Then the precision becomes tenacious. To achieve more accuracy, the supports are scale-fitted. Data is collected in two ways: 70% for training and 30% for testing. They link the accuracy of the machine learning algorithms is tabulated in Table 5.1.

The most accurate approach, logistic regression, has a 92% accuracy rate, and it is used to create a prediction model in Tableau.

An illustration of the algorithm's effectiveness on the dataset is provided by the confusion matrix of logistic regression as in Figure 5.3. It displays the values for the true positive, false positive, true negative, and false negative predictions made by the model. The number of cases that were successfully predicted as positive is represented by the true positive value, while the number of cases that were wrongly forecasted as positive is represented by the false positive value. The true negative value is the number of situations where a negative outcome was

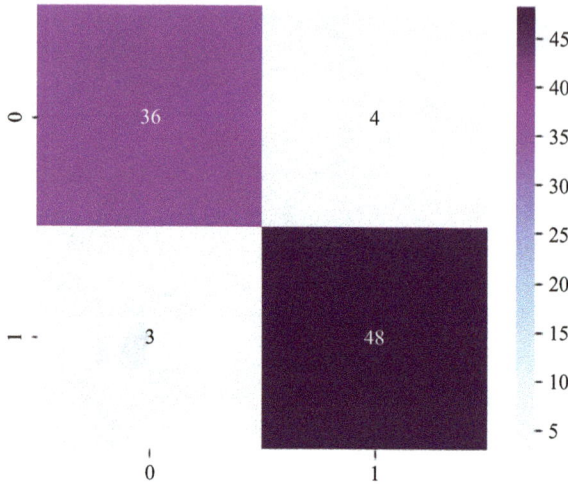

*Figure 5.3    Confusion matrix of logistic regression*

accurately anticipated, while the false negative value is the number of cases where a negative outcome was wrongly forecasted.

Figure 5.3's main findings highlight the critical roles that feature scale and selection play in improving algorithmic performance. The features that are chosen for the algorithm are crucial, and they should be chosen based on how they will affect the outcome variable – in this example, the existence or absence of heart disease. In this study, the most effective classification algorithms, including KNN, naive Bayes, random forest, logistic regression, and decision tree, were employed.

Logistic regression algorithm has proven to be useful in decision making in the field of medicine. In previous studies, Kumar *et al.* had an accuracy of 85%, and Kannan *et al.* had an accuracy of 87% using logistic regression. The accuracy at the end of this research is 92%, which is significantly better than the previous studies. This finding suggests that the algorithm utilised in this study is functioning effectively and may be useful in predicting whether or not heart disease would develop.

In conclusion, Figure 5.3 offers insight into the effectiveness of the algorithm in predicting the existence or absence of heart disease. The results indicate that feature selection and scaling have a significant role in improving the algorithm's accuracy, and the logistic regression algorithm can be helpful in medical decision-making. The accuracy of 92% found in this study is higher than that found in prior studies, showing the potential value of this algorithm in identifying the presence or absence of heart disease.

When it comes to the world of medicine, accuracy is crucial because we are dealing with human lives, and low accuracy is not acceptable. The following formula has been used to calculate the accuracy:

$$\text{Accuracy} = \frac{\text{True Positives} + \text{True Negatives}}{\text{True Pos} + \text{False Pos} + \text{True Neg} + \text{False Neg}}$$

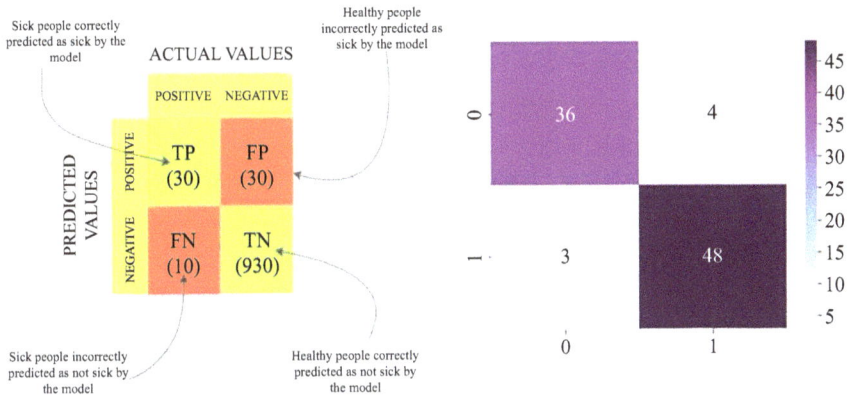

*Figure 5.4    Confusion matrix*

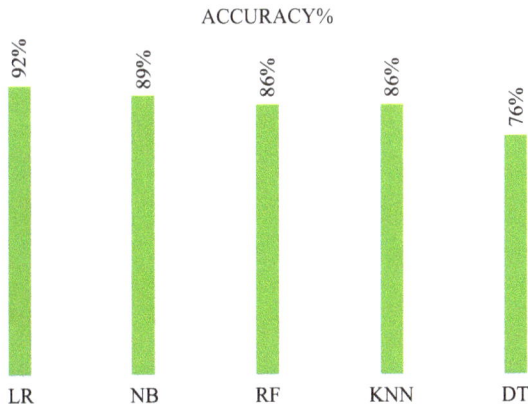

*Figure 5.5    Accuracy*

Confusion matrix has been formulated that depicts the true and false positives and negatives is shown in Figure 5.4.

Figure 5.5 clearly shows that the model is good and can be used for prediction. However, there is room for more improvement.

## 5.11    Predictive dashboard in Tableau

The Python code is executed in Tableau using the TabPy server. A predictive dashboard is built where the user/medical practitioners can enter the values. The model will then predict the presence or absence of heart disease. This will help in timely treatment and save the lives of patients.

Figure 5.6 in the research paper is an example of how Tableau and Python can be used to build a predictive dashboard that can be used by both normal people and medical practitioners to predict the onset of heart disease in the near future.

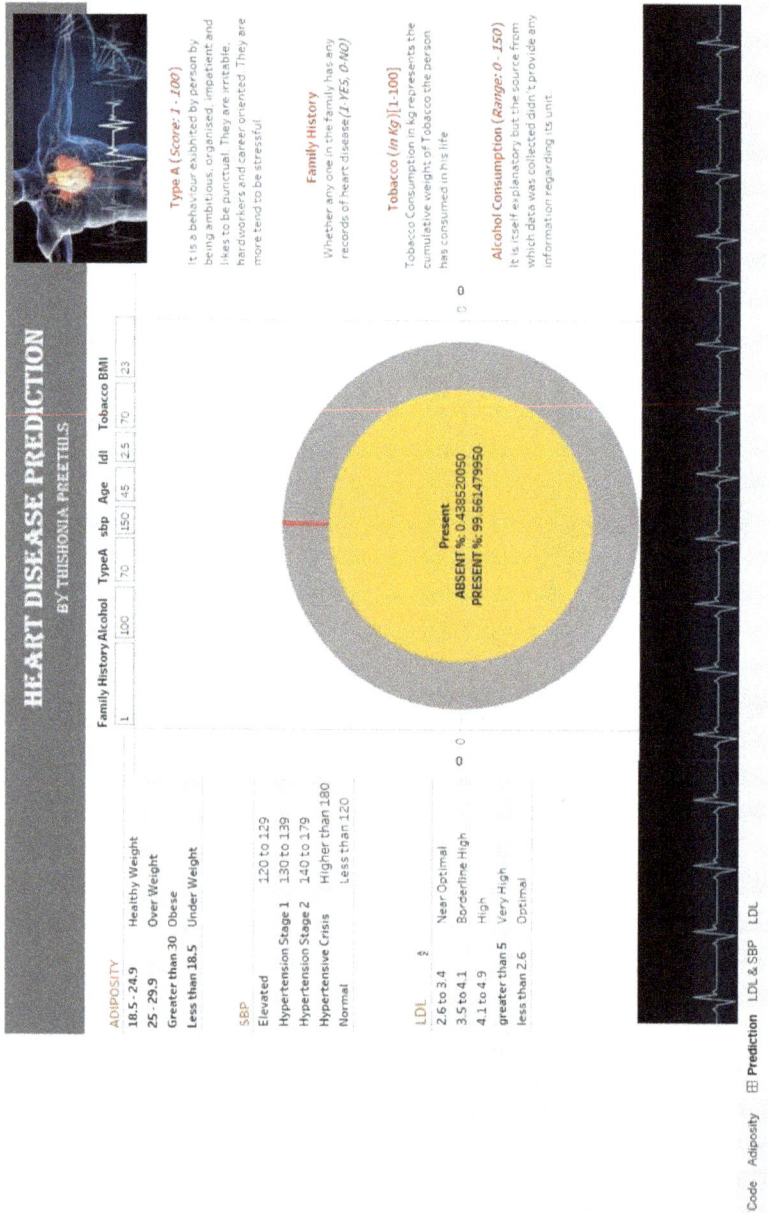

Figure 5.6  Tableau predictive dashboard

The research paper explains that the data was first fed into Tableau, and then the Python code was modified accordingly. This means that the data was pre-processed and cleaned before it was fed into Tableau. Once the data was in Tableau, the linkage between Tableau and Python was done using the TabPy server. This is a way to integrate Python's powerful analytical capabilities with Tableau's data visualisation capabilities.

The result is a predictive dashboard that provides a clear picture of the range of values that give the presence or absence probability of heart disease. The dashboard includes several visualisations, such as scatter plots, histograms, and heatmaps, that can help users explore the data and gain insights into the factors that contribute to the onset of heart disease.

The research paper notes that the predictive dashboard was not built simply to find the highest accuracy but to provide a tool that can be used by both normal people and medical practitioners. The results of the predictive model tie well with previous studies where researchers have made an analysis comparing different machine learning algorithms and finding the best fit.

The research paper also acknowledges that there are limitations to this study, such as the instruments used in the study, including the computer's computing capacity and the time limit available for the study. These limitations may affect the accuracy and reliability of the results. However, the research paper serves as a starting point for learning how to use automated learning to diagnose heart disease and can be expanded for future studies.

Overall, Figure 5.6 demonstrates the power of integrating Tableau and Python to build predictive models that can provide insights and predictions that can be used to improve healthcare outcomes.

## 5.12    Implications

Heart disease is a serious condition that can have significant impacts on one's overall health and quality of life. However, there are steps that can be taken to prevent heart disease and reduce the risk of developing this condition.

Blood pressure should be one of your main considerations. It is crucial to have your blood pressure tested frequently because high blood pressure is a major risk factor for heart disease. The majority of adults ought to have their blood pressure measured at least once each year, and more frequently if they have high blood pressure. If high blood pressure is discovered, lifestyle modifications and medication may be required to control it.

Regarding heart health, cholesterol levels are yet another crucial factor. Clogged arteries and a higher risk of heart attack can result from high cholesterol levels. Healthy cholesterol and triglyceride levels can be maintained by making lifestyle adjustments including eating a balanced diet and exercising frequently. Medication may be required in specific situations.

Maintaining a healthy weight is also important for preventing heart disease. The risk of heart disease, as well as other ailments like diabetes and high blood pressure, increases with obesity and being overweight. By achieving and maintaining a healthy weight, a person's chance of developing heart disease can be significantly reduced.

For heart health, a balanced diet is crucial. Maintaining good blood pressure and cholesterol levels can be achieved by avoiding diets high in salt, added sugars, saturated and trans fats, and other ingredients. Consuming a mix of fruits, vegetables, whole grains, and lean proteins is advised instead. A food plan like this one can offer important nutrients and reduce the risk of heart disease.

Physical activity is also crucial for maintaining heart health. Regular exercise can help to improve circulation, strengthen the heart, and reduce blood pressure and cholesterol levels. Even moderate exercise, such as walking or biking, can have significant benefits for heart health.

Alcohol use should be kept to a minimum to help prevent heart disease. Alcohol abuse raises blood pressure and may result in weight gain, which both raise the risk of heart disease. An individual's risk of acquiring heart disease can be considerably decreased by drinking in moderation or abstaining from alcohol completely.

It is crucial to avoid smoking and limit exposure to second-hand smoke because smoking is a significant risk factor for heart disease. Smoking cessation can have a positive impact on heart health as well as general health and wellbeing.

Stress can also impact heart health, so it is important to manage stress through healthy coping mechanisms such as exercise, relaxation techniques, and social support. Additionally, diabetics need to monitor their blood sugar levels since they can harm blood vessels and raise their risk of heart disease.

In conclusion, maintaining a healthy lifestyle is essential for preventing heart disease and reducing the risk of developing this condition. By making lifestyle changes and taking steps to improve overall health and well-being, individuals can significantly improve their heart health and reduce the risk of heart disease.

## 5.13    Conclusion

The use of machine learning algorithms in healthcare is growing, and they have the potential to significantly improve patient outcomes. In the study you cited, machine learning algorithms are used to forecast patients' risk of CHD based on their medical data. The study's algorithms, which include logistic regression, naive Bayes, decision tree random forest, and KNN, are all well-liked techniques for examining medical data and producing predictions.

One of the advantages of using machine learning algorithms in healthcare is the ability to make predictions based on large amounts of data. By analysing various data points, such as blood pressure, cholesterol levels, and diabetes status, the algorithms can identify patterns that may indicate a higher risk of heart disease. This information can then be used to inform preventative measures and potentially reduce the risk of heart disease in patients.

The study also highlights the importance of family history in predicting the risk of heart disease. By incorporating this information into the algorithms, the accuracy of the predictions can be improved. This is because family history can be a significant factor in developing heart disease, and, by taking this into account, the algorithms can make more accurate predictions.

Overall, the study demonstrates the potential of machine learning algorithms in predicting heart disease risk and improving patient outcomes. By identifying high-risk patients and implementing preventative measures, healthcare providers can potentially reduce the incidence of heart disease and improve patient outcomes.

# References

[1]  WHO (2021). Cardio Vascular Diseases. https://www.who.int/news-room/fact-sheets/detail/cardiovascular-diseases-(cardiovascular diseases).

[2]  S. Kumar and N. Sinha (2020). Cardiovascular disease in India: a 360-degree overview. *Medical Journal Armed Forces India*, 76(1), 1–3.

[3]  D.M. Huffman, D. Prabhakaran, C. Osmond, *et al.* (2012). Incidence of cardiovascular risk factors in an Indian urban cohort. *Journal of the American College of Cardiology*, 57(17), 1765–1774.

[4]  M. Gandhi and S. Narayan Singh (2015). Predictions in heart disease using techniques of data mining. In *International Conference on Futuristic Trend in Computational Analysis and Knowledge Management*.

[5]  J. Thomas and R.T. Princy (2016). Human heart disease prediction system using data mining techniques. In *2016 International Conference on Circuit, Power and Computing Technologies*.

[6]  S. Kumari and R. Viswanathan (2020). Heart disease prediction system. *International Journal of Science and Research (IJSR)*, 9(7), https://www.ijisrt.com/heart-disease-prediction-system.

[7]  S. Abdullah (2012). A data mining model to predict and analyze the events related to coronary heart disease using decision trees with particle swarm optimization for feature selection. *International Journal of Computer Applications*, 55(8).

[8]  H. Sharma and M.A. Rizvi (2017). Prediction of heart disease using machine learning algorithms: a survey. *International Journal on Recent and Innovation Trends in Computing and Communication*, 5, 99–104.

[9]  A. Hazra, S. Kumar Mandal, A. Gupta, A. Mukherjee, and A. Mukherjee (2017). Heart disease diagnosis and prediction using machine learning and data mining techniques: a review. *Advances in Computational Sciences and Technology*, 10(7), 2137–2159. http://www.ripublication.com.

[10]  R. Kaur and P. Kaur (2016). A review – heart disease forecasting pattern using various data mining techniques. *International Journal of Computer Science and Mobile Computing*, 5(6), 350–354.

[11]  A. Rajkumar and G. Sophia Reena (2009). Diagnosis of Heart Disease Using Data Mining Algorithm, ResearchGate, November 2009.

[12]  J. Patel, T. Upadhyay, and S. Patel (2016). Heart disease prediction using machine learning and data mining technique. *International Journal of Computer Science and Communication*, 7, 129–137.

[13] D.E. Salhi, A. Tari, and M-T. Kechadi (2021). Using machine learning for heart disease prediction. In: Senouci, M.R., Boudaren, M.E.Y., Sebbak, F., Mataoui, M. (eds) *Advances in Computing Systems and Applications* (pp. 70–81). Springer, Cham.

[14] A. Garg, B. Sharma, and R. Khan (2021). Heart disease prediction using machine learning techniques. *IOP Conference Series: Materials Science and Engineering*, 1022(1), 012046.

[15] J. Tolles and W.J. Meurer (2016). Logistic regression relating patient characteristics to outcomes. *JAMA*, 316(5), 533–534 doi:10.1001/jama.2016.7653. ISSN 0098-84. OCLC 6823603312. PMID 27483067.

[16] Murtagh (1983). A survey of recent advances in hierarchical clustering algorithms. *The Computer Journal*, 26(4), 354–359, doi:10.1093/comjnl/26.4.354.

[17] A.H. Chen, S.Y. Huang, P.S. Hong, C.H. Cheng, and E.J. Lin (2016). *HDPS: Heart Disease Prediction System*, Tzu Chi University, Hualien City, Taiwan.

[18] B. Bahrami and M.H. Shirvan (2015). Prediction and diagnosis of heart disease by data mining techniques. *Journal of Multidisciplinary Engineering Science and Technology (JMEST)*, 2(2), 164–168.

[19] T.K. Ho (1995). Random decision forests. In *Proceedings of the 3rd International Conference on Document Analysis and Recognition*, Montreal, QC, 14–16 August 1995. pp. 278–282. Archived from the original (PDF) on 17 April 2016. Retrieved 5 June 2016.

[20] B. Kamiński, M. Jakubczyk, and P. Szufel (2017). A framework for sensitivity analysis of decision trees. *Central European Journal of Operations Research*, 26(1), 135–159. doi:10.1007/s10100-017-0479-6. PMC 5767274. PMID 29375266.

[21] A. McCallum (2019). Graphical Models, Lecture 2: Bayesian Network Representation. Retrieved 22 October 2019.

[22] S. Palaniappan and R. Awang (2008). Intelligent heart disease prediction system using data mining techniques. In *AICCSA 08 – 6th EEE/ACS International Conference on Computer Systems and Applications*, pp. 108–115. doi:10.1109/AICCSA.2008.4493524.

[23] S. Kumar, B. Patil, and Y.S. Kumaraswamy (2011). Predictive data mining for medical diagnosis of heart disease prediction. *IJCSE*, 17, 43–48.

[24] V. Chaurasia and S. Pal. (2013). Data mining approach to detect heart diseases. *International Journal of Advanced Computer Science and Information Technology (IJACSIT)* 2(4), 56–66.

*Chapter 6*

# Artificial intelligence integrated approach for healthcare management: a critical analysis

*Gayatri Panda[1], Manoj Dash[2], Anil Kumar[3] and Arvind Upadhyay[4]*

## Abstract

In these turbulent changing conditions, the role of data-driven technologies has increased manifolds. Artificial intelligence (AI) enables understanding the criticalities at a faster rate and provides the required results to the patients for better treatment and results. AI-based models support various healthcare issues such as diagnosis and treatment, radiology, drug design, and dermatology. AI permits emphasis on developing robust solutions to different health-related issues. It focuses on cost minimization, timely delivery, accuracy, and patient-centered services. The sole objective of this present work is to identify the role of AI in healthcare management with a systematic review of literature in terms of its usage, sustenance, and application in future areas of healthcare management. The study implemented a systematic literature review (SLR) and bibliometric visualization process to scrutinize the data from enormous sources. The "SCOPUS database" is used to segregate papers using relevant keywords. Thus, the research work tries to analyze the research questions in terms of leading sources, contributors, and keywords in healthcare management research, to provide topic mapping based on the keyword's co-occurrences, and to develop a model for future researchers. The results focus on understanding the current research trend in terms of the maximum publication of sources and year and significance of AI in healthcare management. This study is beneficial for administration, health consultants, policymakers, and researchers to examine areas where AI can be implemented. The study explores the implication of AI in healthcare management measures through SLR and bibliometric analysis and analyzes the role of AI in

[1]Department of Management, NIST Institute of Science and Technology (Autonomous), Berhampur, India
[2]Department of Management, ABV – Indian Institute of Information Technology and Management, Gwalior, India
[3]Guildhall School of Business and Law, London Metropolitan University, London, UK
[4]International Trade, Supply Chain and Logistics, University of Stavanger Business School, Stavanger, Norway

healthcare measures by diagnosing its practice, application, and potential research directions.

**Keywords:** Artificial intelligence; Healthcare management; Qualitative research; Bibliometric

## 6.1  Introduction

With the growing digitalization and expansion of technological advancement, big data and artificial intelligence (AI) brought a new progression in every sector, including the health sector. AI enables organizations to develop their own data infrastructure to support their own needs typically their computing and storage [1]. AI refers to the ability to emulate human features such as decision-making, knowledge representation, complex task processing, reasoning, communication, vision, and language [2]. AI imbibes to increase the usage in healthcare delivery services for clinical decision support, patient information, and healthcare interventions. It is considered one of the techniques which intervene to understand the role and develop and transform measures in improving universal healthcare services [3]. AI can be attributed to various subset techniques developed such as machine learning, deep learning, and supervised learning through developed algorithms that uncover an understanding of associations between a large amount of data and human expertise.

Although AI has extended to various domains like banking [4,5], education [6,7], supply chain and operations [8,9], and so on. Healthcare management is considered one of the most important pillars of society which proves a major yardstick for societal growth and protects the interest of communities. AI application in the field has gained immense attention for cost-cutting, improving care, and improving efficiency in the health system. The authors of [10] discussed how significantly AI can be utilized in the field of healthcare management to increase clinical diagnosis and ultimately improve healthcare practices through the proper development of the framework for decision-makers and policymakers. Although current literature on the role and application of AI in healthcare management has been addressed by many researchers, a few studies have given a skeptical view on existing studies through visualization and thematic areas analysis. Thus, researchers extracted and analyzed the existing articles with AI in healthcare management from the Scopus database which motivated them to explore the topic and progress the present study. Therefore, "the researchers were stimulated to formulate the current study to find imperative contributions of the technology in the health sector and create pathways for forthcoming researchers which led the researchers to progress the current study based on the stated research questions":

Q1. How can AI be utilized in healthcare management?

Q2: What are the significant sources, productive countries, and authors with maximum research studies on this topic?

Q3: Identifying the significant authors and developing a network map for coauthorship and authorship.

Q4: What are the most used keywords, countries, and clusters on this topic?

Q5: What are the impending research pathways of AI application in the field of healthcare management?

Considering the stated discussion, the following objectives have been articulated such as:

- To explore and examine research studies on the application of AI in healthcare management.
- To formulate a framework to understand the state of research and pave the way for impending researchers.
- To put forward future thrust areas in the application of AI in healthcare management.

The study focused on examining the state of research in AI in the area of healthcare management, as well as determining the future research direction. The present study through a systematic review approach reassesses the selected papers and analyzes the contributions year-wise, authors, countries, and highly cited papers in AI in the healthcare sector. On the other hand, through visualization, the study focused on developing different network maps to understand the contribution of authors and working on identifying the clusters based on keywords occurrence as well as content analysis for identifying the thematic areas of the topic for upcoming researchers.

The current study is divided into seven sections. The beginning segment explains the introduction of the study followed by the stated question and objectives. The background review is explained in Section 6.2. Section 6.3 discusses the schematic representation of the methodological structure, which covers database selection, keywords, and collection of articles. Section 6.4 discusses bibliometric analysis as well as network maps and clustering on AI and its integration into healthcare management whereas Section 6.5 describes the research implications, Section 6.6 enumerates the scope of the study, Section 6.7 includes a discussion of the findings, and lastly, Section 6.8 discusses the conclusion of the present study.

## 6.2 Review of background

The emerging rise of technological applications and techniques brought a revolutionary approach to understanding the relevance of the technique in the healthcare sector for better results [11]. The researchers discussed the benefits in terms of cost reduction, quality, and equity. The major benefit of AI particularly in visual pattern recognition will provide a major advantage in the health sector for speedy detection and treatment. Further, the authors of [12] stated that AI has expanded its wings in the healthcare sector and it has been a tool to be used in routine clinical operations, but still, many stones need to be uncovered to understand the ethical considerations, thus addressing the ethical and regulatory concerns is one of the prime importance for researchers. The authors of [13] discussed the application of AI on multifarious aspects such as health service management, patient data diagnostics, and clinical decision-making. The authors of [14] addressed the application of AI in the treatment of major health problems such as depression, Alzheimer's, and diabetic conditions. The authors of [6] stated that AI can be used for increasing efficiency, safety, and access to value-based health services. The authors of [15] stated that AI is gaining profound importance in handling patient psychology and empathy. It is gaining central importance for proper diagnosis and treatment as well as for creating an interactive learning environment for medical practitioners.

Lastly, the AI technique has expanded its wings in every sector of society, including medicine and healthcare management. Although numerous challenges are witnessed, still their use can be measured for the growth of the people and society at large. The continuous approach towards introducing AI in healthcare became an imperative tool to broaden the possibility of new progress opportunities in this area. Based on the substantiated literature review, the current study identified the resulting gaps such as (1) "Though AI has entered the field of the health sector still amalgamation in the field of healthcare management is very scarce" [16]; (2) "The predominant studies didn't present any prominent thematic areas or future research questions for other researchers" [10,17]. Thus, from the identified gaps, there is a vital need to examine the integration of AI in the health sector, which inspired the formulation of the current research work.

## 6.3    Methodological structure

The schematic diagram discussed the methodology followed in the study as well as highlights the stated research questions, background review, and research contribution.

The study is an integrative approach by researchers to understand the relevance of AI in healthcare management and how far the use of technology provides advanced practices for policymakers and health practitioners to plan, execute, and implement techniques for better and error-free results. Though enough studies have been contributed to the research field where AI has been used, only a few studies carried out their work in bibliometric analysis on AI techniques in the health sector. The present study has opted a step-by-step approach to complete the current study by framing the research questions. The study aims to develop citation, cluster, and future thematic areas to answer the research questions. The study can suggestively determine current and future AI trends in healthcare management. Lastly, the most critical reason AI needs to be endorsed in every area and health system is one of prime importance which is considered as one major research gap which inspired the researchers to develop an amalgamated work that can enhance the value of the field. Figure 6.1 elaborates on the steps followed to select the database, identify the keywords to extract the papers from the database, and elucidate the research contribution of the study.

### 6.3.1    Database used for extracting data

The research work is well-thought-out to use the Scopus database because it is one the most significant databases for aggregation of literature [18] as well as one of the

**Step-1 Research Questions and Objectives**

Q1: How can artificial intelligence be utilized in healthcare management?

Q2: What are the significant sources, countries, and authors with the maximum publications on this topic?

Q3: What are the highly cited articles on this topic specifically in healthcare management?

Q4: What are the most recurrently used keywords and formulating a cluster analysis?

Q5: What are the future-developed thematic areas of artificial intelligence in the field of healthcare management?

**Database selected**

SCOPUS

**Identified keywords**

"Artificial intelligence" OR "AI" OR "Machine Learning" OR "ML" AND "healthcare management" OR "healthcare system"

**Step-2 Background examination**

Analysis and Software: Bibliometric Analysis includes (i) Network maps, (ii) Citation analysis, (iii) Co-citation analysis, (iv) keyword co-occurrence analysis.

Software used: VOS viewer

**Collection of articles**

Criterion for inclusion: publication stage-"final"; language-"English" document type "journal" article type " article" This resulted in the identification of 499 articles for the final study.

**Step 3: Contribution of the study**

- Identified the influential aspects of the literature on artificial intelligence in healthcare management.

- Identifying the thematic areas.

- Identified future research questions for impending researchers.

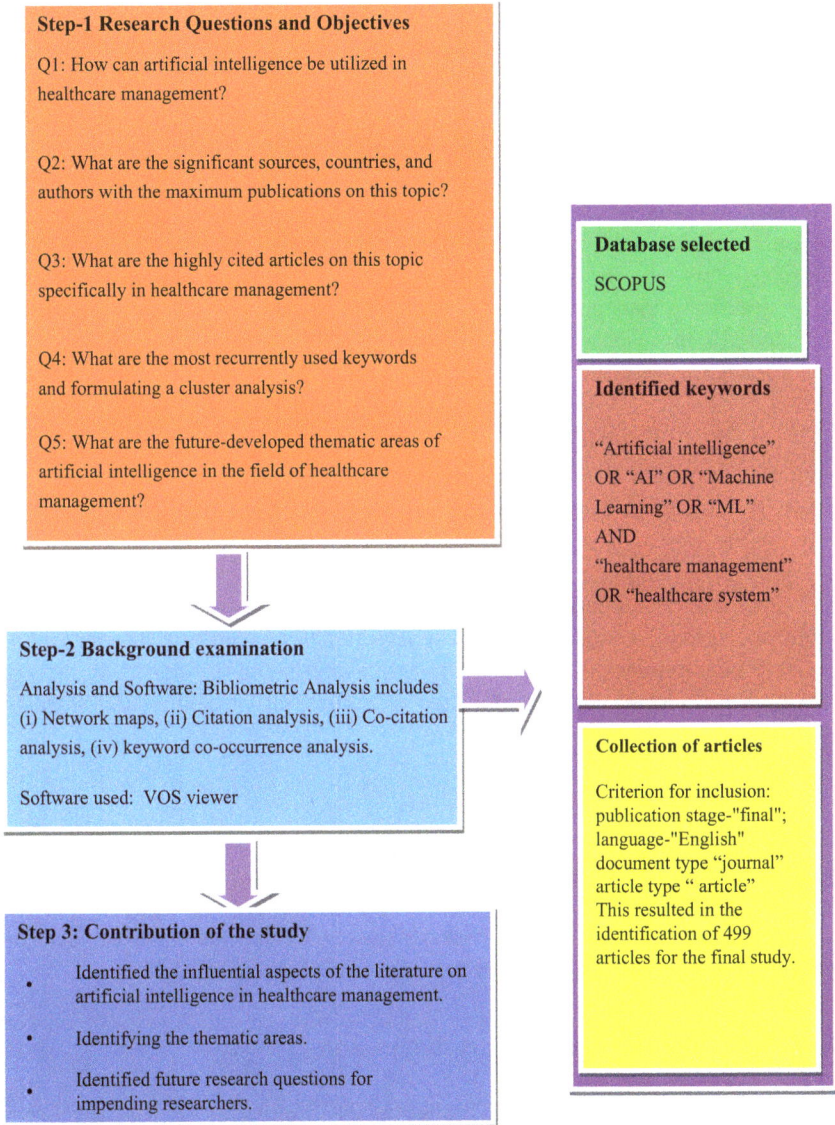

*Figure 6.1   Methodological structure*

databases with profuse abstracts and citations of literature developed in the field and it is also an exhaustive database with comparison to other databases. Thus, the research study considered the database for data assortment because of its inclusive coverage. "To examine a comprehensive range of studies for the study, the researchers followed an assimilation of keywords and discussed in the next sections."

### 6.3.2    Keywords identified and search query

The study focused on identifying literature through the use of relevant keywords; after discussion with two subject experts the researchers considered the required keywords for extracting the data. The whole procedure followed two steps, such as in the first step it considered the keywords relevant to AI whereas in the second part, it considered healthcare management. Thus, the final search query used for extracting the required data for further analysis and developing the network maps and understanding the current state of research as well as developing the future research streams are elucidated ("AI" OR "AI" OR "Machine Learning" OR "ML" AND "healthcare management" OR "healthcare system"). Two operators such as AND and OR are used with the keywords to extract the required data from the Scopus database for further analysis and discussion.

### 6.3.3    Cleaning of articles

The initial extraction of articles using keywords resulted in 1,234 articles, but the researcher adopted the exclusion/inclusion criterion of literature based on the stated step such as first focused on document type: "article," second on article type "journal," third, language "English" whereas lastly on keywords "such as "AI," "AI" OR "Machine Learning" OR "ML" AND "healthcare management" OR "healthcare system" which resulted in an output of 499 documents. The researchers considered the extracted data file for further analysis and developed the network maps and analyze the Scopus extracted data files for presenting the sketch of research in the area.

### 6.3.4    Articles assortment

The researchers after the exclusion/inclusion criteria listed the taken out 499 documents for preparing the study through the use of the extracted CSV (comma-separated values) file from the Scopus database for bibliometric analysis. The files were checked by the researchers manually to recognize the topic of "AI" and "healthcare management" in the abstract, title, and keywords respectively.

## 6.4    Analysis of findings and discussion

The consecutive section discussed bibliographic information such as elucidating the top journals, countries, and authors with maximum publication as well as highlighting the publication trend which provides a focus on expanding the area of research and transferring the

### 6.4.1    Ten identified journal

Figure 6.2 visualizes the top ten journals with maximum publication in the area of AI and healthcare management. Among the top ten journals, *Journal of Biomedical Informatics* is in the first position with nine publications. It belongs to Elsevier publishing house followed by the next journal *Artificial Intelligence in Medicine*

JOURNALS

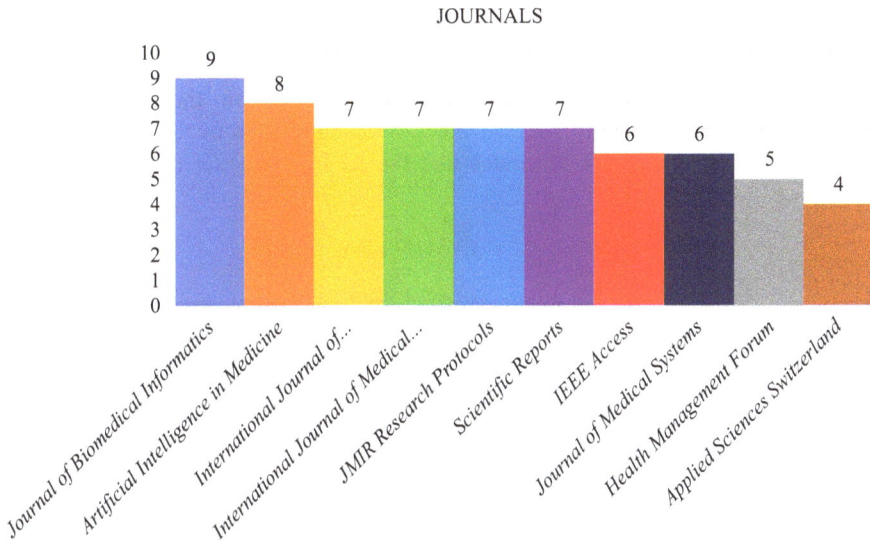

*Figure 6.2    Ten top journals*

with eight papers, next the *International Journal of Environmental Research and Public Health* with seven publications followed by other journals with equivalent publications. Lastly, the *Journal of Applied Sciences Switzerland* is with the least number of publications.

Figure 6.2 indicates that the publications in the field of AI and healthcare management have been restricted to scientific journals so other journals with interdisciplinary approach can be included which enhances the scope of research articles and develops a heterogeneous set of research studies with multiple benefits for researchers.

## 6.4.2    Country statistics

Figure 6.3 discusses the country statistics and identifies the top ten countries with the maximum publications. It conveys the statistics on countries' contributions based on the first author's affiliation. Among the top ten countries, the United States of America is the top priority with the maximum contribution of $n=178$ articles. Next to that the UK, India, and China are the countries with a relatively progressive contribution. The country statistics comprises both developing and developed nations. Thus, Figure 6.3 suggests that the application of AI in healthcare management has gained immense attention. Hence, impending researchers can develop studies by considering the existing state of research and develop more robust strategies which will enable health practitioners, and policymakers to identify cost-effective and secured solutions for data retrieval and management.

## 6.4.3    Publication trend

Figure 6.4 presents the trend in publications on AI in healthcare management. The trend indicates there is steady progress in publication from the year 2015, the researchers have constantly focused on developing studies in the area and contributing. Thus, Figure 6.4 illustrates that the AI in healthcare management is a

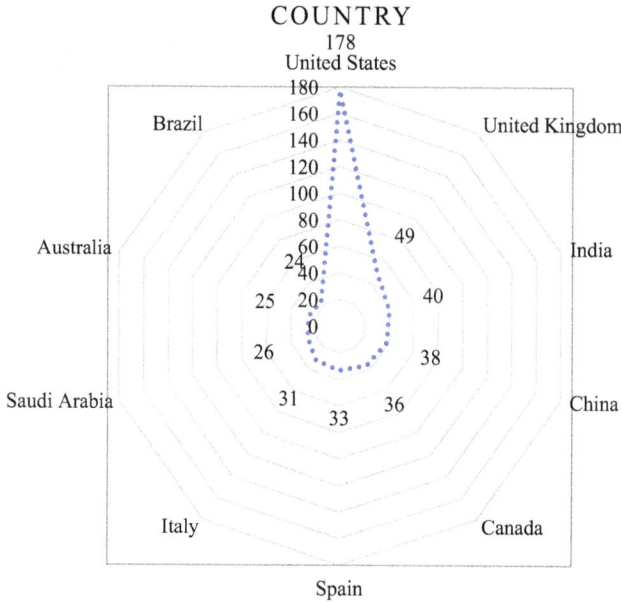

*Figure 6.3    Ten top journals*

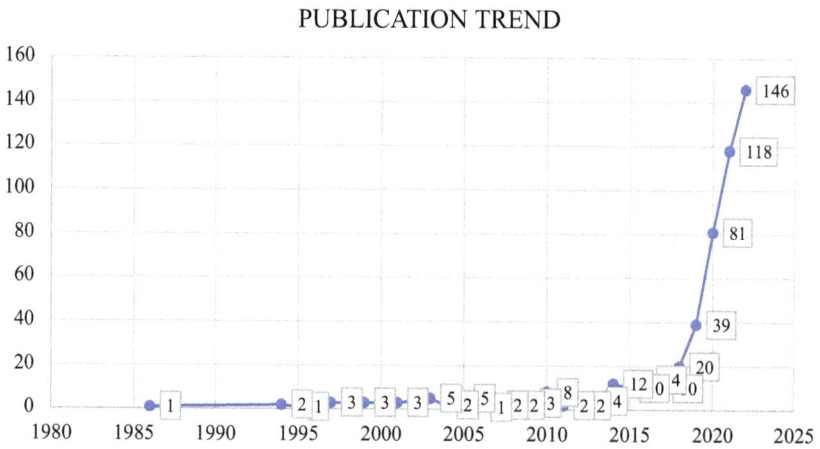

*Figure 6.4    Publication trend*

budding topic, researchers are actively engaging to address various issues and its application for better results. Developing research studies can provoke to understand the benefits as well as challenges in its application and study can be a measurement tool for adding value to the existing research base and expanding the scope of the area in every field of operations.

### 6.4.4   Author statistics

Figure 6.5 illustrates the author contribution and identifies the top ten authors who have the maximum contribution to the field. The extracted 499 articles fit with 159 authors. Among the listed authors Prof. Jaedon P. Avey is the most contributing author with maximum publication ($n=4$). Presently he is associated with south central foundation, his area of interest lies in health disorders, suicide prevention, data science.

Next to that Prof. Vanessa Hiratsuka contributed ($n=4$) articles to the field of AI. She is presently working as an Assistant Professor of Clinical and Translational Research. Her area of interest lies in disability research. The third author Jalal Ai Muhtadi has contributed ($n=3$) papers as per the statistics. He is associated with the college of computer and information sciences, in Saudi Arabia. His area of interest lies with IoT, big data computer network security, healthcare management as well as AI. Taking the statistics into consideration other authors also contributed in a significant manner which shows that the field is gaining momentum among researchers. Thus, the upcoming researchers need to address the research studies in various domains and contribute to the field of healthcare management by integrating AI for better results and optimum solutions.

AUTHOR STATISTICS

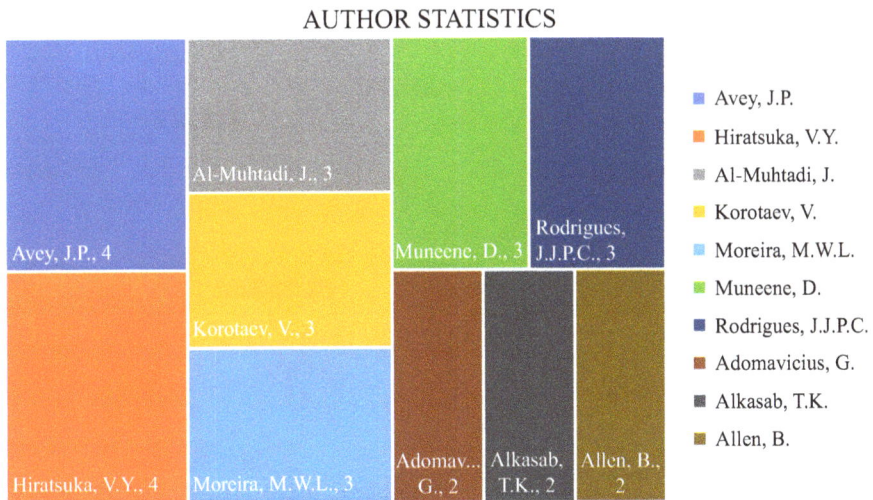

*Figure 6.5    Author statistics*

## 6.4.5  Bibliometric analysis

### 6.4.5.1  Network map on authorship

The present research study advocated the development of network maps based on author–coauthorship using the VOS viewer software. It focuses on developing maps on the basis "authorship, keyword co-occurrence, and intercountry-wise" [19]. The map on author-wise measures the authorship conditions among other authors in the dataset. The present study identified a total of 2,485 authors in the dataset, only those authors who have at least two papers and two citations are considered for further development of the network map. Considering the stated criteria around 111 authors were considered for further analysis.

Figure 6.6 analyzes the generated map based on co-authorship by the software. The authorship map is connected through lines to establish the relationship. The identified authors are grouped in one cluster and the cluster comprises nine items: the cluster stated that all authors have co-authored with other authors and maximum collaborative works have been developed.

### 6.4.5.2  Country statistics map

Figure 6.7 discusses country-wise statistics. The country-wise statistics map identifies the top countries that have explored and developed research papers in the area of AI in healthcare management. The extracted map presents the "United States," the "United Kingdom," and "India" as the countries whose authors have maximum collaboration. The countries are connected through lines and represented through square boxes. The inclusion criteria have been fixed in that at least every country must have two articles and two citations to be included, out of 92 countries 54 countries were included. Thus, the authors of these countries can extend their scope of work and develop advanced and multi-country-wise studies to increase the scope of the field.

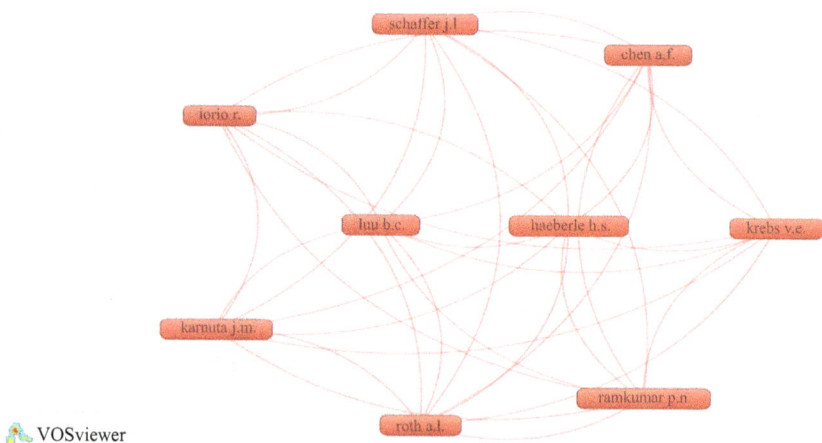

*Figure 6.6    Authorship network map*

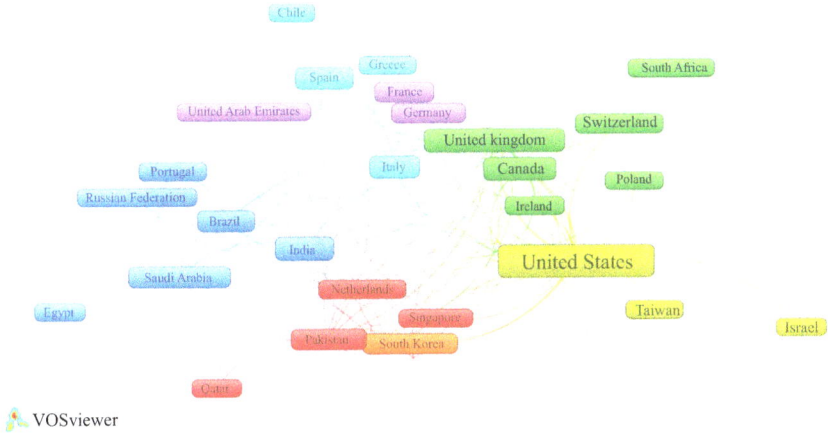

*Figure 6.7   Country wise map*

*Table 6.1   Country-wise statistics*

| Countries | Publications |
|---|---|
| United States | 179 |
| United Kingdom | 49 |
| India | 43 |
| Canada | 36 |
| Saudi Arabia | 27 |
| Australia | 25 |
| Pakistan | 18 |
| Spain | 33 |
| Switzerland | 11 |
| Italy | 31 |

Table 6.1 lists out the top ten countries whose authors have co-authored the highest number of times.

### 6.4.5.3   Keyword wise occurrence

Figure 6.8 demonstrates the statistics of keyword occurrence. Keyword occurrence manifests the frequency of keyword usage and identifies the highly used keywords for the research study. "The prime objective of the keyword co-occurrence map is to classify the keywords that have been repeatedly used in the existing studies and are used in this research work. It provides the upcoming researchers with enough idea about which type of topic and context has been preferred mainly by other researchers. The connection of the terms and the publications' co-occurrences were analysed" [19].

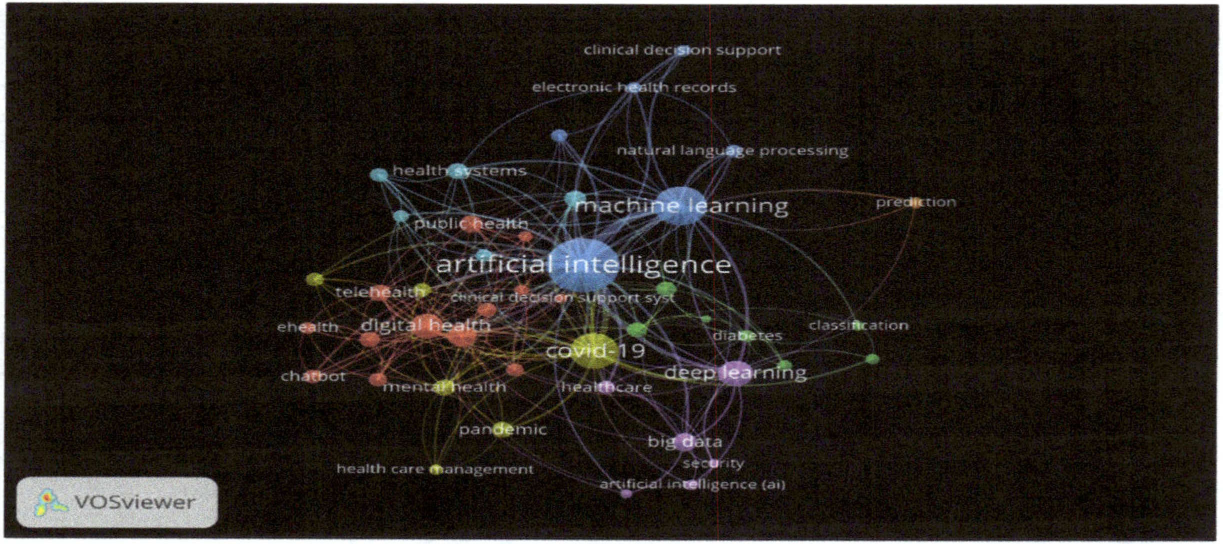

Figure 6.8  Keyword occurrence

The present study identified a total of 1,551 keywords out of which, 45 keywords meet the threshold limit which has been set to 5. The keywords which have been used five times have been considered by the researchers for developing the map. The map presents an idea on the frequency of keywords as well as presenting the upcoming researchers with what are the keywords which are mainly preferred by other researchers. Table 6.2 provides a detail statistic of keywords and their occurrence. It discusses the top ten keywords frequently used in the existing research studies. It will lay down to portray their research studies and understand the occurrence statistics for better management of the present state of research studies.

### 6.4.5.4   Citation analysis

Figure 6.9 presents the citation analysis statistics based on documents. Citation analysis enables us to identify the most influential work on a specific topic or uncover the intellectual base of research in AI in healthcare management [20].

*Table 6.2   Top ten keywords occurrence*

| Keyword | Occurrence |
| --- | --- |
| AI | 126 |
| Machine learning | 66 |
| COVID-19 | 44 |
| Deep learning | 22 |
| Digital health | 16 |
| Telemedicine | 16 |
| Health system | 9 |
| E-health | 9 |
| Technology | 6 |
| Mental health | 6 |

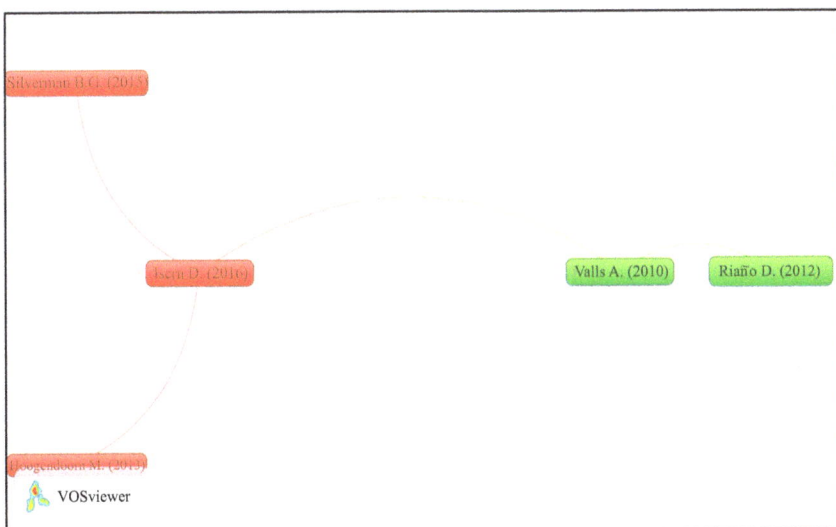

*Figure 6.9   Citation analysis*

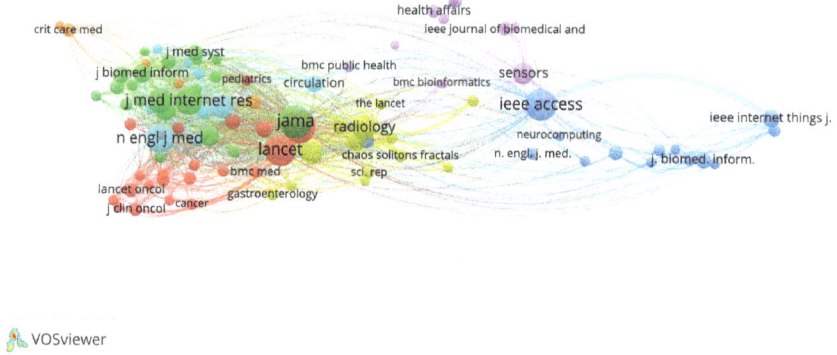

*Figure 6.10   Co-citation analysis*

"Thus, citation analysis analyses the positive alignment of research work in a specific area and how relevant they are" [21]. The present research work developed the citation map based on the documents. The threshold limit has been set to ten to include a research paper in the analysis. Taking the threshold limit into account, it resulted in identification of 156 articles. The identified articles are further considered for analysis. Thus, Figure 6.10 elucidates the identified five research papers which are the most cited papers by other research studies. The identified research articles are [22–26]. The citation map provides with a roadmap for future researchers to identify the literature which are imperative in the field and can be taken as base studies to develop their research work as well understand their role for better developing studies and making a significant contribution to the field for developing strategies and methodologies to deal with health problems and issues.

### 6.4.5.5   Co-citation analysis

Figure 6.10 describes the co-citation map based on sources. Co-citation analysis presents the highly cited sources in the present literature studies. Co-citation analysis measures the significant collaboration of studies and analyses the growth trend of studies [20].

The present study uses the co-citation map to understand the highly cited sources in the existing literature as well as identify the contribution of existing studies and prolific sources to be considered by future impending researchers for addressing various topics and areas in the field of healthcare management through AI integration.

## 6.4.6   Cluster analysis

Figure 6.11 elucidates the identified thematic areas extracted from keyword occurrence. The identified thematic areas are grouped into six clusters. The identified cluster analysis led to the devising of six research propositions such as (1) AI and decision support system; (2) AI and data security; (3) AI and COVID-19 pandemic; (4) AI and public health management; (5) AI and public health mechanism; (6) AI and prediction

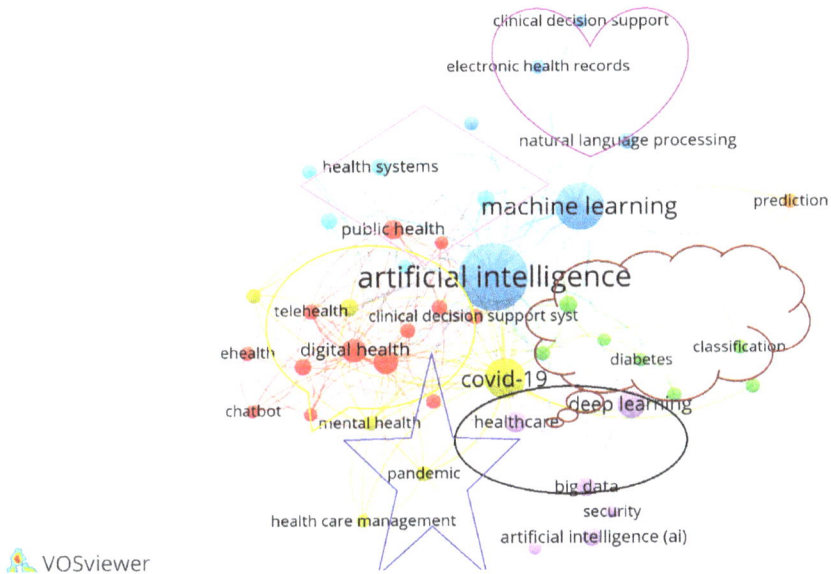

*Figure 6.11 Cluster analysis*

*Table 6.3 Cluster using keywords*

| S. no. | Clusters | Keywords |
|---|---|---|
| 1 | AI and decision support system | "Clinical decision support, natural language processing, electronic health records" |
| 2 | AI and data security | "Big data, Security, deep learning" |
| 3 | AI and COVID-19 pandemic | "Pandemic, healthcare management, mental health" |
| 4 | AI and public health management | "Public health, health system" |
| 5 | AI and public health mechanism | "Chatbot, e-health, digital health, mental health" |
| 6 | AI and prediction of disorders | "Diabetes, classification" |

of disorders using content analysis. "The developed research pathways and research propositions will enable forthcoming researchers to develop studies by understanding the benefits of AI in the health sector, and its application for better results and growth standpoints." Table 6.3 provides a detailed analysis of clusters developed using keywords through VOS viewer. It describes the clusters and their associated keywords for better understanding of readers.

### 6.4.6.1    Cluster 1: AI and decision support system (purple)

The authors of [27] stated that the application of AI enables to synchronize the decisions and provides clinicians to reach effective decisions with reliability and validity. The authors of [28] researchers focused on understanding the application of AI in filtering and treatment of a large amount of information and enabling to get the required information as and when required which improves the effectiveness of information and decisions through the extracted data. Followed with the study by [29] stated that AI became an embedded system in a digital system with and profound impact on decision-making, it strengthens the extraction of data and enhances the performance of data management for better decision-making. The authors of [30] stated that evidence-based record provides efficacy and minimize the pitfalls and assess the risk for taking an effective decision and improving the performance mechanism. The authors of [31] stated that AI enables fair and translucent information processing for a better decision-making approach. The authors of [32] analyzed the optimization of decision-making and analyzed large data sets for predicting prognostic solutions for handling uncertainties and risks. The stated discussion resulted in identifying the imperative role of AI in the decision support system and it led to the formulation of two future stated questions for impending researchers.

### 6.4.6.2    Cluster 2: AI and data security (black)

The authors of [33] in their research study stated that AI application enables the use of neural network development of smart models for malware classification and detecting intrusion which will prevent data and security. The researchers [34] expanded to understand the AI application in cyber-physical systems. The stated discussion resulted in identifying the imperative role of AI in the decision support system and it led to the formulation of two future stated questions for impending researchers.

### 6.4.6.3    Cluster 3: AI and COVID-19 pandemic (blue)

The authors of [35] predicted that the application of AI during COVID enables to identifying, screening, tracking, and predicting patients' details for proper diagnosis and timely treatment as well as detection of infection for developing required measures for the patients. The authors of [36] discussed that AI implementation enables to address the timely detection and quarantine of cases. The authors of [37] discussed that the imposition of AI to deal with the COVID-19 pandemic enables identification, screening, diagnosis, and prediction of the results on a better scale which is one of the major through of AI implementation. The researchers [38] stated that the application of AI enables to handle of the pandemic through proper management of data as well as vaccine development, excluding potential virus carriers, telemedicine service, economic recovery, material distribution, disinfection, and health care services. Thus, the stated discussion enabled us to understand the impending role of AI during COVID-19 and develop measures and strategies to handle the crisis. The stated discussion resulted in the formulation of two future stated questions for impending researchers.

#### 6.4.6.4    Cluster4: AI and public health management (pink)

The authors of [39] stated that the application of AI focuses on how computers learn data and understand the human mind to securely transmit the data and enhance the secrecy of information. AI provides unparalleled opportunities to enhance clinical performance, minimize cost and reduce the health effects for better results [40]. The researchers stated that AI provokes to state that with its infinite power, it can develop more potential to handle patient history and try to identify different cost-effective models for better results [41]. Thus, the stated discussion enabled us to understand the impending role of AI in public health management and also develop measures and strategies to handle the current state of health conditions of the community. The stated discussion resulted in the formulation of two future stated questions for impending researchers.

#### 6.4.6.5    Cluster 5: AI and digital health mechanisms (yellow)

The authors of [42] stated that the digitalization of patient records offers multiple benefits such as ease of data management as well as quick access to real-time treatment of patients. Although data management leverages more benefits at the same time it needs to be protected from cyber threats. The authors of [43] pointed out the benefits of AI integration with health policies. It develops a framework for strengthening different exogenous factors for a collaborative approach to the sustainable development of health practices. The authors of [44] in their research study stated that growth and digitalization enable to transform the health services from reactive to proactive and even preventive measures. Thus, the stated discussion enabled us to understand the impending role of AI in digital health mechanisms and also develop policies to handle health records through digitalization procedures ensuring timely management and security of records. The stated discussion resulted in the formulation of two future stated questions for impending researchers. Table 6.4 developed the future research propositions based on the above discussion, it focuses on developing impending research questions for future researchers and providing a path-way to develop studies adding value to the academic literature.

#### 6.4.6.6    Cluster 6: AI and prediction of disorders (marron)

The researchers stated that AI can redefine the problems in relation to mental health disorders [45]. The authors of [46] in their research study explained the relevance of AI in developing different predictive models which will assist health practitioners in proper diagnosis and fixing the problem for better results. Extending the study by [47] in their research enumerated that AI is one of the premier tools to identify personality disorders, it aims to identify the disorder as well as propagate the most appropriate therapy for personality disorder patients. The authors of [48] stated that AI enables the development of analytical models to identify, predict, diagnose, and treatment of patients through an evidence-based approach and clarify patients' history in a detailed manner. Thus, the stated discussion enabled us to understand the impending role of AI in the prediction of disorders and also develop policies for measuring patient

*Table 6.4    Future research propositions*

| Research streams | Impending research questions |
| --- | --- |
| *AI and decision support system* | What role AI plays to make effective decision-support systems? How to identify effective strategies through AI applications for risk assessment? What strategy should be adopted to deal with future changes in healthcare management? |
| *AI and data security* | How AI effectively measures the data security aspects |
| *AI and COVID-19 pandemic* | What is the role of AI in developing ways in dealing COVID-19 pandemic? What is the impact of AI in the health sector on identifying, screening, and analyzing patients' data in the health sector? |
| *AI and public health management* | What is the role of AI in effectively handling public health management issues? |
| *AI and digital health mechanisms* | How AI can develop cost-effective models to deal with different health treatment mechanisms. |
| *AI and prediction of disorders* | How AI can enable access to real-time information for sustainable development of patient health practices. How AI can process health records and ensure the secrecy of data for better management practices. What role AI plays to deal with mental disorders? How AI can develop different predictive models to deal with patients with appropriate therapy? |

conditions through proper diagnosis and ensuring timely treatment. The stated discussion resulted in the formulation of two future stated questions for impending researchers.

### *6.4.7    Outlined future research propositions*

Thus, upcoming researchers need to examine the stated relationship from the framed propositions and develop research studies that can add value to the existing research state as well as enable to develop of new mechanisms and methods for treatment which will be a yardstick for health practitioners and government to develop solutions with more reliable and focused with error-free operations. Thus, future research propositions give opportunities to impending researchers to add value to the future research agenda through significant contributions to the academic fraternity.

## 6.5    Implications

### *6.5.1    Theoretical implications*

The healthcare sector is confronted with manifold challenges and problems. In the changing scenario, the adoption of new technology and practices is very vital for understanding problems and enabling health practitioners for providing enhanced solutions and predicting problems among patients. Thus, to measure the role of AI techniques in providing health practices and solutions and securely analyzing patient data, the current study aimed to explain and elucidate the benefits of the application of AI in healthcare management systems by reviewing existing research studies. The present research work through visualization analysis tried to identify the relevant contribution made by authors and countries in the research field. The research work enabled us to understand various theoretical dimensions to develop the framework that will help to understand the state of research and advocated that application of AI in healthcare management is a boon for better, patient-centric, and customized services for better performance in the health sector.

### 6.5.2 Practical implications

The research study analyzed the existing literature through a systematic literature review and visualization methodology. The research study adopted a step-by-step approach to understanding the present state of research in the application of AI in healthcare management. Although previous studies explained the application of AI in healthcare management, no study suggested or developed a research proposition after examining the literature studies. The present took a sincere effort to present how AI can be extended not only for handling patient's history or data, but also access real-time information, prediction of disorders as well as in developing drug and vaccination for better treatment of patients. Thus, health practitioners, policy makers, and government agencies should consider that the application of technology towards enhancing better treatment mechanisms, access timely information, and enhancing the management of proper health practices for better patient-oriented results with cost-effective and reliable results.

## 6.6 Scope of the research

The study discussed and elaborated on the application of AI in the field of healthcare management. The study made a progressive approach to understanding the current research state as well as developing network maps which will provide a way forward for upcoming researchers to extend their studies. Although AI has expanded its wings in every domain including healthcare management. The study analyzed the role of AI technology in identifying, analyzing, diagnosing, and predicting patients' problems and providing timely solutions with accurate results as well as handling a large amount of data through patient-centric services. The application of AI has expanded its wing not only in diagnosing but also in developing drugs and predicting disorders for better services.

The present study is a sincere endeavor by researchers to understand the current state of research conditions through network maps on authorship, country, and keyword occurrence as well as developing thematic areas for future researchers. The study can be considered as a base work and explore other domains in the health sector where the application of AI can be combined for concrete results and overcome the gaps in the outmoded record management and problem-solving methods.

## 6.7    Discussion of findings

The findings of the present study indicate that the technology has expanded to every domain and sector, including the health sector but still, there are many areas to be uncovered. The framed research questions enumerate to explain the visualization aspects in terms of identifying the highest source of the journal, countries, authors, and year-wise. The *Journal of Biomedical Informatics* is the highest source with maximum publication in the field of AI in health care management. The publication trend indicates there is a steadily increasing trend, since 2015. The most prolific author is Prof. Jaedon P. Avey. The network maps developed using the visualization software, i.e. VOS Viewer, indicate that the "United States of America" is the country with the maximum publication. Thus, the information is based on authorship and country as well as through the keyword co-occurrences map identified the highest appearing keywords are "AI," "medicine," "digital health," and "telemedicine." Further through clustering, the thematic areas were identified, and develop future pathways. The clustering led to the formation of six clusters such as (1) "AI and decision support system"; (2) "AI and data security"; (3) "AI and COVID-19 pandemic"; (4) "AI and public health management"; (5) "AI and public health mechanism"; (6) "AI and prediction of disorders." Hence, considering the discussion, the developed Figure 6.12 will identify the noteworthy impact of AI on improved perspectives and administration in the health sector.

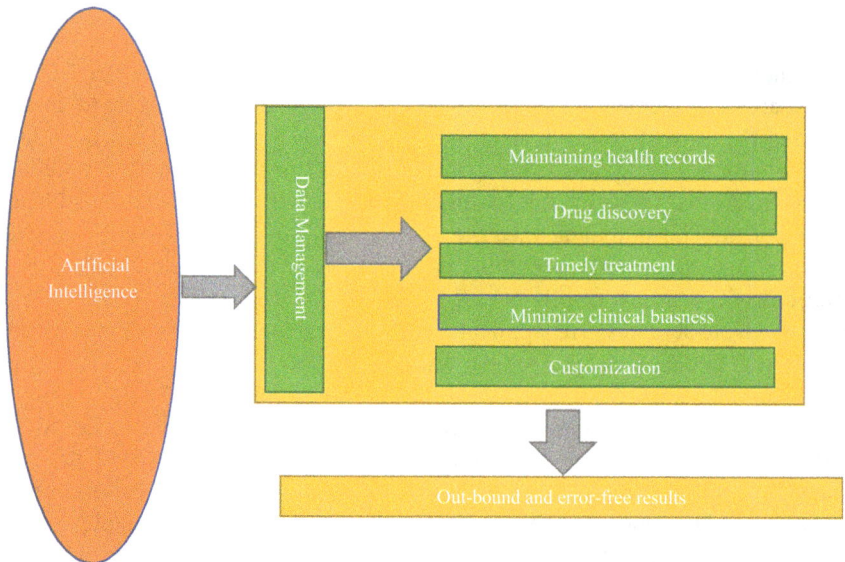

*Figure 6.12    Framework for future research*

## 6.8   Conclusion

The conclusion of the study outlined certain limitations that can be addressed by future researchers and can be considered despite the above discussions. First, AI has entered every domain but still, it is identifying numerous challenges to its security and reliability, thus future studies need a thorough explore-oriented approach towards enhancing the features for better applicability. Second, the research work has been constrained to the database, i.e., Scopus for incisive papers, outlining those published in other journals not indexed in Scopus. Hence, future studies regardless consider the above point in future studies, other databases can be regarded for extracting the required literature and data files for conducting research studies

Third, with the condition to language, only English written papers were considered, whereas other languages were excluded as well as the present study excluded, conference proceedings, and book chapters on AI in healthcare management. "Therefore, the extracted results can include such changes in future research and compare the results. Therefore, the present study is an amalgamated bibliometric paper that has been designed to provide an en route for other researchers. Further, this research was based on, i.e., SLR and bibliometric visualization." Hence, impending researchers may extend the meta-analysis approach and identify the application of the technique in other fields and further authenticate the results of this research and validate the generalizability of the anticipated concepts.

## References

[1]   Panch T, Mattie H, and Celi LA. The "inconvenient truth" about AI in healthcare. *NPJ Digital Medicine*. 2019;2(1):1–3.

[2]   Reddy S, Fox J, and Purohit MP. Artificial intelligence-enabled healthcare delivery. *Journal of the Royal Society of Medicine.* 2019;112(1):22–8.

[3]   Panch T, Szolovits P, and Atun R. Artificial intelligence, machine learning and health systems. *Journal of Global Health.* 2018;8(2):020303.

[4]   Rahman M, Ming TH, Baigh TA, and Sarker M. Adoption of artificial intelligence in banking services: an empirical analysis. *International Journal of Emerging Markets.* 2021.

[5]   Kaya O, Schildbach J, and Schneider S. Artificial intelligence in banking. *Artificial Intelligence.* 2019. https://www.google.co.in/url?sa=i&rct=j&q= &esrc=s&source=web&cd=&ved=0CAIQw7AJah cKEwj4rcTo_6SBAxUA AAAAHQAAAAAQAg&url=https%3A%2F%2Fwww.dbresearch.com%2F PROD%2FRPS_EN-PROD%2FPROD0000000000495172%2FArtificial_inte lligence_in_banking%253A_A_lever_for_pr.pdf&psig=AOvVaw2Di9a1Tb32 Wc TV45fIzNDA&ust=1694605553822144&opi=89978449.

[6]   Chen L, Chen P, and Lin Z. Artificial intelligence in education: a review. *IEEE Access.* 2020;8:75264–78.

[7]   Schiff D. Education for AI, not AI for education: the role of education and ethics in national AI policy strategies. *International Journal of Artificial Intelligence in Education.* 2022;32(3):527–63.

[8]   Toorajipour R, Sohrabpour V, Nazarpour A, Oghazi P, and Fischl M. Artificial intelligence in supply chain management: a systematic literature review. *Journal of Business Research.* 2021;122:502–17.

[9]   Helo P and Hao Y. Artificial intelligence in operations management and supply chain management: an exploratory case study. *Production Planning & Control.* 2021;33:1–8.

[10]  Morley J, Machado CC, Burr C, *et al.* The ethics of AI in health care: a mapping review. *Social Science & Medicine.* 2020;260:113172.

[11]  Emanuel EJ and Wachter RM. Artificial intelligence in health care: will the value match the hype? *Jama.* 2019;321(23):2281–2.

[12]  Reddy S, Allan S, Coghlan S, and Cooper P. A governance model for the application of AI in health care. *Journal of the American Medical Informatics Association.* 2020;27(3):491–7.

[13]  Secinaro S, Calandra D, Secinaro A, Muthurangu V, and Biancone P. The role of artificial intelligence in healthcare: a structured literature review. *BMC Medical Informatics and Decision Making.* 2021;21(1):1–23.

[14]  Guo Y, Hao Z, Zhao S, Gong J, and Yang F. Artificial intelligence in health care: bibliometric analysis. *Journal of Medical Internet Research.* 2020;22(7):e18228.

[15]  Srivastava TK and Waghmare L. Implications of artificial intelligence (AI) on dynamics of medical education and care: a perspective. *Journal of Clinical and Diagnostic Research.* 2020;14:1–2.

[16]  Powell J. Trust Me, I'm a chatbot: how artificial intelligence in health care fails the turing test. *Journal of Medical Internet Research.* 2019;21(10):e16222.

[17]  Rajpurkar P, Chen E, Banerjee O, and Topol EJ. AI in health and medicine. *Nature Medicine.* 2022;28(1):31–8.

[18]  Schotten M, Meester WJ, Steiginga S, and Ross CA. A brief history of Scopus: The world's largest abstract and citation database of scientific literature. In *Research Analytics* (pp. 31–58), 2017. Auerbach Publications.

[19]  Van Eck N and Waltman L. Software survey: VOS viewer, a computer program for bibliometric mapping. *Scientometrics.* 2010;84(2):523–38.

[20]  Hou J, Yang X, and Chen C. Emerging trends and new developments in information science: a document co-citation analysis (2009–2016). *Scientometrics.* 2018;115(2):869–92.

[21]  Üsdiken B and Pasadeos Y. Organizational analysis in North America and Europe: a comparison of co-citation networks. *Organization Studies.* 1995;16(3):503–26.

[22]  Silverman BG, Hanrahan N, Bharathy G, Gordon K, and Johnson D. A systems approach to healthcare: agent-based modeling, community mental health, and population well-being. *Artificial Intelligence in Medicine.* 2015;63(2):61–71.

[23]  Valls A, Gibert K, Sánchez D, and Batet M. Using ontologies for structuring organizational knowledge in home care assistance. *International Journal of Medical Informatics.* 2010;79(5):370–87.

[24]   López-Vallverdú JA, Riaño D, and Bohada JA. Improving medical decision trees by combining relevant health-care criteria. *Expert Systems with Applications.* 2012;39(14):11782–91.

[25]   Isern D and Moreno A. A systematic literature review of agents applied in healthcare. *Journal of Medical Systems.* 2016;40:1–4.

[26]   Becker D, van Breda W, Funk B, Hoogendoorn M, Ruwaard J, and Riper H. Predictive modeling in e-mental health: a common language framework. *Internet Interventions.* 2018;12:57–67.

[27]   Shortliffe EH and Sepúlveda MJ. Clinical decision support in the era of artificial intelligence. *Jama.* 2018;320(21):2199–200.

[28]   Moreira MW, Rodrigues JJ, Korotaev V, Al-Muhtadi J, and Kumar N. A comprehensive review on smart decision support systems for health care. *IEEE Systems Journal.* 2019;13(3):3536–45.

[29]   Duan Y, Edwards JS, and Dwivedi YK. Artificial intelligence for decision making in the era of Big Data – evolution, challenges and research agenda. *International Journal of Information Management.* 2019;48:63–71.

[30]   Sutton RT, Pincock D, Baumgart DC, Sadowski DC, Fedorak RN, and Kroeker KI. An overview of clinical decision support systems: benefits, risks, and strategies for success. *NPJ Digital Medicine.* 2020;3(1):1–0.

[31]   Braun M, Hummel P, Beck S, and Dabrock P. Primer on an ethics of AI-based decision support systems in the clinic. *Journal of Medical Ethics.* 2021;47(12):e3.

[32]   Gupta S, Modgil S, Bhattacharyya S, and Bose I. Artificial intelligence for decision support systems in the field of operations research: review and future scope of research. *Annals of Operations Research.* 2022;308(1):215–74.

[33]   Li JH. Cyber security meets artificial intelligence: a survey. *Frontiers of Information Technology & Electronic Engineering.* 2018;19(12):1462–74.

[34]   Sedjelmaci H, Guenab F, Senouci SM, Moustafa H, Liu J, and Han S. Cyber security based on artificial intelligence for cyber-physical systems. *IEEE Network.* 2020;34(3):6–7.

[35]   Vaishya R, Javaid M, Khan IH, and Haleem A. Artificial Intelligence (AI) applications for COVID-19 pandemic. *Diabetes & Metabolic Syndrome: Clinical Research & Reviews.* 2020;14(4):337–9.

[36]   Kumar A, Gupta PK, and Srivastava A. A review of modern technologies for tackling COVID-19 pandemic. *Diabetes & Metabolic Syndrome: Clinical Research & Reviews.* 2020;14(4):569–73.

[37]   Khan M, Mehran MT, Haq ZU, *et al.* Applications of artificial intelligence in COVID-19 pandemic: a comprehensive review. *Expert Systems with Applications.* 2021;185:115695.

[38]   Yi J, Zhang H, Mao J, Chen Y, Zhong H, and Wang Y. Review on the COVID-19 pandemic prevention and control system based on AI. *Engineering Applications of Artificial Intelligence.* 2022;114:105184.

[39]   Noorbakhsh-Sabet N, Zand R, Zhang Y, and Abedi V. Artificial intelligence transforms the future of health care. *The American Journal of Medicine.* 2019;132(7):795–801.

[40]    Efthymiou-Egleton IP, Sidiropoulos S, Kritas D, Vozikis A, Rapti P, and Souliotis K. AI transforming healthcare management during COVID-19 pandemic. *HAPSc Policy Briefs Series.* 2020;1(1):130–8.

[41]    Nasseef OA, Baabdullah AM, Alalwan AA, Lal B, and Dwivedi YK. Artificial intelligence-based public healthcare systems: G2G knowledge-based exchange to enhance the decision-making process. *Government Information Quarterly.* 2022;39(4):101618.

[42]    Anjum A, Choo KK, Khan A, *et al.* An efficient privacy mechanism for electronic health records. *Computers & Security.* 2018;72:196–211.

[43]    Xu S, Hu C, and Min D. Preparing for the AI era under the digital health framework. In *2019 ITU Kaleidoscope: ICT for Health: Networks, Standards and Innovation (ITU K),* 2019 Dec 4 (pp. 1–10). IEEE.

[44]    Aerts A and Bogdan-Martin D. Leveraging data and AI to deliver on the promise of digital health. *International Journal of Medical Informatics.* 2021;150:104456.

[45]    Graham S, Depp C, Lee EE, *et al.* Artificial intelligence for mental health and mental illnesses: an overview. *Current Psychiatry Reports.* 2019;21(11):1–8.

[46]    Ćosić K, Popović S, Šarlija M, Kesedžić I, and Jovanovic T. Artificial intelligence in prediction of mental health disorders induced by the COVID-19 pandemic among health care workers. *Croatian Medical Journal.* 2020;61(3):279.

[47]    Sulistiani H, Muludi K, and Syarif A. Implementation of various artificial intelligence approach for prediction and recommendation of personality disorder patient. *Journal of Physics: Conference Series.* 2021;1751(1):012040. IOP Publishing.

[48]    Merkin A, Krishnamurthi R, and Medvedev ON. Machine learning, artificial intelligence and the prediction of dementia. *Current Opinion in Psychiatry.* 2022;35(2):123–9.

*Chapter 7*

# Privacy preserving blockchain-based healthcare model for EMR – a study

*N.M. Saravana Kumar[1], K. Hariprasath[2],*
*N. Kaviyavarshini[3] and Ing. Pavel Lafata[4]*

## Abstract

In recent years, data privacy issues have become increasingly prevalent in the healthcare industry. With the increasing amount of data being generated by healthcare providers, there are now more opportunities for sensitive information to be compromised. Electronic medical records (EMRs) are becoming increasingly popular in healthcare management due to their many benefits, such as easier access to patient data, improved patient safety, and increased efficiency. However, implementing and using EMRs also present several challenges, including cost, staff training, data security, and interoperability. An effective healthcare data management requires a holistic approach that addresses the various challenges in collecting, managing, and using healthcare data. The adoption of emerging technologies such as blockchain and the development of interoperability standards and data governance frameworks are critical to achieving this goal. The uniqueness of the chapter is that it discusses the commercial models along with the research models in the survey. This chapter summarizes the challenges in EMR maintenance, a few benchmarking existing approaches, and a brief study of blockchain-based models.

**Keywords:** EMR; Privacy and data management issues; Blockchain-based models

[1]Department of Information Technology, Karpagam College of Engineering (affiliated under Anna University), Coimbatore, India
[2]Department of Computer Science and Engineering, Shree Sathyam College of Engineering and Technology (affiliated under Anna University), Sankari, India
[3]Department of Information and Communication Engineering, Anna University, Chennai, India
[4]Faculty of Electrical Engineering, Department of Telecommunication Engineering, Czech Technical Universit, Prague, Czech Republic

## 7.1    Introduction

The healthcare industry is continuously evolving with the advent of new technologies that have brought significant changes in healthcare data management [1–5]. Healthcare data management involves the collection, storage, and sharing of data related to patient care, medical research, and healthcare operations. Data privacy is a crucial issue in healthcare data management as healthcare data is sensitive and confidential [6–8]. This research chapter discusses the data privacy challenges in healthcare data management and the existing models for data privacy in healthcare data management [9–15].

One of the most significant data privacy issues in healthcare data management was the Anthem data breach in 2015, in which the personal information of nearly 80 million individuals was compromised. More recently, in 2020, there was a data breach at Blackbaud, a company that provides fundraising and engagement software to healthcare organizations [16–19]. Ransomware plagued hospitals in 2020 and 2021, and 2022 will likely be no different. As many as 34% of healthcare organizations experienced a ransomware attack in 2020, and 65% of those attacks were successful. The breach affected millions of individuals, and the stolen data included sensitive information such as social security numbers and healthcare data.

Another significant data privacy issue in healthcare data management is the use of third-party vendors to handle data. In some cases, these vendors may not have adequate security measures in place, which can lead to data breaches. For example, in 2019, Quest Diagnostics suffered a data breach that affected nearly 12 million patients. The breach was caused by a third-party vendor that had access to Quest's systems [20–22].

With the advent of the healthcare industry has been exploring the use of blockchain technology as a means of improving healthcare data management. Blockchain technology offers a decentralized, secure, and transparent way of storing, sharing, and managing healthcare data. This chapter provides an overview of various commercial blockchain-based healthcare data management models and their potential advantages and disadvantages rather than put forth research models alone.

### 7.1.1    Causes of data privacy issues in healthcare data management

There are several causes of data privacy issues in healthcare data management. One is the increasing amount of data being generated by healthcare providers. With more data comes more opportunities for that data to be compromised. Another cause is the use of outdated or inadequate security measures. As technology advances, so do the methods that hackers use to access sensitive information. Healthcare providers must keep up with these advancements to protect their patients' data. A third cause is the use of third-party vendors to handle data. While these vendors may provide valuable services, they may not have the same level of security measures in place as the healthcare provider [23–25].

## 7.1.2    Need for evolved smart healthcare data management systems

There are several solutions to data privacy issues in healthcare data management. One is to implement stronger security measures, such as multi-factor authentication and encryption, to protect sensitive information. Healthcare providers should also regularly review and update their security measures to ensure they remain effective against the latest threats. Another solution is to limit the amount of data collected and stored. Healthcare providers should only collect and store the minimum amount of data necessary to provide quality care to their patients. Finally, health-care providers should carefully vet any third-party vendors they work with to ensure they have adequate security measures in place [26–30].

In summary, data management and privacy issues in healthcare data management are a serious concern. Recent data breaches have highlighted the need for healthcare providers to take stronger measures to protect their patients' data. The causes of these issues include the increasing amount of data being generated, outdated or inadequate security measures, and the use of third-party vendors. To address these issues, healthcare providers should implement stronger security measures, limit the amount of data collected and stored, and carefully vet any third-party vendors they work with. By doing so, they can better protect their patients' sensitive information and maintain their trust. The following chapter is organized in such a way that it briefs electronic medical record (EMR), its challenges in healthcare management. This chapter then deals with data privacy and data management of EMR records with the challenges and existing models. Finally, it suggests the mandate of blockchain-based healthcare data models, the commercial blockchain models in the industry, and various beta research models. Rather than prioritizing any work, this chapter generalizes them in brief and sum-marizes the future research prospects after a serious study of the existing models.

## 7.2    EMR in healthcare management

EMR, or electronic medical records, is a digital version of a patient's paper medical chart. EMRs contain patient medical histories, diagnoses, medications, treatment plans, test results, and other relevant health information. EMRs are becoming increasingly popular in healthcare management, as they provide many benefits over traditional paper-based records, such as easier access to patient data, improved patient safety, and increased efficiency. However, implementing and using EMRs also present several challenges [31–34].

One of the most significant challenges of implementing EMRs is the cost. EMR systems can be expensive to purchase, install, and maintain. Additionally, healthcare providers must often invest in new hardware and software to support the EMR system. The initial cost of implementing an EMR system can be a significant financial burden, particularly for smaller healthcare providers.

Another challenge of implementing EMRs is the training required for health-care staff to use the system effectively. EMRs are complex, and healthcare provi-ders must ensure that their staff is properly trained on how to use the system. This requires additional time and resources, which can further increase the overall cost of implementing an EMR system [35–39].

Data security is also a significant challenge when it comes to EMRs. Patient health information is sensitive, and healthcare providers must ensure that patient data is kept confidential and secure. EMRs can be vulnerable to cyberattacks, which can compromise patient data. Healthcare providers must implement robust security measures, such as encryption and access controls, to protect patient data from unauthorized access.

Finally, interoperability is a significant challenge when it comes to EMRs. Different healthcare providers often use different EMR systems, which can make it challenging to share patient data between providers. This can result in delays in patient care and can make it difficult for patients to receive the coordinated care they need.

## 7.2.1    Existing challenges in EMR data management

1.  Data security: With the increasing amount of healthcare data being generated and stored electronically, data security is a major concern. Cyberattacks and data breaches can result in the theft or misuse of sensitive patient information.
2.  Interoperability: Healthcare data is often siloed in various systems and formats, making it difficult to share and access patient data across different healthcare providers and institutions.
3.  Data accuracy and completeness: Inaccurate or incomplete data can lead to misdiagnosis, incorrect treatment, and compromised patient safety. Ensuring data accuracy and completeness is critical for effective healthcare delivery.
4.  Data privacy: Protecting patient privacy is of utmost importance in healthcare. Health data breaches can lead to identity theft, fraud, and discrimination.
5.  Data governance: Developing and implementing a robust data governance framework is critical to ensure that healthcare data is collected, managed, and used in compliance with regulatory requirements and ethical standards.

## 7.3    Data privacy in EMR healthcare data management

### 7.3.1    Challenges

The healthcare industry faces several data privacy challenges due to the sensitive nature of healthcare data. The following are the data privacy challenges in healthcare data management:

1.  Data breaches: Data breaches are the most common data privacy challenges in healthcare data management. Healthcare organizations often face data breaches due to cyber-attacks, hacking, or unauthorized access to sensitive data. These data breaches can result in significant financial losses, reputational damage, and legal implications.
2.  Lack of encryption: Encryption is a method of securing data by encoding it so that only authorized users can access it. The lack of encryption is a significant data privacy challenge in healthcare data management. Without encryption, data is vulnerable to unauthorized access, hacking, and cyber-attacks.

3. Inadequate access controls: Access controls are security measures that restrict access to sensitive data to authorized users only. The lack of adequate access controls is a significant data privacy challenge in healthcare data management. Without adequate access controls, sensitive data can be accessed by unauthorized users.
4. Data sharing: Healthcare organizations often share data with third-party vendors for research, analysis, or other purposes. However, data sharing can lead to data privacy challenges if the third-party vendors do not have adequate data privacy measures in place.

### 7.3.2 Existing models offering data privacy

The healthcare industry has developed several models for data privacy in healthcare data management. The following are the existing models for data privacy in healthcare data management:

1. HIPAA: The Health Insurance Portability and Accountability Act (HIPAA) is a federal law that provides data privacy and security provisions for safeguarding medical information. HIPAA requires healthcare organizations to implement technical and physical safeguards to protect patient data [40–43].
2. GDPR: The General Data Protection Regulation (GDPR) is a regulation that provides data privacy and security provisions for individuals within the European Union (EU). GDPR requires healthcare organizations to obtain explicit consent from patients before collecting and processing their data [44].
3. Blockchain: Blockchain is a decentralized ledger that provides secure and transparent data sharing. Blockchain technology can be used in healthcare data management to ensure data privacy and security [45]. Blockchain-based models will be discussed later in the future sections.
4. Differential privacy: Differential privacy is a mathematical framework that provides data privacy by adding noise to the data to protect the privacy of individuals. Differential privacy can be used in healthcare data management to ensure that patient data is protected while allowing researchers to access and analyze the data [46].

## 7.4 Data governance issues in healthcare data management

In recent years, healthcare organizations have been increasingly reliant on data to make informed decisions and improve patient care. However, with this increased reliance on data comes a need for effective data governance to ensure data accuracy, consistency, and security [47–49]. This part of the chapter discusses the data governance issues in healthcare data management and the existing models for data governance in healthcare data management.

The following are the data governance issues in healthcare data management:

1. Data quality: Data quality is a significant data governance issue in healthcare data management. Healthcare organizations collect vast amounts of data from

various sources, including electronic health records (EHRs), medical devices, and wearables. This data can often be incomplete, inaccurate, or inconsistent, leading to incorrect or ineffective decision-making.

2. Data security: Data security is another major data governance issue in healthcare data management. Healthcare data is highly sensitive and confidential, making it a prime target for cyber-attacks and data breaches. Healthcare organizations must ensure that data is secured and protected from unauthorized access, both internally and externally.

3. Data ownership: Data ownership is a complex issue in healthcare data management. Multiple stakeholders, including patients, healthcare providers, insurers, and regulators, may claim ownership of healthcare data. Healthcare organizations must define data ownership and ensure that data is shared only with authorized parties.

4. Data integration: Healthcare organizations may have data from various sources, including different EHR systems, medical devices, and wearables. Data integration is a significant data governance issue in healthcare data management, as data must be integrated, normalized, and validated to ensure consistency and accuracy.

## 7.4.1   Existing models

The healthcare industry has developed several models for data governance in healthcare data management. The following are the existing models for data governance in healthcare data management:

1. FAIR data principles: The FAIR (Findable, Accessible, Interoperable, and Reusable) Data Principles provide a framework for data management that promotes data sharing and reuse. The principles help ensure that data is discoverable, accessible, interoperable, and reusable.

2. Data Stewardship: Data Stewardship is a data governance model that assigns responsibility for data management to a designated individual or team. Data stewards are responsible for managing data throughout its lifecycle, ensuring data quality, security, and compliance with regulations.

3. Data governance framework: A data governance framework is a comprehensive model for managing data in an organization. The framework includes policies, procedures, and guidelines for data management, data quality, data security, and data privacy.

4. Data catalog: A data catalog is a central repository that stores metadata about data assets, including EHRs, medical devices, and wearables. The catalog provides a unified view of data assets and facilitates data discovery, data integration, and data governance.

## 7.4.2   Advantages of the existing models

The existing models for data governance in healthcare data management offer several advantages. The following are some of the advantages of the existing models:

• FAIR data principles: The FAIR Data Principles provide a framework for data management that promotes data sharing and reuse. They ensure that data is findable, accessible, interoperable, and reusable, promoting data reuse, reducing data duplication, and improving data quality [50–52].

- Data Stewardship: Data stewardship assigns responsibility for data management to a designated individual or team. This helps ensure that data is managed throughout its lifecycle, improving data quality, security, and compliance with regulations [53].
- Data governance framework: A data governance framework provides a comprehensive model for managing data in an organization. It includes policies, procedures, and guidelines for data management, data quality, data security, and data privacy. It ensures that data is managed consistently, promoting data accuracy, consistency, and security.
- Data catalog: A data catalog provides a centralized repository for metadata about data assets. It facilitates data discovery, data integration, and data governance. It provides a unified view of data assets, reducing data duplication, and improving data quality [54].

## 7.4.3   Disadvantages of the existing models

- FAIR data principles: One of the disadvantages of the FAIR Data Principles is that they may not be applicable to all types of data. The principles were developed primarily for scientific data, and their application to healthcare data may be limited.
- Data Stewardship: The data stewardship model requires the designation of individuals or teams to manage data. This may be a challenge for small healthcare organizations that do not have the resources to hire dedicated data stewards.
- Data governance framework: Developing and implementing a data governance framework can be a complex and time-consuming process. It may require significant resources, including personnel, technology, and financial investment.
- Data catalog: Data catalogs require significant effort to create and maintain. They also require ongoing updates to ensure that they remain accurate and up-to-date.
- Overreliance on technology: Healthcare organizations may become over-reliant on technology to manage data. While technology can help improve data management, it should not be the sole solution. Healthcare organizations must also consider the human element in data governance, including training and education for staff and healthcare providers [55].

## 7.5   Solutions to healthcare data management challenges

1. Blockchain technology: Blockchain technology can help address data security and privacy concerns by providing a secure and tamper-proof way of storing and sharing healthcare data.

2.  Interoperability standards: Developing and adopting interoperability standards can help facilitate the sharing and exchange of healthcare data across different systems and providers.
3.  Data quality management: Implementing data quality management processes can help ensure that healthcare data is accurate, complete, and consistent [56].
4.  Data protection measures: Implementing data protection measures such as encryption, access controls, and monitoring can help prevent unauthorized access and misuse of healthcare data.
5.  Data governance framework: Developing and implementing a comprehensive data governance framework that defines policies, procedures, and standards for healthcare data collection, management, and use can help ensure compliance with regulatory requirements and ethical standards.

## 7.6    Blockchain-based healthcare data management models

Blockchain technology has the potential to revolutionize healthcare data management. The various blockchain-based healthcare data management models have the potential to improve data security, increase efficiency, enhance privacy, and improve interoperability. As blockchain technology continues to mature, it is expected that it will be widely adopted in the healthcare industry, providing patients and healthcare providers with a secure, transparent, and efficient way of managing healthcare data. Figure 7.1 shows the generic blockchain model for healthcare data management [57,58].

There are several blockchain-based healthcare data management models that have been proposed and tested. These models include:

1.  EHRs on the blockchain: This model involves storing patients' medical records on the blockchain in a decentralized manner. Patients can grant access to their medical records to healthcare providers, researchers, or other authorized parties. The use of blockchain technology ensures the privacy and security of the medical data.

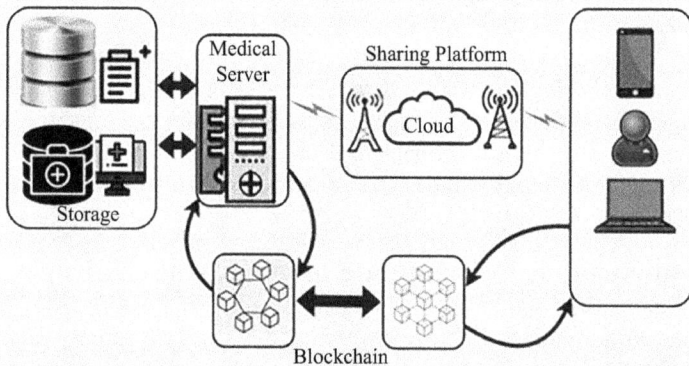

*Figure 7.1    Generic blockchain model for healthcare use case*

2. Personal health records (PHRs) on the blockchain: This model involves patients having control over their medical data by creating their personal health records on the blockchain. Patients can choose who to grant access to their data and can earn tokens or cryptocurrency for participating in research studies.
3. Supply chain management: The use of blockchain technology in supply chain management can help to ensure the authenticity of pharmaceutical products, reduce the risk of counterfeit drugs, and ensure transparency in the drug supply chain.
4. Clinical trials blockchain technology can be used to ensure transparency in clinical trials and prevent data tampering. The use of smart contracts can automate the process of monitoring the progress of clinical trials and ensuring that the data collected is accurate.
5. Telemedicine: The use of blockchain technology in telemedicine can help to ensure the privacy and security of patient data. It can also enable secure and efficient payment transactions between patients and healthcare providers.

### 7.6.1　Potential benefits of blockchain-based models

Blockchain-based healthcare data management models have the potential to offer several benefits. These benefits include:

1. Improved data security: The use of blockchain technology ensures the security and integrity of healthcare data. The decentralized nature of the blockchain network makes it difficult for hackers to attack and compromise the system.
2. Increased efficiency: Blockchain technology can streamline healthcare data management processes and reduce administrative overheads. The use of smart contracts can automate the process of monitoring and enforcing healthcare regulations.
3. Enhanced privacy: Blockchain technology can enable patients to have control over their medical data and who can access it. This can help to ensure privacy and prevent unauthorized access to medical data.
4. Better interoperability: Blockchain technology can facilitate the sharing of healthcare data between different healthcare providers and systems. This can improve healthcare outcomes by providing healthcare providers with a comprehensive view of patient's medical histories.

### 7.6.2　Existing blockchain-based commercial healthcare models

Some significant blockchain-based healthcare models that have been proposed and have emerged in recent years, each with its own unique approach to leveraging blockchain technology to improve the efficiency, security, and transparency of the healthcare industry, are as follows:

- MedicalChain [59]: This is a blockchain platform that allows patients to securely store and share their medical data with healthcare professionals.
- Solve.Care [60]: This platform uses blockchain technology to create a healthcare administration network that connects patients, healthcare providers, and insurance companies.

- Healthereum [61]: This blockchain-based platform incentivizes patients to engage in their healthcare by providing rewards for completing tasks such as attending appointments or taking medications as prescribed.
- HealthChain [62]: This platform is focused on clinical trial management, using blockchain technology to improve the efficiency and transparency of the clinical trial process.
- Shivom [63]: This blockchain-based platform allows patients to securely store and manage their genomic data, and provides tools for researchers and pharmaceutical companies to access this data for research purposes.
- BurstIQ [64]: This platform uses blockchain technology to create a secure, decentralized health data exchange network that allows patients to control and monetize their health data.
- Coral Health [65]: This platform uses blockchain technology to create a decentralized health record system that allows patients to own and control their medical data, and share it with healthcare providers as needed.
- BitMED [66]: This platform uses blockchain technology to create a secure, decentralized telemedicine network that connects patients with healthcare providers around the world.
- Health Nexus [67]: This blockchain-based platform is designed to enable secure and efficient data exchange between healthcare stakeholders, including patients, providers, payers, and regulators.
- Guardtime [68]: This blockchain platform is focused on data integrity and cybersecurity for healthcare, providing solutions for secure data storage, identity management, and audit trails.
- Gem [69]: This blockchain platform enables healthcare organizations to securely share and manage data across different systems and stakeholders, with a focus on improving data interoperability and analytics.
- Medical Token Currency (MTC) [70]: This platform is focused on using blockchain technology to create a healthcare payment and rewards system, allowing patients to earn tokens for healthy behaviors and redeem them for healthcare services.
- Health FX [71]: This blockchain-based platform is designed to improve the efficiency and transparency of healthcare supply chain management, enabling providers to track and trace medical products and devices from manufacturing to patient care.
- HealthChainRx [72]: This platform uses blockchain technology to create a secure, decentralized network for pharmaceutical supply chain management, improving transparency and reducing the risk of counterfeiting.
- MediBloc [73]: This blockchain-based platform enables patients to store and manage their medical data, and provides tools for healthcare providers and researchers to access and analyze this data for improved patient care and medical research.
- Lympo [74]: This blockchain-based platform focuses on incentivizing patients to engage in healthy behavior by rewarding them with cryptocurrency for achieving fitness goals and sharing their data with healthcare providers.

- Patientory [75]: This platform uses blockchain technology to create a secure, decentralized EHR system that allows patients to manage and share their medical data with healthcare providers and insurers.
- TrustedHealth [76]: This blockchain-based platform connects patients with healthcare providers around the world, enabling patients to access second opinions and alternative treatment options for complex medical conditions.
- SimplyVital Health [77]: This platform uses blockchain technology to create a decentralized healthcare infrastructure that enables secure, real-time data sharing and collaboration between healthcare providers and payers.
- HealthChainUS [78]: This blockchain-based platform is focused on improving the transparency and security of the healthcare supply chain, enabling providers to track and trace medical products from manufacturing to delivery.

Table 7.1 shows the comparison of recent consensus algorithms

## 7.6.3 Challenges of adapting blockchain-based healthcare model

While blockchain technology holds great promise for improving the efficiency, security, and transparency of healthcare systems, there are also some potential disadvantages to consider:

- Lack of standardization: There are currently no industry-wide standards for blockchain-based healthcare models, which can lead to interoperability issues between different systems.

*Table 7.1   Comparison of recent consensus algorithms*

| Consensus algorithm | Pros | Cons |
| --- | --- | --- |
| Proof of Work | Secured and provides overall control and power in the network | Consumes high power for processing and requires more electricity |
| Proof of Stake | Provides high rewards and energy efficient | Less secure than Proof of Work |
| Delegated Proof of Stake | Low expense in hardware, Processing speed is high when compared to Proof of Work and Proof of Stake | High chances of attacks, low decentralization |
| Proof of Activity | Reduces 51% attack in network, less transaction cost, highly secured | Hard to implement, users have to sign the transactions dually |
| Proof of Burn | Can be customized, when a new block in a node is mined, the power may be decreased | No recovery is guaranteed, high resource waste |
| Ripple | When compared to proof of work, it requires less power, the path is dependent | Centralized, Node lists are to be maintained |
| Steller Consensus Protocol | Holds high decentralized control, lower in latency | Issues in proposing new argument and difficulties in choosing quorum |

- Limited scalability: Some blockchain platforms have limited capacity and may struggle to handle large volumes of data, which could impact their ability to support complex healthcare systems.
- Complexity: Blockchain technology can be complex to implement and may require specialized technical expertise, which could increase costs and limit adoption.
- Regulatory challenges: The use of blockchain in healthcare raises regulatory and legal questions around data privacy, security, and ownership, which could pose challenges for widespread adoption.
- Security vulnerabilities: While blockchain technology is designed to be secure, there is still a risk of data breaches or other security vulnerabilities, particularly if the platform is not implemented properly.
- Dependence on technology: The reliability of blockchain-based healthcare models is heavily dependent on the underlying technology, which could lead to disruptions or outages if there are technical issues or failures.
- Resistance to change: Implementing blockchain-based healthcare models requires significant changes to existing systems and processes, which could face resistance from stakeholders who are comfortable with the status quo.

## 7.7  Conclusion

In conclusion, data governance is essential for healthcare organizations to ensure data accuracy, consistency, and security. Healthcare organizations face several data governance issues, including data quality, data security, data ownership, and data integration. And data privacy challenges due to the sensitive nature of healthcare data. The healthcare industry has developed several models for data governance in healthcare data management, including the FAIR Data Principles, data stewardship, data governance frameworks, and data catalogs. Also, HIPAA, GDPR, blockchain, and differential privacy for data privacy. Healthcare organizations must adopt these models to manage data effectively and make informed decisions to improve patient care. The healthcare industry has developed several models for data privacy in healthcare data management to safeguard patient data and ensure compliance with data privacy regulations.

### 7.7.1  Future directions of research in blockchain-based healthcare models

1. Blockchain capacity: All the existing blockchain-based healthcare models opted for cloud and IPFS for off-chain storage and conventional hashing technology for on-chain storage to ensure data integrity. To store huge piles of data, blockchain capacity and scalability need to be enhanced.
2. Throughput: The current market standards of throughput and latency of any blockchain model are big factors that delimit the adoption of blockchain across various fields. As of now, the most renowned Bitcoin model is able to process

approximately seven transactions per second yet every transaction consumes more than an hour to commit the transaction. Although the counterpart Ether has improved the throughput significantly, it still cannot stand for real-time transactions as a number of instantaneous rises sharply. To store real-time data and perform real-time transactions, the blockchain throughput needs further improvement.

3. Consensus algorithm: The consensus algorithm acts as the heart of the blockchain platform. A customized consensus algorithm could significantly offer a better security with minimal transaction latency to improve the overall throughput. However, only a fewer percentile of the research works focuses on an improved consensus algorithm.

4. Anonymity: Anonymity is essential in healthcare to protect the privacy of patients' sensitive medical information. Blockchain's inherent transparency makes it difficult to achieve anonymity, as all transactions are recorded on a public ledger that can be accessed by anyone. Blockchain-based healthcare models can possibly adapt a robust identity management protocol that allows patients to control access to their data and determine who can view and access their medical records.

5. Encryption algorithms: Undoubtedly the mechanism of using encrypted medical data offers an improved security, but rather it consumes significant time and demands higher order computing power as the complexity of the encrypting algorithm grows. It is high time to design novel encryption approaches possessing high security still consuming lower computational power.

# References

[1] Alsayegh M, Moulahi T, Alabdulatif A, and Lorenz P. Towards secure searchable electronic health records using consortium blockchain. *Network.* 2022;2(2):239–56. https://doi.org/10.3390/network2020016.

[2] Gordon WJ and Catalini C. Blockchain technology for healthcare: facilitating the transition to patient-driven interoperability. *Computational and Structural Biotechnology Journal.* 2018;16:224–30. https://doi.org/10.1016/j.csbj.2018.06.003.

[3] Sun J, Ren L, Wang S, and Yao X. A blockchain-based framework for electronic medical records sharing with fine-grained access control. *PLoS ONE.* 2020;15(10):e0239946. https://doi.org/10.1371/journal.pone.0239946.

[4] Wenhua Z, Qamar F, Abdali T-AN, *et al.* Blockchain technology: security issues, healthcare applications, challenges and future trends. *Electronics.* 2023;12(3):546. https://doi.org/10.3390/electronics12030546.

[5] Adere EM. Blockchain in healthcare and IoT: a systematic literature review. *Array.* 2022;14:100139. https://doi.org/10.1016/j.array.2022.100139.

[6] Bhattacharya P, Tanwar S, Bodkhe U, Tyagi S, and Kumar N. Bindaas: blockchain-based deep-learning as-a-service in healthcare 4.0 applications.

*IEEE Transactions on Network Science and Engineering*. 2019;8:1242–55. doi:10.1109/TNSE.2019.2961932.

[7] Ngabo D, Wang D, Iwendi C, Anajemba JH, Ajao LA, and Biamba C. Blockchain-based security mechanism for the medical data at fog computing architecture of internet of things. *Electronics*. 2021;10:2110. doi:10.3390/electronics10172110.

[8] Kim JH, Lee JH, Park JS, Lee YH, and Rim KW. Design of diet recommendation system for healthcare service based on user information. In: *2009 Fourth International Conference on Computer Sciences and Convergence Information Technology*. Seoul: IEEE, 2009. p. 516–18.

[9] Kutia S, Chauhdary SH, Iwendi C, Liu L, Yong W, and Bashir AK. Socio-technological factors affecting user's adoption of eHealth functionalities: a case study of China and Ukraine eHealth systems. *IEEE Access*. 2019;7:90777–88. doi:10.1109/ACCESS.2019.2924584.

[10] Plastiras P and O'Sullivan D. Exchanging personal health data with electronic health records: a standardized information model for patient generated health data and observations of daily living. *International Journal of Medical Informatics*. 2018;120:116–25. doi:10.1016/j.ijmedinf.2018.10.006.

[11] Shabbir A, Shabbir M, Javed AR, Rizwan M, Iwendi C, and Chakraborty C. Exploratory data analysis, classification, comparative analysis, case severity detection, and internet of things in COVID-19 telemonitoring for smart hospitals. *Journal of Experimental and Theoretical Artificial Intelligence*. 2022;35:1–28. doi:10.1080/0952813X.2021.1960634.

[12] Mani V, Manickam P, Alotaibi Y, Alghamdi S, and Khalaf OI. Hyperledger healthchain: patient-centric IPFS-based storage of health records. *Electronics*. 2021;10:3003. doi:10.3390/electronics10233003.

[13] Singhal V, Jain S, Anand D, *et al.* Artificial intelligence enabled road vehicle-train collision risk assessment framework for unmanned railway level crossings. *IEEE Access*. 2020;8:113790–806. doi:10.1109/ACCESS.2020.3002416.

[14] Wang Y, Kung L, and Byrd TA. Big data analytics: understanding its capabilities and potential benefits for healthcare organizations. *Technological Forecasting and Social Change*. 2018;126:3–13. doi:10.1016/j.techfore.2015.12.019.

[15] Jaiswal V. A new approach for recommending healthy diet using predictive data mining algorithm. *International Journal of Research and Analytical Reviews*. 2019;6:58–65.

[16] Argaw ST, Bempong NE, Eshaya-Chauvin B, and Flahault A. The state of research on cyberattacks against hospitals and available best practice recommendations: a scoping review. *BMC Medical Informatics and Decision Making*. 2019;19:1–11. doi:10.1186/s12911-018-0724-5.

[17] Egala BS, Pradhan AK, Badarla V, and Mohanty SP. Fortified-chain: a blockchain based framework for security and privacy-assured internet of medical things with effective access control. *IEEE Internet of Things Journal*. 2021;8:11717–31. doi:10.1109/JIOT.2021.3058946.

[18]  Alsufyani A, Alotaibi Y, Almagrabi AO, Alghamdi SA, and Alsufyani N. Optimized intelligent data management framework for a cyber-physical system for computational applications. *Complex & Intelligent Systems*. 2021;9:1–13. doi:10.1007/s40747-021-00511-w.

[19]  Singh P, Masud M, Hossain MS, and Kaur A. Blockchain and homomorphic encryption-based privacy-preserving data aggregation model in smart grid. *Computers & Electrical Engineering*. 2021;93:107209. doi:10.1016/j.compeleceng.2021.107209.

[20]  Li H, Zhu L, Shen M, Gao F, Tao X, and Liu S. Blockchain-based data preservation system for medical data. *Journal of Medical Systems*. 2018;42 (8). https://doi.org/10.1007/s10916-018-0997-3.

[21]  Thwin TT and Vasupongayya S. Blockchain-based access control model to preserve privacy for personal health record systems. *Security and Communication Networks*. 2019;2019:1–15. https://doi.org/10.1155/2019/8315614.

[22]  Wang H and Song Y. Secure cloud-based EHR system using attribute-based cryptosystem and blockchain. *Journal of Medical Systems*. 2018;42(8). https://doi.org/10.1007/s10916-018-0994-6.

[23]  Sahoo MS and Baruah PK. HBasechainDB – a scalable blockchain framework on Hadoop ecosystem. In *Asian Conference on Supercomputing Frontiers* (pp. 18–29), 2018. Springer. https://doi.org/10.1007/978-3-319-69953-0_2.

[24]  Peng C, He D, Chen J, Kumar N, and Khan MK. EPRT: an efficient privacy-preserving medical service recommendation and trust discovery scheme for eHealth system. *ACM Transactions on Internet Technology*. 2021;21:1–24. doi:10.1145/3397678.

[25]  Agrawal S and Jain SK. Medical text and image processing: applications, issues and challenges. In: *Machine Learning with Health Care Perspective*. Cham: Springer, 2020. p. 237–62.

[26]  Johari R, Kumar V, Gupta K, and Vidyarthi DP. BLOSOM: BLOckchain technology for Security Of Medical records. *ICT Express*. 2022;8:56–60.

[27]  Wu H, Dwivedi AD, and Srivastava G. Security and privacy of patient information in medical systems based on blockchain technology. *ACM Transactions on Multimedia Computing, Communications, and Applications*. 2021;17:1–17.

[28]  Liu X, Wang Z, Jin C, Li F, and Li G. A blockchain-based medical data sharing and protection scheme. *IEEE Access*. 2019;7:118943–53.

[29]  Zou R, Lv X, and Zhao J. SPChain: blockchain-based medical data sharing and privacy-preserving eHealth system. *Information Processing and Management*. 2021;58:102604.

[30]  Shahnaz A, Qamar U, and Khalid A. Using blockchain for electronic health records. *IEEE Access*. 2019;7:147782–95.

[31]  Wang M, Guo Y, Zhang C, Wang C, Huang H, and Jia X. MedShare: a privacy-preserving medical data sharing system by using blockchain. *IEEE Transactions on Services Computing*. 2021;16:438–51.

[32] Portugal I, Alencar P, and Cowan D. The use of machine learning algorithms in recommender systems: a systematic review. *Expert Systems with Applications*. 2018;97:205–27. doi:10.1016/j.eswa.2017.12.020.

[33] Elghoul M, Bahgat S, Hussein A, and Hamad S. A review of leveraging blockchain based framework landscape in healthcare systems. *International Journal of Intelligent Computing and Information Sciences*. 2021;21(3):71–83.

[34] Patel V. A framework for secure and decentralized sharing of medical imaging data via blockchain consensus. *Health Informatics Journal*. 2019;25(4):1398–411. doi:10.1177/1460458218769699.

[35] Abdleall NMM, Elalfi AEE, and El-Mougi FA. An intelligent educational system for breast cancer management. *International Journal of Intelligent Computing and Information Sciences*. 2022;22(3):39–53. doi:10.21608/ijicis.2022.136628.1179.

[36] Mohamed MM, Ghoniemy S, and Ghali NB. A survey on image data hiding techniques. *International Journal of Intelligent Computing and Information Sciences*. 2022;22(3):14–38. doi:10.21608/ijicis.2022.130393.1174.

[37] Hasselgren A, Kralevska K, Gligoroski D, Pedersen SA, and Faxvaag A. Blockchain in healthcare and health sciences—a scoping review. *International Journal of Medical Informatics*. 2020;134:104040.

[38] Ding Y, Tan F, Qin Z, *et al.* Deep key gen: a deep learning-based stream cipher generator for medical image encryption and decryption. *IEEE Transactions on Neural Networks and Learning Systems*. 2021;33;4915–29.

[39] Liu X, Zheng Y, Yi X, and Nepal S. Privacy-preserving collaborative analytics on medical time series data. *IEEE Transactions on Dependable and Secure Computing*. 2022;19:1687–702.

[40] Yang Y, Deng R, Liu X, *et al.* Privacy-preserving medical treatment system through nondeterministic finite automata. *IEEE Transactions on Cloud Computing*. 2022;10(3);2020–37.

[41] Huang J, Kong L, Chen G, Wu M-Y, Liu X, and Zeng P. Towards secure industrial IoT: blockchain system with credit-based consensus mechanism. *IEEE Transactions on Industrial Informatics*. 2019;15:3680–89.

[42] Wang S, Ouyang L, Yuan Y, Ni X, Han X, and Wang FY. Blockchain-enabled smart contracts: architecture, applications, and future trends. *IEEE Transactions on Systems, Man, and Cybernetics: Systems*. 2019;49:2266–77.

[43] Fan K, Wang S, Ren Y, Li H, and Yang Y. Medblock: efficient and secure medical data sharing via blockchain. *Journal of Medical Systems*. 2018;42:136.

[44] Zhang A and Lin X. Towards secure and privacy-preserving data sharing in e-health systems via consortium blockchain. *Journal of Medical System*. 2018;42:140.

[45] Cui S, Asghar MR, and Russello G. Towards blockchain-based scalable and trustworthy file sharing. In *2018 27th International Conference on Computer Communication and Networks (ICCCN)*. IEEE, 2018. p. 1–2.

[46]   Uddin MA, Stranieri A, Gondal I, and Balasubramanian V. A patient agent to manage blockchains for remote patient monitoring. *Studies in Health Technology and Informatics*. 2018;254:105–15.

[47]   Griggs KN, Ossipova O, Kohlios CP, Baccarini AN, Howson EA, and Hayajneh T. Healthcare blockchain system using smart contracts for secure automated remote patient monitoring. *Journal of Medical Systems*. 2018;42 (7):130.

[48]   Mohanta BK, Jena D, Panda SS, and Sobhanayak S. Blockchain technology: a survey on applications and security privacy challenges. *Journal of IoT*. 2019;8:100107.

[49]   Zhang P, Schmidt DC, White J, and Lenz G. Blockchain technology use cases in healthcare. *Advances in Computers*. 2018;111:1–41.

[50]   Gordon WJ and Catalini C. Blockchain technology for healthcare: facilitating the transition to patient-driven interoperability. *Computational and Structural Biotechnology Journal*. 2018;16:224–30.

[51]   Medicalchain. Whitepaper, 2019. https://medicalchain.com/Medicalcha in-Whitepaper-EN.pdf.

[52]   Jamil F, Hang L, Kim KH, and Kim DH. A novel medical blockchain model for drug supply chain integrity management in a smart hospital. *MDPI Journal of Electronics.* 2019;8:505–23.

[53]   Nakamoto S. *Bitcoin: A Peer-to-Peer Electronic Cash System.* www. Bitcoin.Org.

[54]   Larimer D. Transactions as Proof of Stake. https://bravenewcoin.com/assets/ Uploads/TransactionsAsProofOfStake10.pdf.

[55]   Larimer D. Delegated Proof of Stake. https://en.bitcoinwiki.org/wiki/DPoS.

[56]   P4Titan. Slimcoin: A Peer-To-Peer Crypto-Currency with Proof-of-Burn. http://www.doc.ic.ac.uk/~ids/realdotdot/crypto_papers_etc_worth_reading/ proof_of_burn/slimcoin_whitepaper.pdf.

[57]   Schwartz D, Youngs N, and Britto A. The Ripple Protocol Consensus Algorithm; Ripple Labs Inc White Paper, 2014. https://ripple.com/files/ ripple_consensus_whitepaper.pdf.

[58]   Mazieres D. The Stellar Consensus Protocol: A Federated Model for Internet-Level Consensus, 2015. https://www.stellar.org/papers/stellar-consensus-protocol.pdf.

[59]   MedicalChain – https://medicalchain.com/.

[60]   Solve.Care – https://solve.care/.

[61]   Healthereum – https://healthereum.com/.

[62]   HealthChain – https://healthchain.co/.

[63]   Shivom – https://shivom.io/.

[64]   BurstIQ – https://www.burstiq.com/.

[65]   Coral Health – https://coral.health/.

[66]   BitMED – https://www.bitmed.io/.

[67]   Health Nexus – https://healthnexus.tech/.

[68]   Guardtime – https://guardtime.com/.

[69]   Gem – https://gem.co/.

[70]   Medical Token Currency (MTC) – https://medicaltokencurrency.com/.
[71]   Health FX – https://healthfx.io/.
[72]   HealthChainRx – https://healthchainrx.com/.
[73]   MediBloc – https://medibloc.org/.
[74]   Lympo – https://lympo.com/.
[75]   Patientory – https://patientory.com/.
[76]   TrustedHealth – https://trustedhealth.com/.
[77]   SimplyVital Health – https://simplyvitalhealth.com/.
[78]   HealthChainUS – https://healthchainus.com/.

*Chapter 8*

# An exploratory review on Internet of Things in healthcare applications

*E. Umamaheswari[1], V. Kanchana Devi[2], A. Karmel[2], A. David Maxim Gururaj[3] and Nebojsa Bacanin[4]*

## Abstract

Internet of Things (IoT) is currently a widely used paradigm owing to its ability to make everyday activities convenient and manageable. The impact of IoT in various sectors is unmistakably a concept of interest. From healthcare to industries, each complex or mundane task is automated. IoT in simple terms refers to the concept of tangible devices (things) that contain sensors, transducers, actuators, etc., and computing capability connected to each other over the Internet. This enables data transmission and storage for the proper functioning of any product. Multiple 'smart' products are built every day using this concept and these devices are connected creating an IoT ecosystem. This chapter describes the various applications of IoT in healthcare.

**Keywords:** Internet of Things; Healthcare; EKG monitors; Sphygmomanometers; Bluetooth low energy

## 8.1 Introduction

The recent innovations in technology paved the way for the IoT to present an opportunity in connecting human beings. To understand the notion of the Internet of Things (IoT) completely, its related concepts should also be briefed. Ubiquitous computing (UbiComp) is yet another area that colludes with IoT. UbiComp simplifies the task of integrating and correlating devices through the internet. This can be done by employing multiple middle-wares or frameworks making the network of devices appear as though they are present everywhere [1]. Although the idea of UbiComp was presented before the idea of the IoT, constructing an IoT environment

[1]Centre for Cyber Physical Systems, Vellore Institute of Technology, Chennai, India
[2]School of Computer Science and Engineering, Vellore Institute of Technology, Chennai, India
[3]School of Advanced Sciences, Vellore Institute of Technology, Chennai, India
[4]Faculty of Informatics and Computing, Singidunum University, Belgrade, Serbia

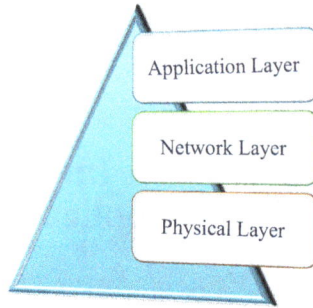

*Figure 8.1    Three-layered IoT architecture*

is far more complicated. These complications arise due to the fact that an IoT environment has a relatively greater number of devices. Other related notions include Industry 4.0 and IIoT for which IoT acts as a foundation. The smallest and basic IoT architecture has three layers namely: physical layer, network layer, and application layer. Figure 8.1 represents the three-layered IoT architecture.

The physical layer is otherwise called the perception layer [2]. It includes all tangible devices or nodes similar to the physical layer in the Open Systems Interconnection (OSI) model. Sensors and transducers come under this layer. The physical layer accepts control information from the layer above it (network layer) to perform the necessary operations. Hence it is also called the control layer. The network layer is in charge of information transfer from the control layer to the application. Hence, it is also called the transmission layer. Communication technologies like Bluetooth, Wi-Fi, ZigBee, etc. are a part of this layer. These technologies will be covered in detail in the following sections. Lastly, the application layer is the final and topmost layer of the three-layered IoT architecture model. It acts as an interface between any IoT device and the end user. It analyses data from the perception layer and the network layer.

For better connectivity and execution, the three layers were later expanded into a five-layered architecture which was more amenable [3]. The three layers were sustained and two additional layers (middleware layer and management layer) were added. These additional layers assist in making decisions and efficient data analysis.

Additionally, IoT devices that operate on account of humans are in the making. However, huge this advancement is, it also has its flip side [4]. In general, IoT devices are susceptible to attack and hence garner privacy concerns. Deployment of these devices also leads to loss of employment in certain areas. Apart from these, the making of these devices also has design issues that have to be handled with complete discretion. In the following sections, the impact of IoT in various sectors has been discussed.

## 8.2    Architecture of IoT in healthcare

Figure 8.2 represents the architecture of IoT. It includes the components such as product infrastructure, Sensors, application platform, analytics, and connectivity.

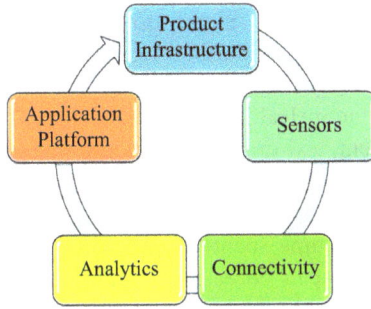

*Figure 8.2 Architecture of IoT*

## 8.2.1 Product infrastructure

The hardware and software components of IoT product infrastructure read the sensor signals and display them on a specific device. A study published in 2011 used a wearable sensor system to identify mental stress and analyse physiological signs. ECG, respiration, EMG, skin conductance of the trapezius muscles were monitored during the surgery. These signals yielded a total of 19 physiological characteristics which were reduced to 7 principal components. The accuracy of categorisation between stress and non-stress circumstances was found to be almost 80% using these PCs and several classifiers. This indicates that a promising feature subset for the future development of a customised stress monitor has been discovered.

## 8.2.2 Sensors

Nowadays, one of the most important aspects of our daily lives is Internet It has been adapted to the ways in which people live, work, play, and learn. The Internet is used for a variety of purposes, including education, finance, business, industry, recreation, social networking, shopping, and so on. In this pandemic, the remote treatment has increased and for the doctors managing remote patients and analysing their results is not organised as there are many patients at the same time, they need to track which sometimes becomes difficult.

For the elderly patients, staying alone and managing their medicines and taking a remote treatment are challenging tasks. Along with this for chronic disorders where the condition needs to be monitored on a regular basis becomes difficult in a remote manner and due to this pandemic, it is not preferred to visit the doctors periodically for follow-up of the treatment. Doctors, having privileged access to medical instruments and knowledge, have traditionally been the doorway for the improved diagnosis and treatment. Today with the advanced technology, people have instant access to e-Health resources, medical guidelines, and online courses; through the personal health portals and e-Health monitoring and self-management apps on their smartphones and other wearables have catered their attention to health management and its importance.

As per statistics in the United States, up to 85% of people look for health information online on a daily basis. Furthermore, the number of mHealth platforms in the healthcare domain has increased dramatically over the years. As per the Global Market Insights, the mHealth industry will reach $289.4 billion in 2025.

Effective and efficient real-time health monitoring systems are proposed to improve management that can report potential health threats associated with environmental conditions, support individuals' long-term health monitoring, and reduce the cost, effort, and time spent on traditional hospital visits, and provide digitalised information that can be easily accessed across the world. For older persons who live alone, a health monitoring system is nested with infrared sensors in each room to track their in-house movements. Medicine reminders, emergency notifications, and contact with physicians and hospitals nearby can all be quite beneficial. In addition, having immediate access to e-Health information is critical for chronic illness self-management. Self-management has grown in prominence as an important aspect of care and support for persons with chronic diseases, both within health service organisations and outside of them.

### 8.2.3   Connectivity

Better connectivity between devices or sensors from the microcontroller to the server and back is made possible by IoT systems.

### 8.2.4   Analytics

To determine the patient's health parameters, the healthcare system analyses data from sensors and correlates the same. Based on the results of the analysis, patient's health can be improved. There are four primary types of IoT analytics namely, descriptive analytics, diagnostic analytics, predictive analytics, and prescriptive analytics.

Analyses of the IoT that are descriptive primarily concentrate on the past. To create a report that details what happened, when it happened, and how frequently it did, the historical data collected from devices is processed and analysed. This kind of IoT analysis is helpful for supplying solutions to specific queries about the behaviour of things or people and can also be used to spot any anomalies.

Diagnostic IoT analytics, in contrast to descriptive analytics, go further to address the question of why something occurred by delving deeper into the data to pinpoint the underlying cause of a particular problem. The most sophisticated form of IoT analytics, called prescriptive IoT analytics, not only forecasts future events but also makes recommendations for how to proceed to achieve the desired business outcomes.

### 8.2.5   Application framework

IoT systems give healthcare practitioners access to data for all patients with full details on their monitor devices. IoT application framework includes hardware, software, networking elements (IoT protocols), device management, security, data management, application development, and cloud-based platform. Together, these elements make it possible for systems and IoT devices to be seamlessly integrated. For updating and keeping track of the device's performance, for instance, device management is essential. Different connections between devices and the Internet are made possible by protocols. Data must be processed and stored on a cloud platform that connects to a platform or application that is in charge of displaying the data and enabling other features or services.

## 8.3   IoT in healthcare

The healthcare sector is in a terrible condition of despondency. While technology cannot rearward population aging or completely remove chronic diseases, it can at least modify healthcare by supplying users with low-priced medical services. A significant portion of hospital expenses are for medical diagnostics. The routines of medical examinations can be moved by technology from a hospital (which is hospital-centric) to the patient's home (home-centric). Figure 8.3 shows the effects if IoT in healthcare.

The cost of hospitalisation will be decreased if patients receive the proper outcomes. There are unmatched advantages to exploit this technology-based healthcare approach, which could intensify the quality and effectiveness of therapies and, also intensify the health of elderly patients.

## 8.4   Case study

### 8.4.1   *IoT in patient healthcare monitoring*

#### 8.4.1.1   Remotely monitoring the patients

Residents of numerous regions of the global reside many kilometres from the closest hospital. As a result, it may consume the time for them to get to the medical

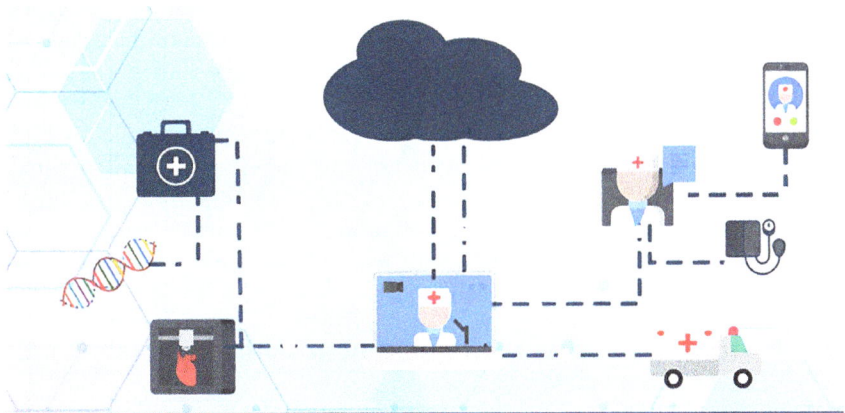

*Figure 8.3   Effect of IoT in healthcare*

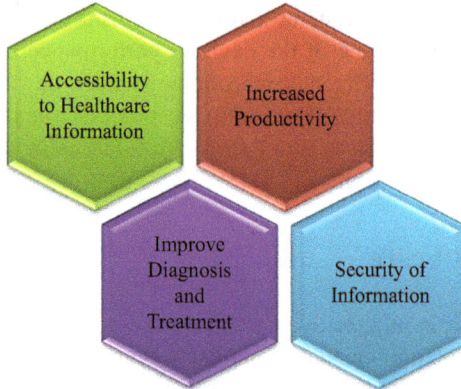

*Figure 8.4    Benefits of medical charting*

readiness in an emergency. In a similar vein, it becomes challenging for medical professionals to visit patients with chronic diseases regularly. Monitoring the patients remotely is powered by the IoT that can address the issue of the lengthy journey. Healthcare professionals may be able to assist patients with prescriptions and medication in addition to measuring their biometrics with the aid of sensors and remote equipment. Patients are able to link up any wearable device to the cloud to modify the data in real time. Figure 8.4 lists the benefits of medical charting.

A few IoT gadgets can enable face-to-face communication all over the cyberspace. This can give medical staff the knowledge they need to make treatment ideas patch the patients are travelling to the healthcare facility. Or perhaps they would not even require going to the hospital in the first place! This makes it easier to compile a list of chronic patients' most recent health updates.

### 8.4.1.2    Critical conditions

The promptness, accuracy, and accessibility of contextual information are essential for emergency care to be effective. Additionally, it depends on how accurately the data was gathered both during the exigency call and when the patient was taken to the hospital for providing contiguous care.

Furthermore, gathering, processing, storing, and retrieving the data over that instance frame requires a significant amount of time and effort. IoT can help in the accurate collection of data that emergency care workers or staff in the ER, can approach for more rapid and effective medical aid. The ability to share this information with ER staff in real-time will help hospitals provide better care while the patient is being transported to the facility.

### 8.4.1.3    Keeping a daily track of patients, and other hospital-related parameters

The main goals of healthcare companies are to boost employee productivity and cut expenses. This holds true for both little and big institutions with lots of employees, clients, and inventory. Using wireless ID cards, the hospitals can regulate admissions, enhance security, and evaluate staff productivity. Staff members can trail the localisation of the inventory using RFID tags and Bluetooth Low Energy (BLE) beacons in case of an emergency. Asset tracking can also be facilitated by real-time location systems (RTLS) and IoT. The staff can therefore devote more time to patient care because it is an affordable way to keep trail of the tools, medications, and autonomous resources.

### 8.4.1.4   Surgeries through augmentation

The IoT has gotten into operating rooms when it comes to healthcare. Consider the utilisation of linked, artificially intelligent robotic devices for various surgical procedures. The main goal of these procedures is to increase precision with the use of surgical robots. Additionally, connected devices and IoT applications can absolutely contour the pre- and post-operative medical staff's tasks. In both instances, IoT sensors can be used to transmit, collect, and analyse data. This makes it easier to record even the smallest details, which helps prevent surgical challenges. Figure 8.5 shows the devices used for daily monitoring of patient's health.

### 8.4.1.5   Monitoring of critical hardware through virtualisation

It goes without saying that all contemporary healthcare facilities need cutting-edge gear and software to operate. The hardware might present a number of dangers and concerns if these are not taken care of in the greatest way feasible. Consider system malfunctions, power outages, or even cyberattacks. Healthcare organisations choose the best IoT-driven solutions because they don't want these accidents to happen. A good example is Philips' e-Alert, which can remotely monitor essential medical equipment. The solution notifies hospital workers of any anomalies in any equipment so that preventive maintenance can be performed in order to avert a failure.

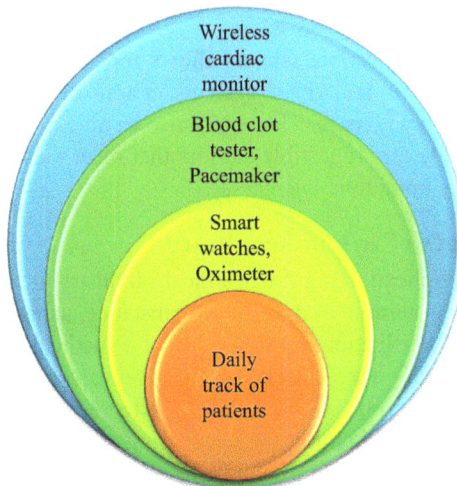

*Figure 8.5   Daily monitoring of patients – IoT in biomedical*

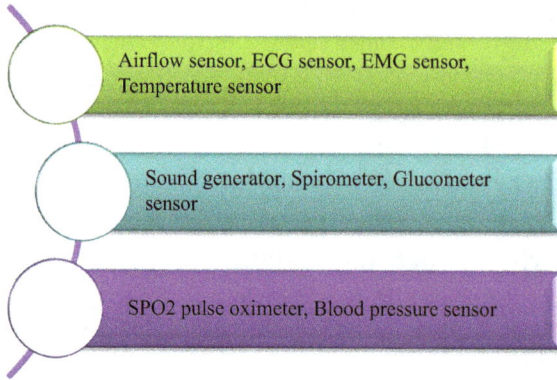

*Figure 8.6    Sensors used in IoT healthcare*

### 8.4.1.6    Managing pharmacy

The multimillion-dollar pharmacy industry is very complex. Due to the numerous steps required to transport and maintain pharmaceuticals from a plant to depository readiness in a hospital, there may be a number of preservation concerns. IoT can assist in fusing the best safety practices with cutting-edge technology to ensure quicker medication delivery, better patient care, and safer operations. Consider smart refrigerators as an illustration, which can be used to store vaccines and prevent their harm during handling, transfer, or storage. IoT-enabled pharmaceutics may guarantee increased operational effectiveness and efficiency, secure medicine dispensing free of mistakes, and overall higher patient happiness. Figure 8.6 shows the sensors used in IoT healthcare system.

### 8.4.1.7    Sensors

It is typically messy and quite disruptive to collect data from inside the human body. No one, for instance, enjoys having a camera or probe placed inside their digestive system. Using ingestible sensors allows for much less invasive data collection from the digestive and other systems. These devices must be compact enough to be swallowed with ease. They must also be able to neatly depart the body on their own or disintegrate. Ingestible sensors that meet these needs are the focus of intense research by numerous businesses.

### 8.4.1.8    Advantages of IoT in healthcare

The benefits of IoT applications in the healthcare industry are found in distant use cases. Real-time patient remote monitoring, for instance, using IoT devices that are connected and smart notifications in the event of a medical emergency, can find illnesses, save lives, and treat diseases. Smart sensors keep track of life-style decision-making, the environs, and health status to recommend preventive measures which will lessen the likelihood of developing acute conditions and diseases. Access to medical data enables individuals to obtain high-quality aid while also supporting medical professionals in devising the best choices. Figure 8.7 shows the advantages of IoT in the healthcare domain.

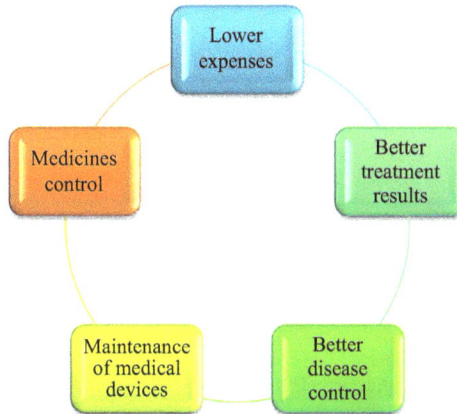

*Figure 8.7   List of advantages of IoT in healthcare*

### 8.4.1.9   Disadvantages of IoT in healthcare

Although there are many benefits, as evidenced by examples of the IoT in healthcare, there are drawbacks as well. Frequently, healthcare professionals are charged with maintaining the security of numerous sites and sizable data warehouses. However, transitioning a whole facility to create a new system and practice may take time, and the first investment funds and installation expenses can be exorbitant, especially for smaller medical installations and clinics in remote areas.

### 8.4.1.10   Importance of IoT in healthcare

A network of ubiquitous computing that primarily manages external operations can be imagined as an IoT healthcare facility. IoT-based healthcare systems in the medical field collect a variety of patient data and solicit input from doctors. All of these devices have the capacity to communicate with one another and carry out crucial operations that might be used right away to save someone's life. An IoT healthcare gadget would communicate this crucial data to the cloud after gathering it so that doctors could act on it.

From this, we may conclude that the potential use of IoT in healthcare can enhance patient health as well as the productivity of healthcare professionals and hospital procedures. Figure 8.8 shows the disadvantages of IoT in healthcare domain.

### 8.4.1.11   Scope for IoT in healthcare

A device with a sensor and the ability to communicate with the outside world and upload data to the Internet is what is known as an Internet of Things (IoT) device. These IoT-based medical devices can connect and yield important state that could rescue a life and provide prompt assistance. In order for doctors to take action on it, IoT healthcare devices would transmit this important information to the cloud later collecting inactive data. IoT-based healthcare services improve patient well-being as a result, offer support in times of need, and improve workflow efficiency for healthcare organisations.

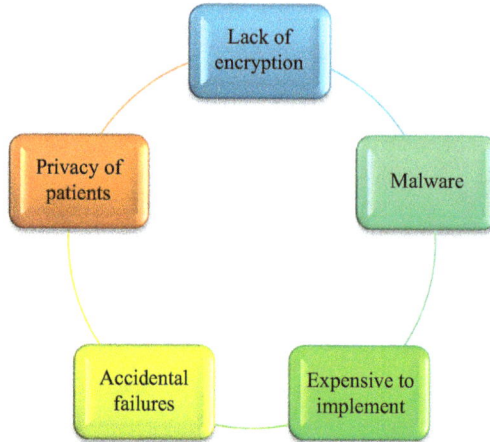

*Figure 8.8    Disadvantages of IoT in healthcare*

## 8.4.2    IoT in multifaceted remote health monitoring system

Although it is typically done with physical documentation in hospitals and other healthcare facility centres, patient health monitoring is a crucial aspect of the healthcare domain. With the development of technology, electronic health records (EHR) are now kept, which reduces the amount of time and money needed to complete the process. In recent years, there has been an increase in the collection of health-related data using technologies like wearable health devices, smartphone apps, remote monitoring devices, portable devices with embedded sensors, and other technologies. Chronic illnesses like diabetes, organ transplants, and heart conditions require ongoing patient monitoring and follow-up, which is typically done in person.

### 8.4.2.1    IoT health monitoring

The system's fundamental idea is to transmit data via a web page to enable continuous patient monitoring over the Internet. A device of this kind would continuously monitor vital physiological indicators like temperature and pulse rate, compare them to a predetermined range, and alert the physician if the values went above a predetermined limit. In this setup, the data is transmitted using a microcontroller. It is connected to the IoT, which sends data to a doctor or caretaker. The patient's health data is saved in the cloud. Sensors detect environmental conditions, and GPS data is used to calculate the patient's location and time [5].

The goal is to develop some criteria that will aid in the identification of relevant relationships between various datasets, which will be beneficial in determining the impact of environmental factors on asthmatic patients' health [6]. ECG sensor, temperature sensor, blood pressure sensor, and pulse oximeter sensor are among the sensors used. The GSM device sends a message to the mobile phone if any of the health metrics reaches or exceeds the threshold value.

ThingSpeak allows users to see real-time visualisations and analysis of shared data over the cloud. When a patient hits a button while feeling uneasy in an emergency, the system sends an EMERGENCY SMS message to the patient's phone [7]. These systems were implemented using the Crossbow MICA2 mote (MPR400CB), Thermal Sensor [National Semiconductors LM92 Precision Centigrade], Crossbow MDA300CA Interface Board, and Ipod (Nonin Integrated Pulse Oximetry Device). The thermal sensor was included in the MICA2 mote via the I2C interface. The data from the LM92 sensor is wirelessly transferred to the base station successfully.

Before being displayed on the host computer, the data was double-checked [8]. Since the treatment and rehabilitation of chronic diseases is a continuous process, a full range of IoT sensors are used to support bodily and environmental monitoring as part of a comprehensive strategy that enables data linkages from various locations in preparation for potential TeleHealth virtual consultations. On the basis of this, a doctor's and patient's consultation can include not only lab results but also a history of data that was remotely measured while the patients were at home using wearables and in-home remote patient monitoring apps.

The doctor can make a better diagnosis and deliver individualised therapy using the available data and decision support tools that have admittance to huge data. This kind of breakthrough technology might have a huge impact on global healthcare systems, lowering healthcare costs and improving diagnosis speed and accuracy. The quality of services in terms of Performance, Reliability, Security, Functional Stability, Privacy, Law and Ethics, Scalability, and Interoperability has been examined, and it has been discovered that these technologies are not widely adopted in the medical community. They still have reservations about adopting remote monitoring technology, even though they see it as an aid to current medical approaches rather than a replacement [4].

### 8.4.2.2  HER-based health monitoring

The impact of EHR on current clinical documentation was examined using doctors, nurses, interns, and patient person hours observation time for documentation studies. There are not many studies examining how the adoption of an EHR will affect staff documentation time in a hospital setting, it was found. The system's full adoption may eventually result in a decrease in documentation time, improved work and information flow, a significant decrease in multitasking, and increased patient safety [2]. In terms of time pressure, technostress, and workflow-related concerns, the influence of an EHR integrated with health data on physician burnout is clear. Algorithm-based clinical decision assistance, artificial intelligence, human–computer interface mechanism, visualisation format, financial reimbursement, and workflow optimisation are all mentioned as ways to reduce burnout. Quality control is crucial in an EHR-integrated PGHD. The AI-enabled system may detect and warn physicians of incorrect diagnostic and therapy items, as well as the particular reasons for the advice. If a specific drug is not prescribed or the dosage is not correct, this can be easily modified. The AI-enabled solution can also provide fast feedback to hospital stakeholders on the healthcare quality control report. Clinical tests are included in the EHR, and certain health systems may also have unstructured biomedical data or patient-to-provider electronic messages [3].

To strengthen population stratification efforts and assess the additional values of various medication adherence indices in forecasting hospitalisation and annual healthcare total cost, risk stratification models are constructed based on EHR data and insurance claims. Medication possession ratio (MPR) measures of adherence did not significantly improve model performance, while prescription fill rate (PFR) measures added only minor gains. The drug regimen complexity index (MRCI) and MPR measures were found to improve usage risk classification models in a study, although their effects need to be validated. Hence, the Patient's Medication Adherence Indices' predictive effects in EHR have been examined, and future improvements are suggested for incorporating in improving utilisation prediction in subpopulations that benefit the most from medication adherence interventions [1].

### 8.4.2.3   Tele-health monitoring

During the COVID-19 pandemic for chronic disease patients, the role of telehealth, eHealth, and telemedicine has primarily emerged, demonstrating the need for tele-health in current medication systems. Research was carried out for various chronic diseases to gain the proper insight, but there is a lack of study in the area of providing medical consultations to patients and their implications. For highlighting the importance and benefits of e-Health during and after the pandemic for chronic diseases, the authors employed the PRISMA flow model and electronic databases (PubMed, Science Direct, Google Scholar, and Web of Science Core Collection) [5].

Studies on the use of telehealth in the case of paediatric transplant patients have also been conducted, which include interventions such as remote visits using mobile apps. Telehealth treatments may provide the potential to provide care that overcomes many of the drawbacks of in-person care, making it more convenient and feasible for patients and caregivers alike. Because there is a widespread dearth of evidence on long-term usage, mHealth platforms have reported high approval rates in the short term. Before telehealth therapies may be widely adopted, a multi-centre RCT with strong measurements of medication adherence and other outcome variables, as well as longer term follow-up, is required [9]. With the increased usage of eHealth tools, studies have been done to see how e-health has affected people's self-management and wellness through time. The focus on self-management has evolved in tandem with a larger view of health, merely the relationship between the two notions is complicated.

A theory on the relationship between motivation, self-regulation, and well-being is planned as a broader definition of health, claiming that eudaimonia – or living well – can be achieved by (a) following intrinsically valuable goals and (b) processes that are characterised and associated with various wellbeing outcomes. There is a need for clarity and confirmable evidence on the good and negative effects of eHealth technologies on these relationships. However, with direct access to self-management assistance and a network of peers, web-based communities developed on these platforms can mitigate isolation, loneliness, and negative emotions, allowing individuals to express themselves and improve their health [10]. Web applications, Mobile applications, and Smart TV applications are created to provide remote monitoring which can be useful for patients and health centres.

These applications can incorporate the patient and doctor communication interfaces along with set of reminders and a user-friendly interface that can be easily accessed by the elderly population for monitoring chronic ailments, and conditions are therapy. These can be used to track and visualise the process [11]. These tele-monitoring platforms are also cloud computing compatible. Medical data such as sugar levels, blood pressure, and other medical signals are measured by pervasive devices or medical sensors attached to specific parts of patients' bodies, and the ascertained medical information is sent to medical advisors via wireless media such as cellular networks, where the medical information is received and examined for further diagnosis. ECG analysers are also integrated in to the telemonitoring system for real-time medical data processing. This allows for the collection of real-time data from patients who are far away, and the medical data is then communicated via the Internet to allow for enhanced medical diagnosis and treatment in real time [12]. Adaptive designs can be used by the AI expert system to model both daily behaviour and the way people react to changes over time.

An elderly person who prefers to live at home and not in a nursing home can lead a more autonomous life if smart home engineering science and its supporting infrastructure are completely developed. The automated decision-making and alerting system may be beneficial to those who need 24-hours monitoring. The Technology Assisted Friendly Environment for the Third Age [TAFETA] group developed a smart home system, especially for the elderly that is being studied and evaluated in light of its potential use by the elderly [13]. Infrared sensors installed in each room might persist monitoring longer than other sorts of monitoring since their movements were uncontrolled. Through this monitoring, a distinct movement pattern was identified.

The health status was calculated by comparing the length of time they spent in various places, such as the restroom, to previously collected data. Features like alerting the family of the incident if an unexpected status was discovered after analysis. As a result, both the elderly subjects who lived alone and their family members had less worry as a result of this system [14,15]. Overall, there are various IoT-based implementations for health monitoring system using sensors, could computing, EHRs telehealth interfaces, and many more. However, it observed that telehealth and EHR are low-cost and widely adopted systems.

## 8.5  Conclusion

As seen from this chapter, IoT has been developing and causing a number of changes to our daily lives. This in turn serves to make our lives convenient and pleasant. IoT by itself has many applications in multiple sectors proving its ver-satility. In this chapter, the main two case studies, IoT in patient healthcare mon-itoring and IoT in multifaceted remote health monitoring system, are analysed along with various aspects such as Remotely Monitoring the Patients, Critical Conditions, Keeping a Daily Track of Patients, and Other Hospital Related Parameters and HER-based health monitoring. Other domains in this concept are employed including energy, construction, mobility, manufacturing, etc. On the other side of these numerous benefits, it also has its downsides. The method of using this concept is the most required ability of everything to ensure that we receive all of its impeccable benefits.

# References

[1]  Andrade, R. M., Carvalho, R. M., de Araújo, I. L., Oliveira, K. M., and Maia, M. E. (2017, July). What changes from ubiquitous computing to internet of things in interaction evaluation? In *International Conference on Distributed, Ambient, and Pervasive Interactions* (pp. 3–21). Springer, Cham.

[2]  Zhu, Z. and Huang, R.-G. Study on the IoT architecture and access technology. In *2017 16th International Symposium on Distributed Computing and Applications to Business, Engineering and Science (DCABES)*, IEEE, 2017.

[3]  Choudhary, G. and Jain A. K. Internet of Things: a survey on architecture, technologies, protocols and challenges. In *2016 International Conference on Recent Advances and Innovations in Engineering (ICRAIE)*, IEEE, 2016.

[4]  Fischer, J. E., Colley, J. A., Luger, E., *et al.* (2016, September). New horizons for the IoT in everyday life: proactive, shared, sustainable. In *Proceedings of the 2016 ACM International Joint Conference on Pervasive and Ubiquitous Computing: Adjunct* (pp. 657–660).

[5]  Wang, M., Callaghan, V., Bernhardt, J., White, K., and Peña-Rios, A. (2018). Augmented reality in education and training: pedagogical approaches and illustrative case studies. *Journal of Ambient Intelligence and Humanized Computing*, 9(5), 1391–1402.

[6]  Slavova, Y. and Mu, M. (2018, March). A comparative study of the learning outcomes and experience of VR in education. In *2018 IEEE Conference on Virtual Reality and 3D User Interfaces (VR)* (pp. 685–686). IEEE.

[7]  Kuyoro, S., Osisanwo, F., and Akinsowon, O. (2015, March). Internet of things (IoT): an overview. *In Proceedings of the 3rd International Conference on Advances in Engineering Sciences and Applied Mathematics (ICAESAM)* (pp. 23–24).

[8]  Rajurkar, C., Prabaharan, S. R. S., and Muthulakshmi, S. (2017, March). IoT based water management. In *2017 International Conference on Nextgen Electronic Technologies: Silicon to Software (ICNETS2)* (pp. 255–259). IEEE.

[9]  Al-Emran, M., Malik, S. I., and Al-Kabi, M. N. (2020). A survey of internet of things (IoT) in education: opportunities and challenges. In: Hassanien, A., Bhatnagar, R., Khalifa, N., and Taha, M. (eds), *Toward Social Internet of Things (SIoT): Enabling Technologies, Architectures and Applications* (pp. 197–209), Springer, Cham.

[10]  Saini, M. K. and Goel, N. (2019). How smart are smart classrooms? A review of smart classroom technologies. *ACM Computing Surveys (CSUR)*, 52(6), 1–28.

[11]  Beer, W. and Wagner, A. (2011). Smart books: adding context-awareness and interaction to electronic books. In *Proceedings of the 9th International Conference on Advances in Mobile Computing and Multimedia*.

[12]  McRae, L., Ellis, K., and Kent, M. (2018). *Internet of things (IoT): Education and Technology. Relationship Between Education and Technology for Students with Disabilities in Their Learning* (pp. 1–37). Perth, Western Australia: National Centre for Student Equity in Higher Education.

[13]  Tew, Y., Tang, T. Y., and Lee, Y. K. (2017, December). A study on enhanced educational platform with adaptive sensing devices using IoT features. In *2017 Asia-Pacific Signal and Information Processing Association Annual Summit and Conference (APSIPA ASC)* (pp. 375–379). IEEE.

[14]  Lenz, L., Pomp, A., Meisen, T., and Jeschke, S. (2016, March). How will the Internet of Things and big data analytics impact the education of learning-disabled students? A concept paper. In *2016 3rd MEC International Conference on Big Data and Smart City (ICBDSC)* (pp. 1–7). IEEE.

[15]  Burd, B., Barker, L., Divitini, M., *et al.* (2018, January). Courses, content, and tools for internet of things in computer science education. In *Proceedings of the 2017 ITiCSE Conference on Working Group Reports* (pp. 125–139).

*Chapter 9*

# Augmented reality/virtual reality for detecting anxiety disorder

*K. Suganthi[1], Sathiya Narayanan[1], Krithika alias Anbu Devi M.[1] and Ammasai Sengodan Ganapathi[2]*

## Abstract

The objective of this review is to provide an overview of biomedical applications of augmented reality (AR) and virtual reality (VR). The main focus will be on AR and VR methodologies for dealing with patient anxiety disorders. As a traditional approach, music was used to remove anxiety in certain patients. However, the music-based approaches could not provide an immersive experience to patients. To circumvent this challenge, AR/VR-based methods came into existence. AR-based approaches were used to treat phobias. In recent years, due to the advent of VR headsets, VR-based approaches are preferred in a variety of applications ranging from healthcare education to patients anxiety management.

**Keywords:** Augmented reality; Virtual reality; Anxiety disorder

## 9.1 Introduction

In the world of healthcare, augmented reality (AR) and virtual reality (VR) have given a top technical support. Healthcare professionals and patients can interact with simulated settings designed for medical education (including training in simulative surgery), pain treatment, or rehabilitation to VR solution. The interior organs of the human body must frequently be simulated and visualized in the medical field. With CT, MRI, and other medical scans, computer technology can be utilized to create simulated 3D models of the organs. The extraction and modeling of organs and bones with various densities is not entirely obvious in a 3D model produced by a medical image analysis system. The AR and VR system may provide 3D images, real-time interaction, and a great deal of aggregate function detail.

[1]School of Electronics Engineering, Vellore Institute of Technology, Chennai, India
[2]School of Science, Engineering and Environment, The University of Salford Manchester, Manchester, UK

Patients can receive various clinical services in their homes or other non-clinical settings, including some that are often only provided in clinics and hospitals. The ability to access necessary healthcare services when doing so in person would otherwise be challenging for patients, including those from socioeconomically vulnerable and underserved communities, the elderly, or those with disabilities, could make it simpler and more likely for patients to comply with treatment and monitoring regimens.

By 2024, it is anticipated to increase on an average of 30.7%, reaching $2.2 billion.

When simulated digital imagery is combined with the physical world as seen through a camera or display, such as a smart phone or head-mounted or heads-up display, it is known as AR. It is possible for digital graphics to interact with the real world (often controlled by users). It's also known as combined reality or mixed reality.

To entirely replace the user's field of vision with a simulated and interactive virtual environment, VR may be necessary. VR is frequently a viable option when doing something in reality would be expensive or unfeasible.

There are numerous review articles that discuss the use of AR and VR in healthcare. The impact of VR pain treatment on various age groups is evaluated [1]. The article [2] gives a general summary of AR/VR in healthcare. The survey [3] focuses on the usage of AR/VR in surgery and its potential applications. This paper [4] explains the role of VR in the healthcare and well-being of older persons. This article [5] outlines how technology is generally used in medicine. One of the most recent surveys [6] provides the application of metaverse in healthcare. VR restorative environment comprising 3D VR interactive scenes was shown to have a good effect on the cognitive and emotional recovery of individuals having mild or moderate levels of anxiety [7]. The study reported in [7] was carried out for 195 patients and the approach had a good recovery effect (i.e. healing effect) in 26 patients resulting in the reduction of negative emotions. The scenes created included forest, plants-related paintings, lawn and water-related features.

In [8], the effects of VR exposure on claustrophobic patients were reported. The study revealed the fact that variation in the intensity of scenes will provide better senses of closeness. It was reported in [9] that the AR can be used to overcome medical distress, improve surgical success and promote patient's well-being. AR has a reasonable impact in patient education as well [10]. The impact of VR on ICU patients was reported in [11]. VR-based anxiety treatment approaches on patients suffering from post-intensive care syndrome resulted in reduced post-traumatic stress disorder and depression scores [11]. VR has the potential to change the hospital atmosphere from scary to fun/informative [12]. A review of how VR technologies should be improved to treat modern-day anxiety disorders is presented in [13]. Over review is especially based on overview of AR/VR in biomedical applications and the main focus is to analyze the use of AR/VR methodologies to treat patients with anxiety disorders.

## 9.2    Overview of AR/VR

Emerging technologies like AR and VR are altering the way we interact with the digital world. There will be a substantial increase in the global market for AR and

VR in healthcare. Techniques utilizing AR and VR are being employed more frequently in surgery and diagnosis. Technologies like touch surgery use VR to give doctors in the operating room a glimpse of the patient's anatomy and physiology. The markets for VR and AR are then anticipated to grow more quickly as a result. Both patients and doctors benefit from VR technology. This makes it possible for the patient to visit a doctor, which is highly practical. Many applications for healthcare services are available in AR and VR.

This improves remote consultation and treatment. Connecting with international experts for advanced care can significantly assist those who have little access to specialty care. Headset and screenshots in VR bring the real-world environment to the humans. These headsets also incorporate head tracking technology, which allows users to spin their heads physically to see the area around them from every angle. In AR, the physical world around is having superimposed digital graphics. Two AR headsets are currently available on the market: the Microsoft HoloLens and the Magic Leap. They are currently more expensive than VR headsets. A PC, a phone, or a laptop can use AR without a headset.

There are several AR apps available; some of them allow to read text using camera, recognize stars in the sky, and even visualize how various plants would look in the garden. AR is helping in surgical processes, which enhances physician efficiency and, subsequently, clinical results. The first AR knee operation in the world to receive FDA approval, performed by France-based medical business Pixee Medical with the aid of the Vuzix M400 AR smart glasses (shown in Figure 9.1), represents an important development in surgical technology. A growing number of conditions, including depression, addiction, phobias, obsessive-compulsive disorder, psychosis, even post-traumatic stress disorder pain management, and, anxiety disorders, are being treated with VR exposure therapy (VRET) and AR exposure therapy (ARET). There are behavioral therapies and psychotherapies with digital support that deal with how a patient reacts to traumatic events. It has helped people who are battling acrophobia and arachnophobia as well as burn patients and veterans with PTSD.

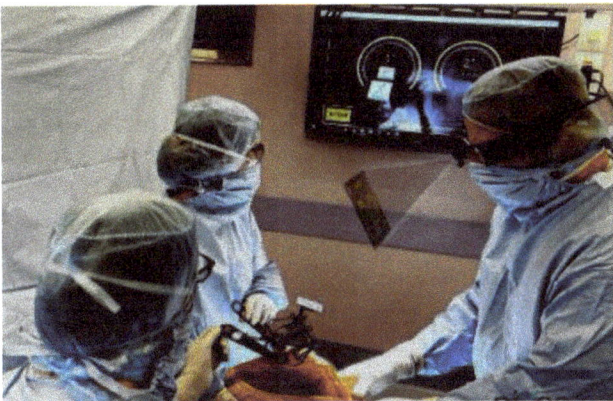

*Figure 9.1   Knee surgery with VuzixM400 AR smart glasses [14]*

AR and VR systems provide practical solutions for visualizations provide more efficient solutions for preventive health care and enhance the recovery time of physical theory. The use of AR and VR in training and education has grown significantly. For example, VR healthcare training effectively teaches human anatomy by clearly portraying each layer and the mechanics of the human body. Moreover, VR environments provide a location for patients to meditate in relaxing activities.

With the aid of technology, patients struggling with the disagreeable side effects of chronic illnesses can also discover a secure setting to get through mental obstacles.

## 9.3    Benefits of AR/VR in healthcare

### 9.3.1    Mental health and psychological therapy

VR/AR is used in clinical psychology to treat disorders and improve well-being. It gives a different environment [15] to the people.

It has been demonstrated that using VR in conjunction with olfactory displays can lessen stress, anxiety, and discomfort in psychiatric inpatients [16]. Playing games, fitness, watching movies, and meditation are the recreational activities reported by participants. The findings support that recreational use of VR can have a good impact on mental and physical health during periods of forced COVID lockdown [17] and that health professionals should consider VR therapy for mitigating the deleterious effects of long periods of isolation. Depression level among the people is increasing because of the shortage of resources during the COVID-19 pandemic period. The AR/VR benefits the effective treatment and diagnosis of mental health [18]. Patient with mental disorders and anxiety uses the AR/VR computer-generated situation using special high-end googles. It is used to treat dementia. The abnormal behavior of a patient with dementia is controlled in VR therapy.

### 9.3.2    Beats phobias

One of the most prevalent mental illnesses is phobias. The treatment with AR/VR reduced the participants' fear of facing their target. Because the elements that the patient is afraid of are virtual, they cannot harm them. The virtual elements in AR or VR scenes can appear whenever the therapist desires. It is as simple as running the program to gain access to the scene. The therapist controls the generation of stimuli, which can be repeated as many times as necessary. The order in which virtual elements appear can also be changed. The therapist has the ability to start and stop the program at any time. The therapist chooses the location of the program so he has complete control over all options. It can be very useful to treat patients with dental phobia [19] and blood-injury-injection phobia [20]. Guided imagery is a type of intervention where clients are informed to picture the situation and stimulate the entire experience. Then, under strict observation of their physical changes, they are instructed to work towards it.

### 9.3.3    Helping to train healthcare professionals

AR and VR overcome the limitations in the medical industry as it provides the 3D model for all the organs in the human body, wherein medical students can effectively practice and learn the medical procedures. Figure 9.2 depicts the 3D model of the heart for surgical training created by VR. Professors can expose new therapies and visualize the diagrams of bones and muscles in the form of VR. Anatomical information (shown in Figure 9.3) helps the healthcare worker to analyze the different categories of patients. This helps in understanding the level of injury. The anatomy of the brain and revolution in ophthalmology surgical training in VR is shown in Figures 9.4 and 9.5, respectively.

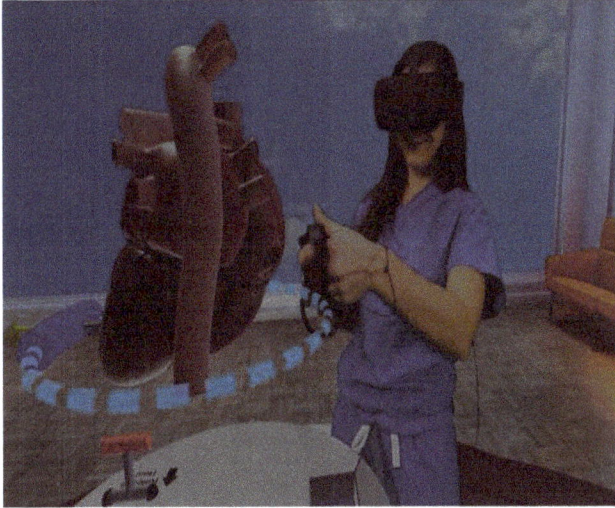

*Figure 9.2   3D model of heart for surgical training [21]*

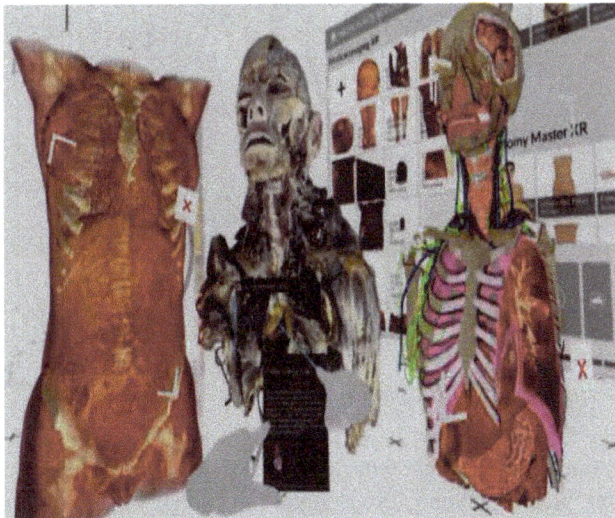

*Figure 9.3   Anatomical information [22]*

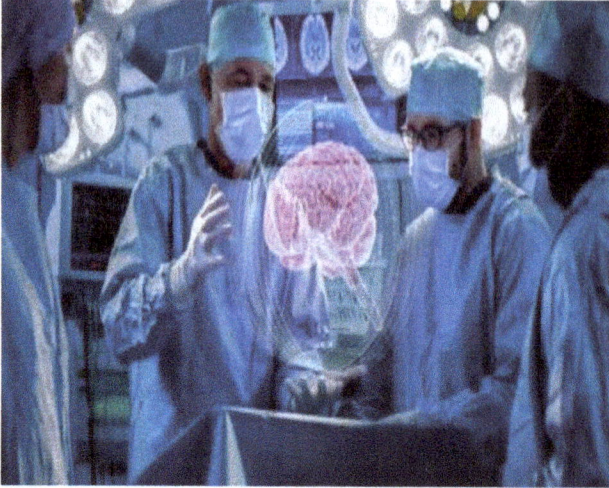

*Figure 9.4   Anatomy of the brain created by AR [23]*

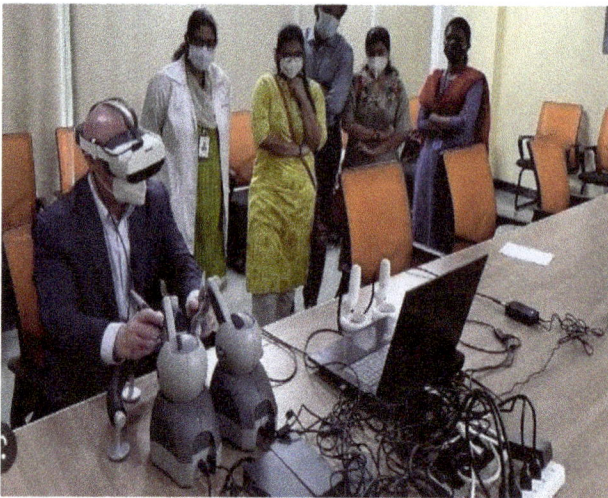

*Figure 9.5   Ophthalmic surgery training with VR [24]*

## 9.3.4   Assistance tool for surgeons

The procedure for the surgery is well trained in the virtual environment before being done to the patient hence it will reduce the mortality rate [25,26]. AR and VR assist surgeons in pre-planning procedures and better visualizing complex surgeries. 3D models improve surgeons' understanding of the anatomy and spatial relationships of organs, allowing them to better prepare for complex procedures

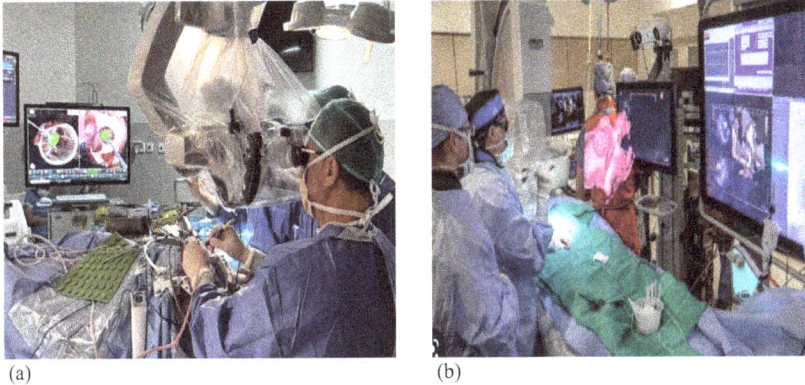

*Figure 9.6 (a) AR in neurosurgery [27]. (b) 4D hologram AR-guided structural heart procedure [28].*

that require access to difficult-to-reach areas. Because they are better prepared for what they will face, this improves patient outcomes and reduces risks during surgery. VR gives them an immersive experience, which can lead to more accurate diagnoses and fewer mistakes. AR and VR technologies can be used in any surgical field (shown in Figure 9.6), but their primary applications are in cardiothoracic surgery, orthopedic surgery, neurosurgery, and ophthalmology.

## 9.3.5 Pain management

The management of pain is becoming an increasingly important issue in healthcare. WHO is extremely worried about the opioid overdose problem in the USA as well as the risks and negative effects that can result from the abuse of painkillers worldwide. Painkiller drugs have inadequate analgesic effects and prominent side effects. VR therapy can potentially reduce acute pain (burn dressing change pain, needle-related procedural pain, postoperative dressing change pain, and thermal pain stimulus) than chronic pain (total knee arthroplasty pain, chronic low back pain, and cancer-related pain). Patients with chronic or difficult-to-treat pain are finding that AR and VR along with mindfulness training and stress reduction is a viable option. Through an immersive experience, AR/VR can help patients to forget about their discomfort and release endorphins, which last longer-lasting pain alleviation.

The fact that AR/VR therapy has few, if any, negative effects is a plus. VAS score measured during acute pain gets low, but this score cannot be differentiated in chronic pain. The application of VR is a useful tool for pediatric kids undergoing various medical procedures to control their pain. Psylaris [29] developed the readily available Oculus Go VR headset (Meta, California, USA). Participants using a VR headset, they are placed in a novel, relaxing, and diverting environment and asked to complete tasks that will help them unwind when anxious before and/or during a medical operation or throughout their hospital stay. The FPS-R scale is

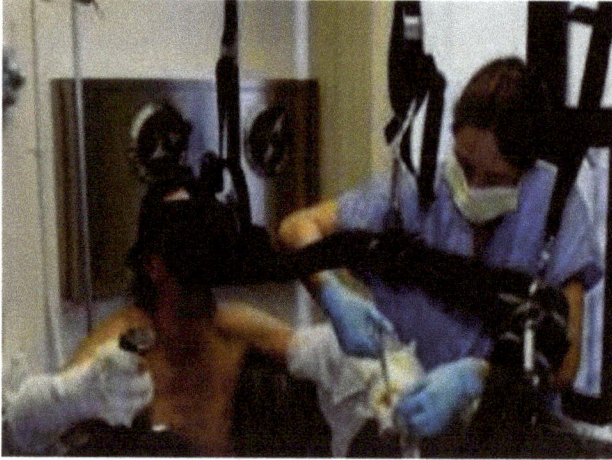

*Figure 9.7   Pain reduction using VR [31]*

used to assess the intensity of a child's acute pain from the ages of 4 or 5 [30]. The fiberoptic9 VR headset (Figure 9.7) enables patients to experience VR as they get wound care, debridement, and bandage changes in a hydro tank that is half submerged in water. The neurological correlates of VR pain can be examined.

## 9.4   Anxiety detection

Anxiety disorder is a sub-type of mental disease. Social anxiety disorders, specific phobias [32,33], panic disorders, separation anxiety disorders, and generalized anxiety disorders (GAD) are some of the most prevalent disorders [34].

### 9.4.1   GAD

It was crucial to look at the effects of a single exposure on anxiety levels to explore the use of VR as an affordable intervention for general anxiety. The effects of a VR experience created by StoryUp VR have numerous elements intended to lower anxiety. In particular, the design aspects were developed based on how mindfulness exercises and exposure to nature can help people relax and reduce anxiety. Additionally, there is mounting proof that stress and anxiety can be alleviated by mindfulness-based techniques.

GAD using a VR experience centered on nature and got encouraging results. This is in accordance with research that demonstrates how being in nature consistently lowers the stress response. This result was drawn from numerous studies and was acceptable when nature was depicted as plants, posters, presentations, movies, etc. A few physiological monitoring techniques, including detecting muscular tension, skin conductance, pulse transit time, cardiac reaction, and hormone levels, have been used to quantify these alterations in the stress response. During periods of rest or the VR intervention, self-reported anxiety symptoms and resting-state EEG were monitored. The analysis of EEG activity changes in Alpha and Beta activities as well as estimations of the current source densities in the relevant cingulate cortex areas are measured using sLORETA [35]. Findings showed that both the VR meditation and the quiet rest control condition dramatically raised alpha power and decreased subjective perceptions of anxiety.

The anterior cingulate cortex's wide and beta activity was dramatically lowered by the VR intervention, which had the unusual effect of moving proportional power from higher beta frequencies into lower beta frequencies. These outcomes are in line with a physiological decrease in anxiety. When exposed to VR images, the patient may experience a relaxation state, but in traditional therapy, the therapist would vocally identify this state. The peaceful and stressful environments are created via the VR environment programmed NeuroVR (version 1.5) [36] (shown in Figure 9.8). Several physiological monitoring techniques, such as measuring muscular tension, skin conductance, pulse transit time, cardiac reaction, and hormone levels, have been used to quantify the changes in the stress response. To track the person's progress, information is gathered via the electromyography sensor, blood volume pulse sensor, skin conductance response sensor, and respiration sensor.

## 9.4.2   Social anxiety disorder (SAD)

It is a type of mental disorder with a high level of suffering and stress and being in an embarrassed state during social gatherings. Social interaction provokes and safety behavior are the main characteristics of SAD. Patients are instructed to forego avoidance or safety behaviors and face the feared situation during exposure-based behavioral experiments to test their pathogenic beliefs and modify

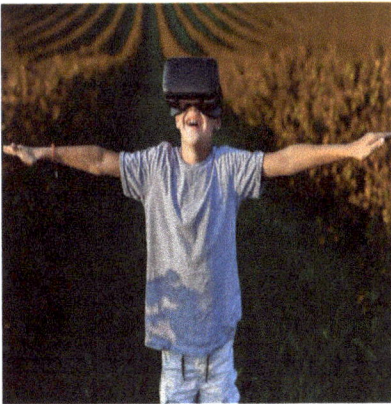
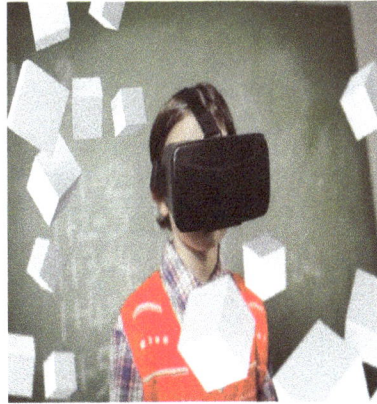

(a)                                           (b)

*Figure 9.8   (a) NeuroVR facilitates relaxation environment. (b) NeuroVR facilitates stressful environment.*

dysfunctional cognitive processes [37]. Average waiting time of 20 weeks for psychiatric treatment and pre-treatment latencies are the drawbacks of SAD therapy. VR can overcome these drawbacks. This therapy includes behavioral experiments which improve the quality of life and reduce social anxiety. VRET has emerged as an important therapeutic tool for simulating relevant social situations within a therapeutic context, and it has been shown to have the potential to elicit the social distress that patients experience. Human interaction with virtual system lowers the level of social anxiety and improves self-efficacy within 3 months [38].

### 9.4.3   *Specific phobias*

AR and VR are used to treat many kinds of phobias (pathological fear) including the fear of natural environment, small animals (cockroaches, spiders, lizards, and rats), mutilation/medical treatment and situations. AR Toolkit 2.65 software with VRML support [39] creates the virtual images of small animals. In a session of AR exposure, the patient was extremely anxious. AR exposure (Figure 9.9) was effective in treating aversion to small animals. Prior to the AR cockroach exposure session, the patient was unable to get close to a terrarium that contained an active cockroach. After the therapy, the patient was able to approach a live cockroach and kill. Subjective unit of discomfort scale (SUDS) is used to measure the anxiety level. SUDS score changes from 10 to 0 after the exposure therapy [41].

Claustrophobia is the fear of a closed or small space. VR develops the interconnected room to increase the symptoms of claustrophobia. The first room created by VR is a small, dark, and windowless room and the second room is bright and spacious.

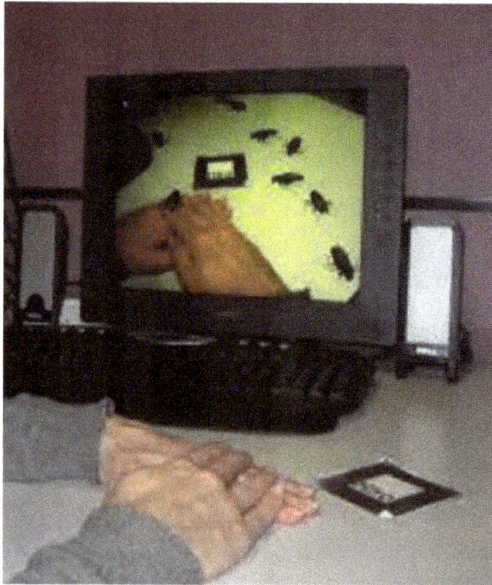

*Figure 9.9   AR exposure to cockroach [40]*

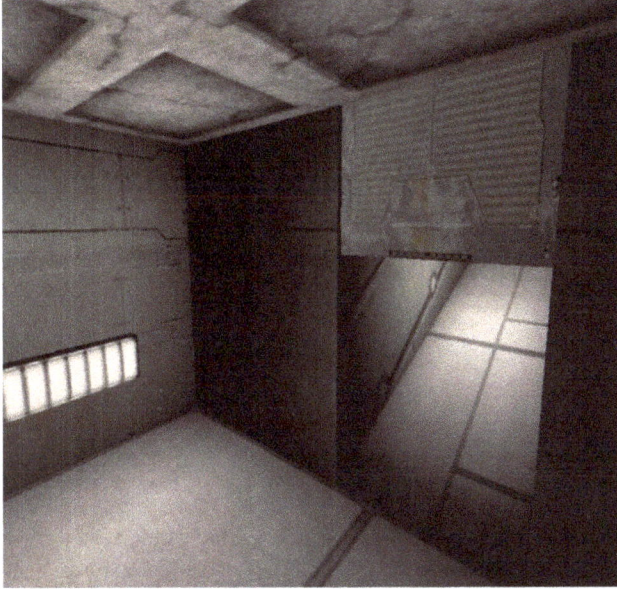

*Figure 9.10    User view in HMD [43]*

The door gets closed while the patient enters the room [42]. The images shown in VR software in HMD (head-mounted device) are depicted in Figure 9.10.

## 9.5    AR/VR-based approaches for anxiety management

It is quite common that a patient will be nervous about the procedures to be carried out, particularly in the case of a surgery. Bringing down the anxiety level of a patient is of paramount importance. There were scenarios where surgeries were delayed due to high blood pressure levels of patients. To bring down the anxiety levels of patients, it is important to study the patients' mindset and understand whether they are in a state of mind to understand the medical procedures to be carried out. In case they are capable of understanding the procedure, they can be subjected to VR scenes depicting the procedures. Features like audio and labeling of parts will pave the way for a better immersive experience. In case the patients are not capable of understanding the procedures, they need to be distracted with VR scenes depicting natural scenes based on their personal choice. This practice is outlined in Figure 9.11.

## 9.6    Technological tools for AR/VR-based patient-anxiety management

After deciding the scenes required for providing an immersive experience for patients, the scenes should be modeled in software. Notable software are Unreal

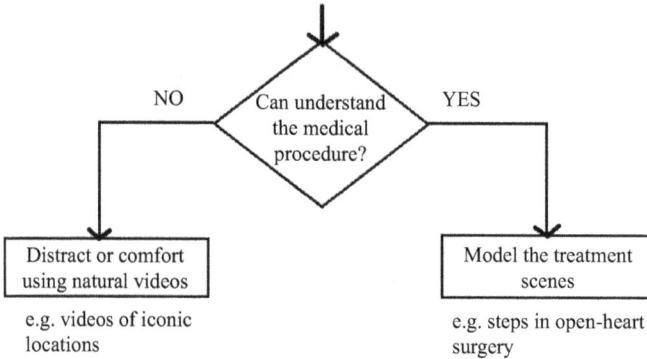

*Figure 9.11    Anxiety management using AR/VR*

Engine (UE) and Unity. Unreal is the video gaming software published GT Interactive for Microsoft Windows in 1998. There were several versions of the software released in regular intervals, with the recent one being Unreal Engine 5 released in 2021. Unity, cross-platform gaming software was first released in 2005. A professional version of Unity's products known as Unity Pro is available in the market. The choice of software is dependent on the type of scenes to be created. Similarly, the choice of hardware depends on the complexity of the scene to be modeled. Notable VR kit manufacturers are HoloLens headset by Microsoft, VR headset by Oculus, Playstation VR by Sony, and AR kit by Apple [44].

## 9.7    Conclusion

In this chapter, we have given impact and well-being of AR/VR in health care. Some of the software and hardware used in AR/VR technology are explored. Most of the prevalent anxiety disorder detection and management using AR/VR are discussed. An immersive experience through AR or VR in many biomedical applications is depicted. It is becoming clear that AR is a viable tool for the treatment of psychological problems.

## References

[1]   Q. Huang, J. Lin, R. Han, C. Peng, and A. Huang, Using virtual reality exposure therapy in pain management: a systematic review and meta-analysis of randomized controlled trials. *Value Health*. 2022;25(2):288–301.

[2]   R. Buettner, H. Baumgartl, T. Konle, and P. Haag, A review of virtual reality and augmented reality literature in healthcare. In: *IEEE Symposium on Industrial Electronics & Applications (ISIEA)*, 9 September 2020; 19950257:1–6.

[3]   J. Roessel, M. Knoell, J. Hofmann, and R. Buettner, A systematic literature review of practical virtual and augmented reality solutions in surgery. In:

*IEEE 44th Annual Computers, Software, and Applications Conference (COMPSAC)*, Madrid, Spain, 22 September 2020;0730-3157:489–498.

[4]  J. Carroll, L. Hopper, A.M. Farrelly, R. Lombard-Vance, P.D. Bamidis, and A. Konstantinidis, Scoping review of augmented/virtual reality health and wellbeing interventions for older adults: redefining immersive virtual reality. *Front Virtual Real.* 2021;2:655338.

[5]  A.W.K. Yeung, A. Tosevska, E. Klager, *et al.*, Virtual and augmented reality applications in medicine: analysis of the scientific literature. *J Med Internet Res.* 2021;23(2):e25499.

[6]  G. Bansal, K. Rajgopal, V. Chamola, Z. Xiong, and D. Niyato, Healthcare in metaverse: a survey on current metaverse applications in healthcare. *IEEE Access*, 2022;10:119914–119946.

[7]  H. Li, W. Dong, Z. Wang, *et al.*, Effect of a virtual reality-based restorative environment on the emotional and cognitive recovery of individuals with mild-to-moderate anxiety and depression. *Int J Environ Res Public Health.* 2021;18(17):9053.

[8]  G. Mayer, N. Gronewold, K. Polte, *et al.*, Experiences of patients and therapists testing a virtual reality exposure app for symptoms of claustrophobia: mixed methods study. *JMIR Ment Health.* 2022;9(12):e40056.

[9]  M. Fiorentino, M. Dastan, S. Ajroudi, A. Boccaccio, and A.E. Uva, Addressing vicious cycle of medical distress with augmented reality: state-of-the-art review. In K. Subburaj, K. Sandhu, and S. Ćuković (eds.), *Revolutions in Product Design for Healthcare: Advances in Product Design and Design Methods for Healthcare*, Springer, 2022:35–51.

[10]  J. Urlings, S. Sezer, M. terLaan, *et al.* The role and effectiveness of augmented reality in patient education: a systematic review of the literature. *Patient Educ Counsel.* 2022;105(7):1917–1927.

[11]  R.R. Bruno, N. Bruining, C. Jung, M. Kelm, G. Wolff, and B. Wernly, & The VR-ICU Study group, Virtual reality in intensive care. *Intensive Care Med.* 2022;48(9):1227–1229.

[12]  Webpage: https://www.northshore.org/healthy-you/from-googles-to-giggles/ (last accessed: 27 March 2023).

[13]  T. Oing and J. Prescott, Implementations of virtual reality for anxiety-related disorders: systematic review. *JMIR Serious Games.* 2018;6(4):e10965.

[14]  Webpage: https://www.prnewswire.com/ (last accessed: 5 February 2023).

[15]  S. Ventura, R.M. Baños, and C. Botella, Virtual and augmented reality: new frontiers for clinical psychology. *State of the Art Virtual Reality and Augmented Reality Knowhow.* 2018;10:74344.

[16]  D. Tomasi, H. Ferris, L. Enman, E. Reyns, P. Booraem, and S. Gates, Olfactory virtual reality (OVR) for wellbeing and reduction of stress, anxiety and pain. *J Med Res Health Sci.* 2021;4(3):1212–1221.

[17]  A. Siani and S.A. Marley, Impact of the recreational use of virtual reality on physical and mental wellbeing during the Covid-19 lockdown. *Health Technol.* 2021;11(2):425–435.

[18]   S.B. Goyal, P. Bedi, and N. Garg, AR and VR and AI allied technologies and depression detection and control mechanism. In: S. Kautish, S.L. Peng, and A.J. Obaid (eds.), *Computational Intelligence Techniques for Combating COVID-19. EAI/Springer Innovations in Communication and Computing.* Springer, Cham, 2021;395:203–229.

[19]   K.R. Gujjar, R. Sharma, and A. De Jongh, Virtual reality exposure therapy for treatment of dental phobia. *Dent. Update.* 2017;44(5):423–424, 427–428, 431–432, 435.

[20]   M.Y.W. Jiang, E. Upton, and J.M. Newby, A randomised wait-list controlled pilot trial of one-session virtual reality exposure therapy for blood-injection-injury phobias. *J Affect Disord.* 2020;276:636–645.

[21]   Webpage: www.stanfordchildrens.org (last accessed: 10 February 2023).

[22]   Webpage: www.viveport.com (last accessed: 15 February 2023).

[23]   Webpage: https://provenreality.com/ (last accessed: 4 March 2023).

[24]   Webpage: https://www.alcon.com/ (last accessed: 10 March 2023).

[25]   M. Larobina and L Murino, Medical image file formats. *J Digit Imaging.* 2013;2:200–206.

[26]   E.L. Wisotzky, J.-C. Rosenthal, P. Eisert, *et al.*, Interactive and multimodal-based augmented reality for remote assistance using a digital surgical microscope. In *IEEE Conference on Virtual Reality and 3D User Interfaces (VR)*, 15 Aug 2019:1477–1484.

[27]   Webpage: https://neuronewsinternational.com/ (last accessed: 17 March 2023).

[28]   Webpage: www.dicardiology.com/ (last accessed: 19 March2023).

[29]   Psylaris. www.psylaris.com (last accessed: 22 March 2023).

[30]   S. Bernaerts, B. Bonroy, J. Daems, *et al.*, Virtual reality for distraction and relaxation in a pediatric hospital setting: an interventional study with a mixed-methods design. *Front Digit Health.* 2022;4:866119.

[31]   Webpage: https://depts.washington.edu/ (last accessed: 26 March 2023).

[32]   M.C. Juan, M. Alcaniz, C. Monserrat, C. Botella, R.M. Banos, and B. Guerrero, Using augmented reality to treat phobias. *IEEE Comput Grap Appl.* 2005;25(6):31–37.

[33]   Juan, M. C., & Pérez, D. (2010).Using augmented and virtual reality for the development of acrophobic scenarios: Comparison of the levels of presence and anxiety. *Computers & Graphics,* Dec 2010;34(6):756–766.

[34]   A. Gorini and G. Riva, The potential of virtual reality as anxiety management tool: a randomized controlled study in a sample of patients affected by generalized anxiety disorder. *Trials.* 2008;9:25.

[35]   J. Tarrant, J. Viczko, and H. Cope, Virtual reality for anxiety reduction demonstrated by quantitative EEG: a pilot study. *Front. Psycho.* 2018;9:1280.

[36]   G. Riva, A. Gaggioli, D. Villani, *et al.*, NeuroVR: an open source virtual reality platform for clinical psychology and behavioral neurosciences. *Stud Health Technol Inform.* 2007;125:394–399.

[37]  F. Schreiber, C. Heimlich, C. Schweitzer, and U. Stangier, Cognitive therapy for social anxiety disorder: the impact of the "self-focused attention and safety behaviours experiment" on the course of treatment. *Behav Cogn Psychother*. 2015;43(2):158–166.

[38]  N. Morina, W.P. Brinkman, D. Hartanto, I.L. Kampmann, and P.M.G. Emmelkamp. Social interactions in virtual reality exposure therapy: a proof-of-concept pilot study. *Technol Health Care*. 2015;23(5):581–589.

[39]  ARToolkit version 2.65vrml, http://www.hitl.washington.ed/artoolkit, 2004.

[40]  Webpage: www.technologyreview.com/ (last accessed: 26 March 2023).

[41]  F. Fatharany, R.R. Hariadi, D. Herumurti, and A. Yuniarti, Augmented reality application for cockroach phobia therapy using everyday objects as marker substitute. In *International Conference on Information & Communication Technology and Systems (ICTS)*, 27 April 2017, 2:49–52.

[42]  M. Bruce and H. Regenbrecht, A virtual reality claustrophobia therapy system – implementation and test. In *2009 IEEE Virtual Reality Conference*, Lafayette,7 April 2009:179–182.

[43]  Webpage: https://karellen.artstation.com/ (last accessed: 26 March 2023).

[44]  S. Narayanan, N.N. Ramesh, A.K. Tyagi, L. Jani Anbarasi, and B. Edwin Raj, Current trends, challenges, and future prospects for augmented reality and virtual reality. In A. Tyagi (ed.), *Multimedia and Sensory Input for Augmented, Mixed, and Virtual Reality*, 2021:275–281.

*Chapter 10*

# Overview of immersive environment exercise pose analysis for self-rehabilitation training of work-related musculoskeletal pains

*Vijayakumar Ponnusamy[1], Dilliraj Ekambaram[1], T.N. Suresh[2], S.F. Mariyam Farzana[2] and Tariq Ahamed Ahanger[3]*

## Abstract

Exercise therapy is a protracted, difficult, and tiresome procedure in rehabilitating various physical disabilities due to recent working conditions in software, health-care professionals, teaching communities, etc. From the perspective of self-rehabilitation training, the technological impact creates numerous solutions to analyze whether the patient/human is performing the exercises properly without any mistakes, as the physicians expect. In this chapter, initially, we explore a variety of physical disabilities due to the working environment, which is elaborated in existing works of literature. Second, review the various implementations of augmented reality (AR) and virtual reality (VR) and how it predicts the correctness of various exercise poses, pose estimation techniques, pros, and cons, and summarize the techniques employed in the immersive visual exercise pose analysis and the outcomes of its experiments through implications of different deep learning algorithms. The system's performance can be increased by optimizing depth analysis to result in the identification of more petite body part movements, adding more features, such as contour identification and more meta-attributes for particular points in 3D reconstruction on participants, scaling up the computational power, and focusing on the current model's refinement to achieve more accuracy and development of a multi-stage ensemble process. Without large datasets for analysis, the system's efficiency is relatively low. To maximize accuracy, real-time enhancement is necessary. More real-time data are required for training and testing to improve the best-effort solutions for classifying the user's exercise pose as

[1]Department of Electronics and Communication Engineering, SRM Institute of Science and Technology, Chennai, India
[2]SRM College of Physiotherapy, SRM Institute of Science and Technology, Chennai, India
[3]College of Computer Engineering and Sciences, Prince Sattam bin Abdulaziz University, Saudi Arabia

proper or improper. To assist the research methodology on imperfections analysis in developing a new plan for future investigations, the correctness of exercise pose mistakes is visualized, and instructing the participants do it properly through audio feedback also.

**Keywords:** Musculoskeletal pain; Microsoft HoloLens; AR-robot; Wearable sensor devices; AR & VR rehabilitation training

## 10.1    Introduction

The largest impacted population is 44.1 crores in high-income countries, 42.7 crores in the WHO Western Pacific Region, and 3.69 crores in the WHO Region of South-East Asia [1]. Currently, the population with musculoskeletal health issues is ~1.71 billion around the globe, as reported by the World Health Organization (WHO) [2]. From birth to old age, musculoskeletal disorders are relevant to everyone. They range from acute, transient diseases (like fractures, sprains, and strains, which cause pain and functional restrictions) to severe illnesses such as osteoarthritis and persistent primary low back pain. Soft tissues, skeletons, joints, and surrounding connective tissues must all be in good shape for the locomotor system to function properly. Musculoskeletal issues affect people of all ages, although the prevalence varies with age and diagnosis.

Musculoskeletal impairments, characterized by muscles, bones, joints, and adjacent connective tissue abnormalities, can be brought on by more than 150 medical illnesses. Along with increasing the chance of developing noncommunicable diseases like cardiovascular disease, musculoskeletal disorders frequently co-exist with other non-communicable conditions. These problems can cause temporary or permanent limits in human activity. Pain (often persistent) and mobility and dexterity restrictions are the usual symptoms of musculoskeletal problems, which may hinder people's ability to work and participate in social activities.

Additionally, those who have musculoskeletal diseases are more likely to experience mental health problems. The most significant portion of the world's rehabilitation needs for musculoskeletal disorders. They account for over two-thirds of all adults who require rehabilitation and are one of the biggest contributors to the need for services for children. For instance, low back discomfort is the primary cause of early retirement from the workforce, whereas pediatric autoimmune inflammatory disorders like juvenile arthritis impact children's development. Early retirement has a significant negative social impact on direct and indirect healthcare expenses (such as lost productivity at work). According to projections, the number of persons who suffer from low back pain will rise in the future, and this increase will happen significantly more quickly in low- and middle-income countries. In Section 10.1.1, we deliberated the work-related health issues and rehabilitation exercises, and Section 10.1.2 shows the summary of augmented reality (AR)/virtual reality (VR)-based rehabilitation systems.

### 10.1.1 *Work-related health issues and their rehabilitation exercises*

Occupational health problems risk factors include working with hands above shoulder height or below knee height, carrying heavy loads, and lifting objects that weigh more than a certain amount. Strain injuries are the primary cause, as are repetitive motion injuries, cumulative trauma disorders, worker age, and working with hands in these positions. Figure 10.1 shows the mapping of various work-related health issues and the prescribed rehabilitation training by physiotherapists.

In Indian societies, the specific incidence of MSDs is 20%, and the occupation-based prevalence is 90% [1]. Musculoskeletal disorders brought on by employment result in lost workdays, decreased productivity, and poor quality of life (QoL). Work-related MSDs can harm employees' quality of life (QoL) and significantly burden businesses and organizations due to lost productivity, the need to educate new employees, and compensation costs.

### 10.1.2 *Summary of AR/VR-based rehabilitation systems*

AR has recently caught the public's interest as a potential alternative for conventional computer–human interfaces in a number of industries, including manufacturing, education, training, the aerospace and military sectors, gaming, and medicine. This is because of their user-friendly design and ongoing interaction with the consumers' actual surroundings.

The AR interaction keeps people immersed in their actual surroundings by superimposing perception data created by a computer over a real-world setting. A touchscreen, keyboard, and mouse-based desktop environment is less natural and more intuitive than AR technologies' user interfaces. Table 10.1 summarizes the various existing AR/VR rehabilitation system's inferences, hardware and software tools used, measured parameters, and each system's research findings.

An intelligent video surveillance system based on tiny implants will be used to address the problems focused on a human aberrant scenario [12]. "Human posture estimate," a popular AI technique, determines the location and orientation of the

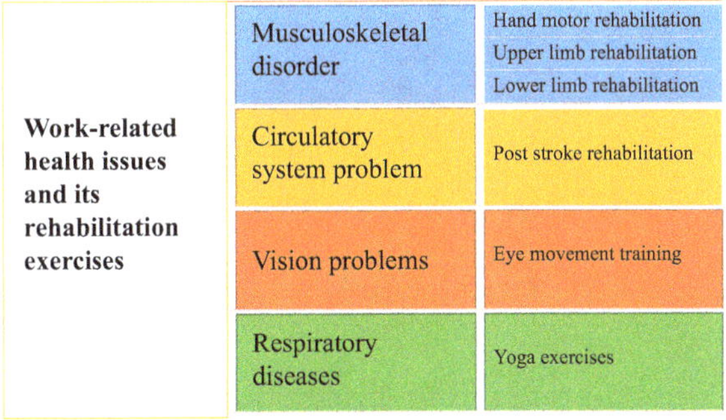

*Figure 10.1 Mapping of work-related health issues and its rehabilitation exercises*

*Table 10.1  Summary of various existing AR/VR rehabilitation systems*

| Reference | Inferences | Hardware and software used | Parameters measured | Research findings |
|---|---|---|---|---|
| Kim et al. [3] | The main characteristic of the system is to provide the self-report discomfort analysis for neck and shoulder human body parts through a biomechanical stress sensor system via AR interaction | Microsoft Kinect, biomechanical stress sensors with Ag/AgCl electrodes, and eight cameras were used to collect kinematic data with 100 frames per second | Right ulnar styloid, right wrist radial styloid, right acromion, right elbow lateral epicondyle, and right middle finger second metacarpal head | Biomechanical stress sensor-based systems cannot afford to provide accuracy on particular exercises performed by the user |
| Xiao et al. [4] | For patients with movement disorders who are at or above Brunnstrom Stage III and have certain motor abilities through a VR rehabilitation system with Kinect sensor | Kinect sensors and Unity SDK | Elbow flexion/extension, shoulder flexion/extension, and shoulder abduction/adduction | To motivate the participants to do more exercises by implementing the system in an interactive environment |
| Cavalcanti et al. [5] | Assessing the success rate of the ARknoidAR tool through a questionnaire and System Usability Score (SUS) | Kinect sensor and canvas game engine | Arm movements | Determining the system response time will improve the SUS score, and providing positive exercise feedback encourages the participants to enhance their volunteer participation |
| Martins et al. [6] | Implementing neurological disease rehabilitation through the serious game with image processing technique | Kinect Sensor and Unity SDK | Exercise program selected for the Physioland Game.(a) Hip joint abduction and adduction; (b) radioumeral joint flexion and extension; (c) Glenohumeral joint abduction and adduction; (d) Cross movement; and (e) Pulleys | This serious gaming in VR platform helps the participants to make them comfortable to attend the traditional physiotherapy training. This framework only aids the participants in playing the various rehabilitation exercises in a virtual environment, but how accurate the participants perform the exercise pose was not assessed. |

*(Continues)*

| Reference | Description | Technology | Application | Future work/limitations |
|---|---|---|---|---|
| Alves et al. [7] | With the adaptation of a virtual gaming approach for physical upper-limb rehabilitation training to patients via a visual feedback user interface | Built-in optical motion tracker GUI with Kinect sensor | Upper-limb abduction/adduction and flexion/extension | Patients with difficulty adjustment problem were not included in this study and display is shown in small screen, so participants cannot visualize the feedback properly |
| Hooks et al. [8] | Usability acceptance study for the two different approaches, namely, flat based or bowl based, was compared and the final result was evaluated | FODT Cyberith Virtualizer and the BODT VirtuixOmni with oculus rift and Unity SDK | User walking experience on FODT and BODT in VR environment | User movement detection has to be incorporated with the system to analyze the accuracy of particular task performed by the user |
| Powell et al. [9] | Through the use of machine learning (XG Boost) and patient observation, an immersive VR (iVR) pipeline may replicate the success metrics for physical therapy | Microsoft Kinect, biomechanical stress sensors with Ag/AgCl electrodes, 8 Cameras used to collect kinematic data with 100 frames per seconds and Unity SDK | Shoulder internal/external/abducted rotation, side/forward arm raise, mixed press/circle | Comparison of accuracy and other performance metrics like time complexity and computational speed with other machine learning algorithms need to be done |
| Tannous et al. [10] | To create and assess a new engineering system as a remedy for home functional rehabilitation. | Network of inertial sensors mounted on various body parts as well as a Kinect camera | Upper and Lower limb rehabilitation exercises | Investigation of data privacy and security needs to be ensured by the investigators |
| Heiyanthuduwa et al. [11] | Making a virtual reality home-care physiotherapy system for seniors that focuses on full-body rehabilitation | Max30100 and temperature sensor, Microsoft Kinect sensor and MPU9250 sensors are utilized to record body movements | Upper/lower limb rehabilitation exercises | System to be enhanced for remote session access by the user from home |

*Table 10.2    Pros and cons of pose estimation techniques*

| Pose estimation techniques | Pros | Cons |
|---|---|---|
| OpenCV | Very simple and inbuilt image processing tools | Poor real-time performance and lack of customization options available |
| OpenPose | Real-time full body key points detection can be done | Perform well GPU compared CPU and it is used only for non-commercial purpose |
| PoseNet | Lightweight model for multi-person detection and fast inference | Insufficient for some pose analysis use cases and provide moderate accuracy for pose detection |
| Detectron2 | Provide high accuracy and large number of models available | Not supportive to real-time applications especially in CPU environment |
| AlphaPose | Provides multi-person detection in high speed and accuracy | Not run well on a CPU in real-time and is for non-commercial use |

human body based on a photograph of a person. An image of a person is used by pose estimation, one of the most used AI techniques, to establish the bodily positioning and orientation. Table 10.2 shows the pros and cons of various pose estimation techniques used for human pose estimate system [13].

## 10.2    AR/VR rehabilitation systems

Users can interact with other things in real time using AR and VR environments. There are three common methods implied in the immersive rehabilitation systems. In the first method, individuals with damaged respiratory systems can regain proper breathing by using a GUI-based trainer. To increase the patients' lung capacity, feedback and instructions are given using the user data collected from the pulse monitor attached to the patients. The second method offers a thorough visualizing method for looking into intricate medical processes. The third endoscopic method under consideration eliminates the requirement for a second physician by using foot control rather than hands to operate some of the equipment [14]. The following subsection deliberated the various existing AR/VR rehabilitation approaches.

### 10.2.1    Biomechanical stress sensor-based system

One of the biomechanical stress sensor systems constructed with the eight cameras captures the 3-D optical motion of a human. The kinematics data are collected from the optical motion system with a frame rate of 100 fps. The muscle activities of humans as EMG data are acquired through surface electrodes Ag/AgCl. An experimental setup shows that the 13 different biomechanical sensors were placed in upper human body parts to identify the tasks (Tasks include the 3-D Cube, Omni-directional Pointing, and Web Browsing) performed by the users [3]. To construct AR interfaces and interactions, the wearable head-mounted device named Microsoft HoloLens [15] or Redmond was employed. Figure 10.2 depicts the experiment procedure for the biomechanical stress sensor-based AR task-performing system.

## 10.2.2　Kinect sensor-based system

Most of the immersive system for rehabilitation training utilizes Microsoft Kinect capture system for collecting the action performed by the patients/users [3–7,9–11]. Patients do not need to wear any form of markers when utilizing Kinect because the data is sufficient. It increases the system's autonomy so that anyone can use it at home without prior knowledge. If not, the system would need to be installed in training facilities where patients would have to travel and waste time while the therapists installed the markers. Figure 10.3 shows the Microsoft Kinect-based system process.

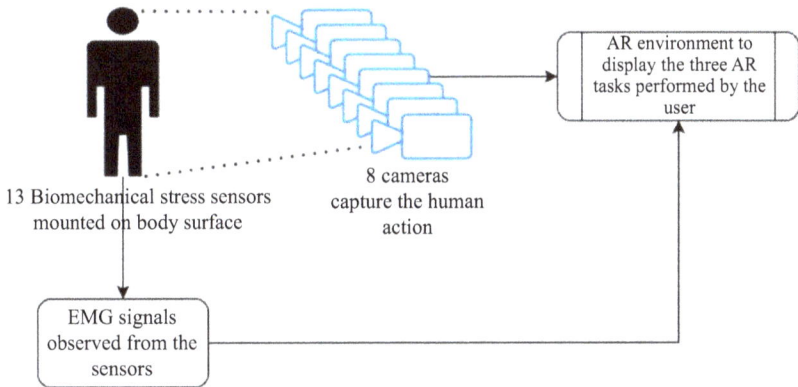

*Figure 10.2　Biomechanical stress sensor-based AR task system [15]*

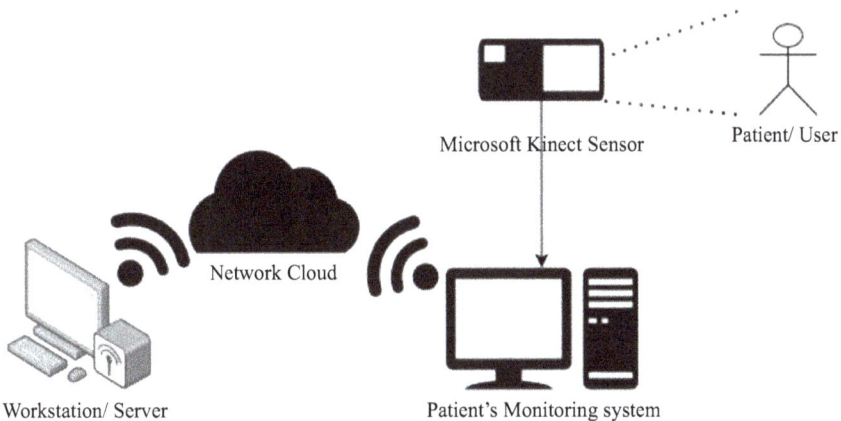

*Figure 10.3　Microsoft Kinect-based system process [16]*

In fact, some elderly and young patients find it difficult to wait while the markers are being set. Leaning, squatting, reaching, and jumping are all actions that might be helpful in the rehabilitation gait, balance, motor control, and strength/flexibility in many popular Xbox Kinect games. Microsoft's depth-sensing camera, Kinect, provides us with data about depth, color, and the skeletons of persons who are in front of it [16]. Each person's angles and poses are calculated using this information.

## 10.2.3    VR walking simulator system

Treadmills are a key component of the system used to navigate humans interacting in virtual environments. Given that the majority of researchers use linear treadmill systems in their deployment strategies. However, this treadmill device allows us to experience linear motion in a virtual setting. But given the diverse rehabilitation scenarios, walking is one of the promising exercises to recover from diseases that cause lower limb discomfort [17]. Walking in a straight path will only make the user or patient more bored and prevent them from experiencing the virtual world. To provide the experience of the virtual world in an immersive environment, one of the researchers presented the system in an omnidirectional treadmill. The device named, BODT-Virtuix Omni and FODT-Cyberith Virtualizer VR [8], will give the virtual real-time experience in an immersive view.

## 10.2.4    Wearable sensors-based rehabilitation

EEG feeling assessment could aid in the diagnosis or recovery of particular illnesses. With the use of three different deep-learning models that can categorize emotions, four emotions – happy, surprised, angry, and sad – were created as positive and negative emotions. Accelerometer is very useful in tracking human linear motion compared with wiimote sensors [18]. Mobile devices will be gathered and tested on a range of materials, mostly from input and output, in order to conduct 2D research [19]. EEG-based signal processing system provides feedback to the users by placing the electrodes in the body joint parts of the human body. In the past ten years, electroencephalography (EEG) [20], which examines the electrical movement of the brain, has produced convincing results among the different techniques for measuring emotion.

## 10.2.5    Robot-AR

Robotic therapy is increasingly being used frequently due to robots' strength, capacity for repetitive action, capacity for reprogramming, and potential adaption to new tasks. These characteristics enable the use of robots in therapy disciplines like physical therapy and emotional therapy [21]. Figure 10.4 shows the flow diagram of AR robot. The user is given a real paint roller to apply paint to a moveable physical wall that is put in the same space as the virtual wall in the robot-AR scenario. To the right of the display is where the robot's end-effector is located. This setup reduces occlusions on the projection display brought on by the user's arm and robot motions and provides the user with an intuitive comprehension of the simulated work.

## 10.2.6    Serious games for exercise rehabilitation (SGER)

Physical therapy called "exercise rehabilitation" uses exercise to help patients regain their motor, cognitive, and emotional abilities. Patients who require exercise

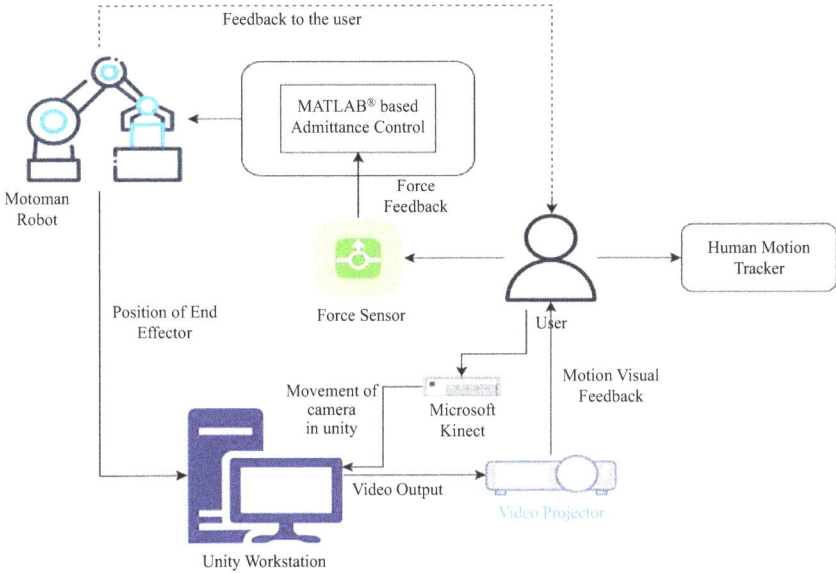

*Figure 10.4   Flow diagram of AR robot [21]*

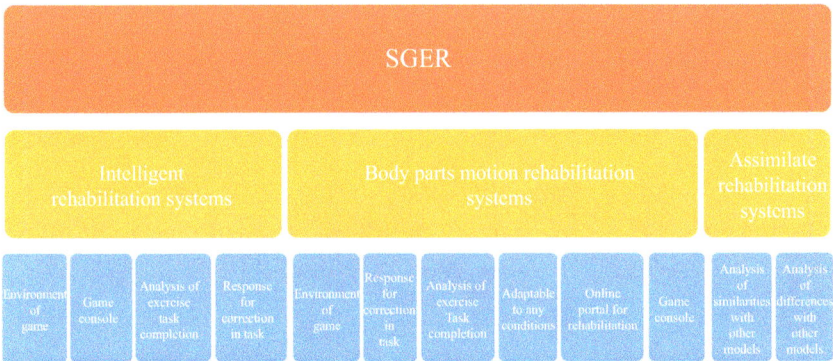

*Figure 10.5   Categories of SGER for rehabilitation training [22]*

therapy frequently have dyskinesia and cognitive impairment to variable degrees, which requires the creation of games with a development on player–game interaction. Additionally, we examined the traits of various user groups and the particular features of the games that catered to them. The solitary functioning of the game is utterly undermined by the 3D motion camera known as Kinect. Dynamic capture, influence identification, microphone input, voice recognition, and social interaction are some of the features of Kinect [22]. Figure 10.5 shows the categories of SGER for exercise-based rehabilitation.

## 10.3    Deep learning approaches for visual exercise pose analysis

In this section, we described the various approaches of deep learning-based exercise pose analysis systems for various images or video classification and prediction system.

### 10.3.1    Baseline convolutional neural network (CNN)

The process in this architecture comprises various layers namely, Input, Convolutional, Max Pooling, Rectified Linear (ReLu), Batch Normalization, Softmax, and Classification layers. The input is fetched in this CNN model with the size of 18 × 10 × 1, then the convolutional block uses 8 filters to produce the output feature maps with the size of 3 × 3.

Max_Pooling reduces the dimension of the input as 2 × 2 from convolution layer. ReLu activation function pulls out the maximum value of an input. By modifying and scaling the activations, the batch normalization layer normalizes the input layer.

Using batch normalization lessens the covariance shift. By dividing by the batch standard deviation and removing the batch mean, batch normalization normalizes the output of a prior activation layer.

The total output from the neurons is fetched to the input of softmax from a fully connected layer. Then, finding the probabilities of each input with values varies from 0 to 1. This process helps to classify the input image which is shown in Figure 10.6.

Considering the expression for baseline, CNN 2D convolution layer is written as,

$$f[x,y] = (g * k)[x,y] = \Sigma\Sigma k[m,n]g[x-m, y-n]nm \tag{10.1}$$

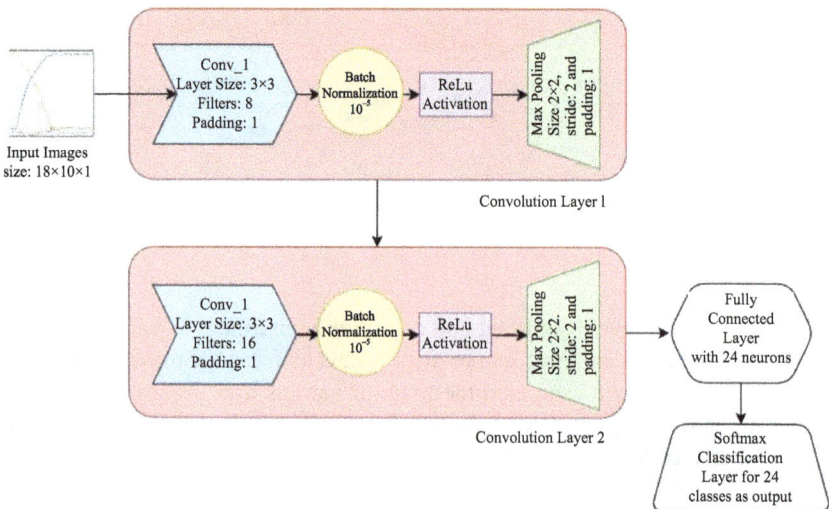

*Figure 10.6    CNN architecture for exercise status identification system*

The symbol for the input picture is "*g*," and the symbol for the kernel is "*k*." The convolution kernel's "*x* and *y*" and the output matrix's "*m,n*" rows-and-column indexes.

## 10.3.2    CNN – long short-term memory (LSTM)

The CNN-LSTM is a hybrid deep learning CNN model category to strengthen the output prediction through LSTM. Extracted features from CNN are given to the LSTM; the LSTM captures the temporal dependencies from the input images and provides the classification output with the help of the softmax activation function. Figure 10.7 displays the structure of video-based exercise pose classification using CNN-LSTM.

According to CNN-LSTM, the memory cell in the architecture is difficult to remodel. LSTM unit [18] done by using the following equation in CNN architecture:

$$ft = \sigma(Wf.[ht-1, xt] + bf) \tag{10.2}$$

$$it = \sigma(Wi.[ht-1, xt] + bi) \tag{10.3}$$

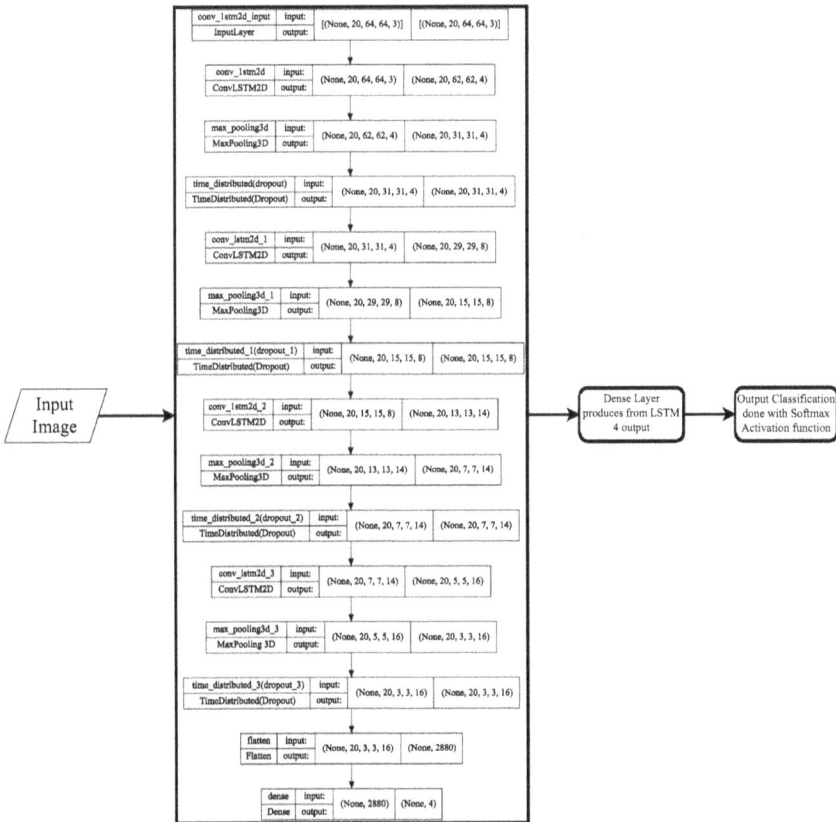

*Figure 10.7    CNN-LSTM architecture for four types of human activity recognition [18]*

$$Ctemp = \tanh(WC.[ht-1,xt]+bC) \tag{10.4}$$

$$Ct = f1 * Ct - 1 + it * Ctemp \tag{10.5}$$

$$Ot = \sigma(W0.[ht-1,xt]+bo) \tag{10.6}$$

$$ht = ot * \tanh(Ct) \tag{10.7}$$

where $i$ – input gate, $C$ – cell activation vectors, O – output gate, f – forget gate, $W$ – matrix weight for different gates, and WC – weights activation cell.

## 10.3.3  *Spatial transform – attention-based multiscale CNN*

Using the spatial transformer network (STN) as an alignment module, ST-AMCNN was able to extract multi-scale properties from a person's stance. The results were then displayed for Grad-CAM matching [2]. It offers the learner's pose corrected assistance in addition to the correct and incorrect positions and a matching score between the two input poses. As shown in Figure 10.8, the process of identifying the class of the actual exercise performed by the user is done with pair-based matching system.

Eventually, this system requires image data for the best score prediction and provides the output. Through visualization, the feedback for correcting the pose mentioned in the output image. The following equations are the most common performance measures for the deep learning approaches.

The spatial transform attention-based multi-scale convolutional network (ST-AMCNN) [2] expressions are as follows:

Standard pose and the output features of the standard pose is expressed as,

$$Ia,s \in \mathbb{R}H'xW'xC' \text{ expression for standard pose} \tag{10.8}$$

$$F \in \mathbb{R}HxWxC \text{ expression for output feature} \tag{10.9}$$

$$fc = kc * Ia,s = \Sigma kcn * inC'n = 1 \tag{10.10}$$

where $kc$ – cth filter parameter; $kc = kc1,2,...,kcc';Ia,s = i1,i2,...,ic'$ and $fc \in \mathbb{R}HxW$.

Then, by decreasing $F$ through its spatial dimensions $H \times W$, a statistic $z \in \mathbb{R}C$ was obtained using adaptive average pooling, allowing us to determine the cth element of $z$ by:

$$zc = 1H \times W\Sigma\Sigma\Sigma(i,j) \, 3s = 1Wj = 1Hi = 1 \tag{10.11}$$

Scale factor "l" calculated as,

$$l = (W2\delta(W1z)) \tag{10.12}$$

where $\delta$ – SELU activation function; $\sigma$ – Sigmoid activation function; $W1,W2$ are the parameters of the CNN.

The output of the AMC module determined by rescaling $F$ and l be like,

$$\tilde{fc} = lc\Sigma fcs3s = 1 \tag{10.13}$$

where $\tilde{fc}$ – find from multiplication of scalar $lc$ and sum of $fcs$ for the three different convolutions.

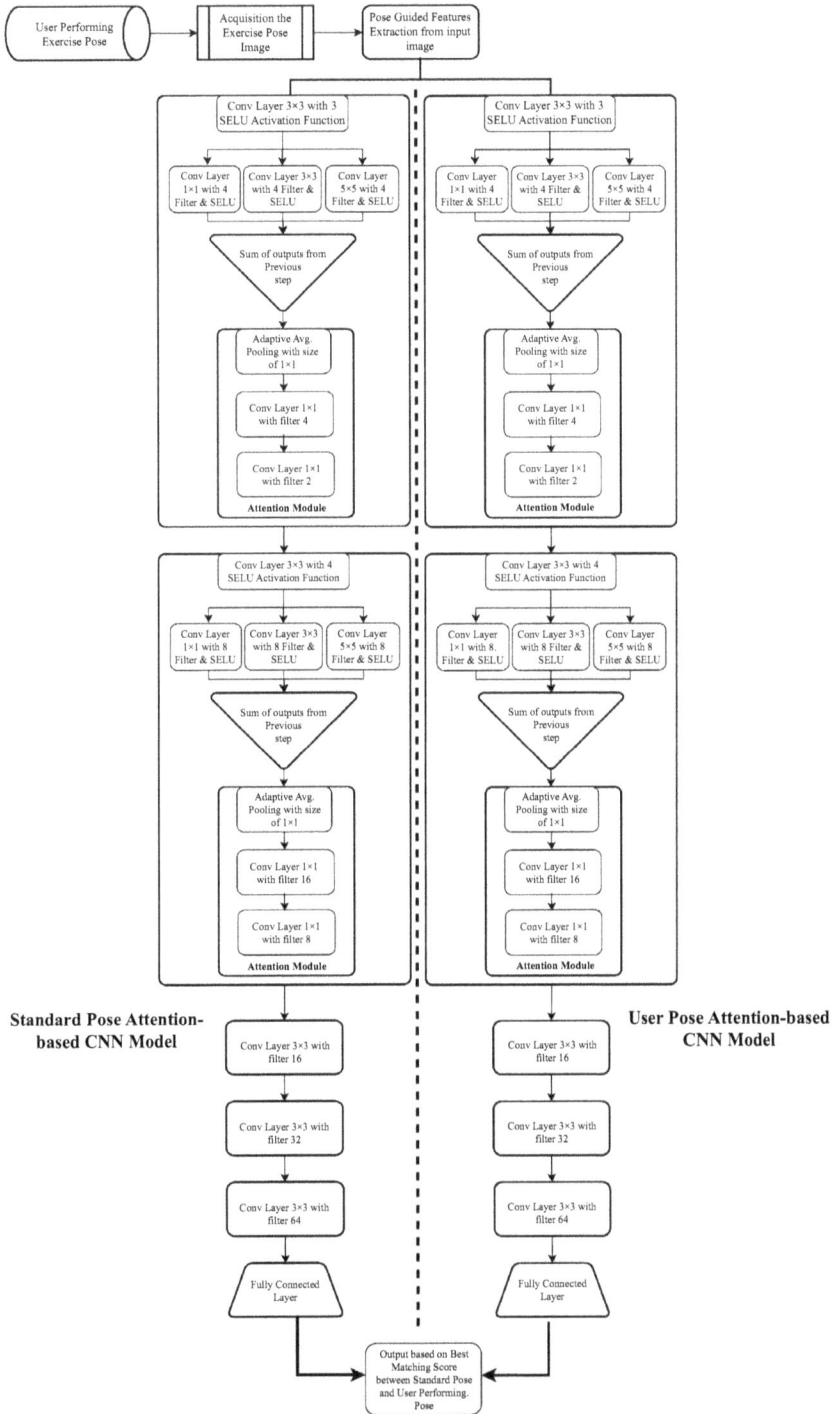

*Figure 10.8   Overview ST-AMCNN architecture [2]*

## 10.4    Discussion

Through the use of virtual objects that integrate motions, trajectory guidance, closed-loop graphics, and other features, virtual environment practice heavily emphasizes assisting patients in completing the task prescribed by the doctors and helping them overcome a variety of paralytic conditions. Patients greatly appreciate participating in the training thanks to the immersive environment-based recovery process. Even though AR/VR-based rehabilitation system creates interest in doing rehabilitation exercises, we deliberate notable research gaps in the existing systems and challenges to be solved in the future.

### 10.4.1    Research gaps

- Evaluating the accuracy of the complex exercise task, performed by the user is the primary performance metrics of a system.
- Real-time feedback in animated gifs that depict the necessary adjustment can be used as movement assistance for rehabilitation applications, as this can be audio or visual text directions [4].
- Determining the system response time will improve the SUS score and providing the positive feedback on exercise encourages the participants to improve the volunteer participation [5].
- Physioland framework only aids the participants to play the various rehabilitation exercises in virtual environment, but how accurately the participants are performing the exercise pose was not assessed [6].
- Patients with difficulty adjustment problem were not included in this study and display is shown on small screen, so participants were not able to visualize the feedback properly [7].

### 10.4.2    Challenges

(a) Evaluating the muscle fatigue for the user, while usage of AR interaction for longer duration.
(b) Providing feedback to the patients when they perform the exercise wrongly makes the participants feel guilt. Instead, providing positive feedback also motivates the users to continue the exercises.
(c) Development of home-based rehabilitation system with low cost and commercially available for the user.
(d) Visual and aural signals, as well as an adjustable level of difficulty, should be possible in the created games, and the therapist should be able to supervise them remotely.
(e) The system needs to have an automatic or semi-automatic calibration mechanism that can match the patient's range of motion to the user's range of motion in a virtual environment.
(f) Ensuring the security and safety of the patients and their health-related information during the progression of analysis of exercise pose analysis.

## 10.5    Conclusion

Considering occupational illness throughout the globe drastically reduces the gross domestic product (GDP). To provide a better solution to avoid this situation, the researchers around globe provide various solutions through technological impart. One of the most important processes to reduce or prevent occupational illness is to undergo rehabilitation training. This chapter overviews the immersive-based rehabilitation system for musculoskeletal pain. Some major accomplishments have been attributed to the employment of AR and VR over the past ten years. However, there is still a shortage of both laboratory-based research and real-world application for AR and VR devices for musculoskeletal rehabilitation.

The introduction of interactive technologies that allow users to move the upper and lower limbs has led to an evolution in musculoskeletal rehabilitation techniques. These devices have proven to be useful for patients of all ages and genders and capable of addressing musculoskeletal problems brought on by various illnesses. Game development is influenced by the findings presented in the evaluated studies, which are focused on systems efficiency evaluation. Patients' adherence and motivation are influenced by three factors: challenge, feedback to the patients, and individually increased difficulty. Automated tracking, simple integration into the home environment, and the collection of precise data may boost the system's scalability and make it easier for healthcare experts to make assessments.

## References

[1] Rajan Sreeraj, S. and Chheda, P. (2020). Prevalence of musculoskeletal symptoms and quality of life in housekeeping workers of a tertiary care hospital in Navi Mumbai, India: a descriptive study. *MGM Journal of Medical Sciences*, 7(3), p. 133. https://doi.org/10.4103/mgmj.mgmj_26_20.

[2] WHO (2021, February 8). *Musculoskeletal conditions*. Who.int; Geneva: WHO. https://www.who.int/news-room/fact-sheets/detail/musculoskeletal-conditions.

[3] Kim, J.H., Ari, H., Madasu, C., and Hwang, J. (2020). Evaluation of the biomechanical stress in the neck and shoulders during augmented reality interactions. *Applied Ergonomics*, 88, p. 103175. doi:10.1016/j.apergo.2020.103175.

[4] Xiao, B., Chen, L., Zhang, X., *et al.* (2022). Design of a virtual reality rehabilitation system for upper limbs that inhibits compensatory movement. *Medicine in Novel Technology and Devices*, 13, p. 100110. doi:10.1016/j.medntd.2021.100110.

[5] Cavalcanti, V.C., Ferreira, M.I. de S., *et al.* (2019). Usability and effects of text, image and audio feedback on exercise correction during augmented reality based motor rehabilitation. *Computers & Graphics*, 85, pp. 100–110. doi:10.1016/j.cag.2019.10.001.

[6] Martins, T., Carvalho, V., and Soares, F. (2020). Physioland – a serious game for physical rehabilitation of patients with neurological diseases. *Entertainment Computing*, 34, p. 100356. doi:10.1016/j.entcom.2020.100356.

[7]    Alves, T., Carvalho, H., and Simões Lopes, D. (2020). Winning compensations: adaptable gaming approach for upper limb rehabilitation sessions based on compensatory movements. *Journal of Biomedical Informatics,* 108, p. 103501. doi:10.1016/j.jbi.2020.103501.

[8]    Hooks, K., Ferguson, W., Morillo, P., and Cruz-Neira, C. (2020). Evaluating the user experience of omnidirectional VR walking simulators. *Entertainment Computing,* 34, p. 100352. doi:10.1016/j.entcom.2020.100352.

[9]    Powell, M.O., Elor, A., Robbins, A., Kurniawan, S., and Teodorescu, M. (2022). Predictive shoulder kinematics of rehabilitation exercises through immersive virtual reality. *IEEE Access,* 10, pp. 25621–25632. doi:10.1109/ACCESS.2022.3155179.

[10]   Tannous, H., Istrate, D., Perrochon, A., *et al.* (2021). GAMEREHAB@HOME: a new engineering system using serious game and multisensor fusion for functional rehabilitation at home. *IEEE Transactions on Games,* 13(1), pp. 89–98. doi:10.1109/TG.2019.2963108.

[11]   Heiyanthuduwa, T.A., Nikini Umasha Amarapala, K.W., Vinura Budara Gunathilaka, K.D., Ravindu, K.S., Wickramarathne, J., and Kasthurirathna, D. (2020). VirtualPT: Virtual Reality based Home Care Physiotherapy Rehabilitation for Elderly. *IEEE Xplore.* doi:10.1109/ICAC51239.2020.9357281.

[12]   Vijayakumar, P. and Dilliraj, E. (2022). A comparative review on image analysis with machine learning for extended reality (XR) applications. In: Karuppusamy, P., García Márquez, F.P., and Nguyen, T.N. (eds.), *Ubiquitous Intelligent Systems. ICUIS 2021. Smart Innovation, Systems and Technologies*, vol. 302. Singapore: Springer. https://doi.org/10.1007/978-981-19-2541-2_24.

[13]   Challenges of Human Pose Estimation in AI-Powered Fitness Apps. (2020). *InfoQ.* https://www.infoq.com/articles/human-pose-estimation-ai-powered-fitness-apps/

[14]   www.proquest.com. (n.d.). *Exploring the Technological Benefits of VR in Physical Fitness – ProQuest.*

[15]   Ponnusamy, V., Coumaran, A., Shunmugam, A.S., Rajaram, K., and Senthilvelavan, S. (2020). Smart glass: real-time leaf disease detection using YOLO transfer learning. In *2020 International Conference on Communication and Signal Processing (ICCSP).*

[16]   Pedraza-Hueso, M., Martín-Calzón, S., Díaz-Pernas, F.J., and Martínez-Zarzuela, M. (2015). Rehabilitation using kinect-based games and virtual reality. *Procedia Computer Science,* 75, pp. 161–168. doi:10.1016/j.procs.2015.12.233.

[17]   Thinh, N.T., Quoc, N.A., Tam Toan, N.V., and Luc, T.T. (2021). Implementation of rehabilitation platform based on augmented reality technology. *IEEE Xplore.* doi:10.23919/ICCAS52745.2021.9650059.

[18]   Paraskevopoulos, I.T., Tsekleves, E., Craig, C., Whyatt, C., and Cosmas, J. (2014). Design guidelines for developing customised serious games for Parkinson's disease rehabilitation using bespoke game sensors. *Entertainment Computing,* 5(4), pp. 413–424. doi:10.1016/j.entcom.2014.10.006.

[19] Zhang, Y., Sun, W., and Chen, J. (2022). Application of embedded smart wearable device monitoring in joint cartilage injury and rehabilitation training. *Journal of Healthcare Engineering*, 2022, pp. 1–11. doi:10.1155/2022/4420870.

[20] Delvigne, V., Facchini, A., Wannous, H., Dutoit, T., Ris, L., and Vandeborre, J.-P. (2022). A saliency based feature fusion model for EEG emotion estimation. arXiv:2201.03891 [cs]. https://arxiv.org/abs/2201.03891.

[21] Fong, J., Ocampo, R., Gross, D.P., and Tavakoli, M. (2019). A robot with an augmented-reality display for functional capacity evaluation and rehabilitation of injured workers. *IEEE Xplore*. doi:10.1109/ICORR.2019.8779417.

[22] Ning, H., Wang, Z., Li, R., Zhang, Y., and Mao, L. (2022). A Review on serious games for exercise rehabilitation. arXiv:2201.04984 [cs]. https://arxiv.org/abs/2201.04984.

*Chapter 11*

# IoT-enabled digital revolution of the healthcare system

*R. Srinivasan[1], M. Kavitha[1], R. Kavitha[1], Saravanan Muthaiyah[2], Ramanathan Lakshmanan[3] and Rajeshkannan Regunathan[3]*

## Abstract

In modern civilization, healthcare is a significant problem. The Internet of Things (IoT) technology is appealing to everyone because it has the ability to change the present healthcare system and address the problems that the aging population and the steady rise in chronic sickness are posing for the healthcare system. This chapter focuses on the conventional healthcare system that has been used in the past to deliver healthcare services as well as the integration of IoT, a new technology, into the healthcare system to modernize patient care. To provide services more quickly and effectively, this chapter illustrates how IoT has changed the conventional approach to monitoring healthcare. Finally, a study on different IoT-based healthcare monitoring systems will be conducted, along with a comparison of numerous IoT-based healthcare systems to show their advantages and disadvantages. The industry's digital transformation is piquing the curiosity of academics and healthcare practitioners alike. In this work, we attempt to examine the research question about the management and commercial uses of digital technology by different stakeholders. This chapter examines IoT applications for medical purposes, the different ways it is affecting the healthcare industry, and some potential future routes for its growth, such as Bio-IoT and Nano-IoT or the Internet of Nano Things. From the perspective of monitoring patients' vital signs, wireless body area networks (WBANs) are crucial components of a system. The WBANs consist of tiny smart devices that communicate wirelessly and are implanted within or on top of the patient. We analyze the literature on digital transformation in healthcare to answer this question. According to our findings, previous research can be grouped into five clusters: organizational characteristics, patient-centered approaches, operational efficiency of healthcare

[1]Department of Computer Science and Engineering, Vel Tech Rangarajan Dr. Sagunthala R&D Institute of Science and Technology, Chennai, India

[2]Department of Information Technology, Multimedia University, Selangor, Malaysia

[3]School of Computer Science and Engineering, Vellore Institute of Technology, Vellore, India

providers, and research techniques. These clusters are linked to illustrate how various technology adoption approaches enhance service providers' operational effectiveness. Research in a variety of directions is recommended, with implications for management as well.

**Keywords:** IoT; Healthcare; Diseases; Services; Security; Technologies

## 11.1    Introduction

Every day, new technologies are developed with the intention of making our lives simpler. This technical innovation has had a significant positive impact on the healthcare business. It facilitates the completion of any protracted and tiresome process and enables doctors and other medical professionals to safely use this incredible instrument. Before technology was brought to the healthcare sector, workers and patients both had to wait a long time to receive an examination. Only hospital visits, phone calls, and texts were used by patients to communicate with clinicians. It was unable to maintain a continuous eye on the patient's condition to deliver a precise and prompt diagnosis. Internet of Things (IoT) and artificial intelligence (AI) have the ability to fundamentally alter medical research, disease detection, and patient care [1].

Recent years have seen a major development in the healthcare industry, which has resulted in huge increases in employment and revenue [2]. Prior until a few years ago, a hospital physical examination was necessary to identify diseases and other bodily irregularities. For the course of their treatment, the majority of patients were required to remain in the hospital. As a result, healthcare costs increased and hospitals' capacity in remote and rural regions was under pressure. Using small gadgets like smartwatches, technological advancements over the years have made it possible to diagnose a number of ailments and track one's health. A hospital-centric healthcare system has also been replaced by a patient-centric one thanks to technology [3,4].

For instance, a number of clinical analyses may be completed on home-based deprived of the assistance of a healthcare expert, such as monitoring blood pressure, blood glucose levels, pO2 levels, and other parameters. Furthermore, clinical data may be sent from distant areas to healthcare institutions with the use of cutting-edge telecommunication technologies. Healthcare facilities are now more accessible because of the use of communication services and fast-evolving IoT, cloud computing, mobile computing, wireless sensing, and machine learning technologies. IoT has made it possible for people to interact with the outside world in a number of ways that have increased their freedom. The IoT connects a range of devices, wireless sensors, home appliances, and electrical equipment to the Internet, considerably advancing contemporary communication protocols and algorithms.

## 11.2    Background

The development and state of the healthcare system in the past are the main topics of the history of the sector.

## 11.2.1   The growth of the healthcare system

An ideal healthcare organization needed to be developed from the outdated conventional healthcare system that existed in the 19th century. Patients were not involved in decision-making regarding their own health and the management of their ailments under the conventional healthcare system. The information, setting, practices, and judgments of healthcare professionals and the system are fully dependent on the patients for their treatment [5,6]. The increased prevalence of chronic illnesses and the aging population were two of the primary drivers of the healthcare system's development. To successfully treat and manage chronic disorders, patients' and doctors' collaboration is essential. Another explanation might be that patients can actively participate in their own care and self-monitoring of their physical health thanks to sensors and linked technologies.

In the current healthcare system, a patient must visit the doctor's office; it receipts an extended period and causes the patient a ratio of stress towards discovering anything about their health. The information may show on either the patient's or the doctor's phone, and if required, they may organize a meeting anywhere. This is because the current healthcare system does not need the patient to visit the doctor's office every time he wants to learn about his health state. Utilizing a personalized health management system, the perfect healthiness maintenance organization would offer services to somebody, wherever, at somewhat period. It is important to identify the cutting-edge technologies that have been created for the healthcare system to achieve this aim. For a more effective healthcare system, advanced technology such as network, sensor, and data processing might be very important.

A healthcare system that incorporates IoT components might be enhanced. As every device in the environment is connected, IoT connections enable "anytime, anywhere with anything and anyone" interactions. It is the IoT that has completely changed the passive style of healthcare service into the ubiquitous mode, which is patient-centric rather than career-centric. The increasing usage of wireless sensor-based devices makes it possible to collect patient health data and analyze it to give patients better care than ever before. The development of these technologies to enhance healthcare services is still ongoing. By increasing accessibility and care quality, the IoT-driven solution lowers costs while also improving health [5,6]. In Table 11.1, a comparison of the conventional and contemporary healthcare systems is shown.

*Table 11.1   Comparison of the conventional and modern healthcare systems [5,6]*

| Traditional healthcare | Modern healthcare |
| --- | --- |
| According to populations | Depending on the person |
| Accentuate the prevention and treatment of diseases | Personalized health management should be emphasized |
| Clinic or lab is the focal point of care | Patient is at the center of care |
| Expensive | Less costly |
| Data that belong to the organization | Data that patients own and share |
| Short time | Any time |

## 11.3    Major smart healthcare system components

Adopting new technology in all areas of life now, when they are rapidly developing, makes life simple and straightforward. A smart healthcare system provides effective medical care to others in distant places in real time. It makes use of the most recent technology, known as IoT, to function as a smart healthcare system. Based on this novel approach, the healthcare system has evolved into an IoT-based healthcare system that comprises five key elements arranged in a circular structure [5], as seen in Figure 11.1. The patient wears several sensors on their body or has them implanted, and sensor technology is the initial part of the system that collects data from these sensors.

Intelligent networks are the name for the second component. To connect with the system, the intelligent network receives data from several sensors and sends it. A network that allows for communication between various entities involved in the healthcare system is known as an intelligent network. Data saved in the cloud via an intelligent network is the third component. The cloud is mostly used for storage since a large amount of patient personal information and health-related data are generated and need to be kept somewhere for future study.

Big data analysis is the fourth component, which comes after the data has been checked for a suitable option and kept in the cloud. For the optimal analysis of the data and output, a variety of data mining techniques must be applied. Once the right choice has been made, the findings are sent to modern hospitals. The IoT healthcare system's smart hospitals make up its fifth component, and they continuously gather data to make sure the system has accurately diagnosed and is treating the patient. To keep the system moving in a circle, it goes back to the first part.

## 11.4    The IoT and healthcare

The potential request of the IoT in healthcare is currently a largely unexplored area of research. This section examines the IoT and emphasizes how well-suited it is to

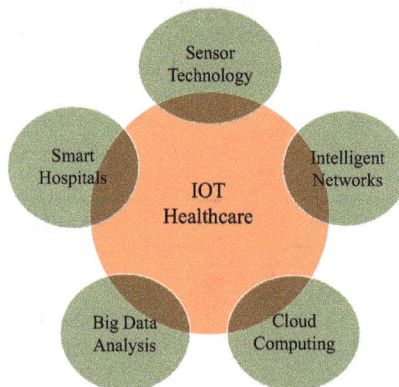

*Figure 11.1    Components of IoT healthcare system [5]*

the healthcare industry. Several ground-breaking initiatives to create IoT solutions for healthcare are mentioned. Future end-to-end IoT healthcare systems are envisaged using a general and standard paradigm based on repeated themes from these initiatives.

### 11.4.1   The IoT

Although the IoT has numerous definitions, at its most basic level, it can be summed up as a network of devices connecting with one another through machine-to-machine (M2M) connections to allow the collection and exchange of data [7–9]. Large-scale data collection and automation are made possible by this technology across many sectors. The many functions of IoT in the healthcare sector are depicted in Figure 11.2. Precision agriculture, smart parking, and water usage monitoring are just a few of the areas where the IoT is already being used commercially and has been hailed as the catalyst for the Fourth Industrial Revolution [10]. In-depth study has also been done [12–17] on how to use IoT to develop intelligent systems for things like lowering traffic congestion, keeping track of the structural health, developing crash-avoidance cars, and smart grids.

Despite what would seem to be their apparent differences from healthcare, the research done in the fields demonstrates the potential of a healthcare organization based on the IoT. Systems deployed in many sectors have shown the practicality of remote object monitoring with data gathering and reporting.

### 11.4.2   IoT architecture for health monitoring

For healthcare, IoT has a four-step design that may be thought of as phases in a process. All four phases are linked together in a way that data acquired or processed at one stage contributes to the next. By incorporating values into a process, you may gain knowledge and create exciting new business prospects. The four levels of IoT for health monitoring are depicted in Figure 11.3.

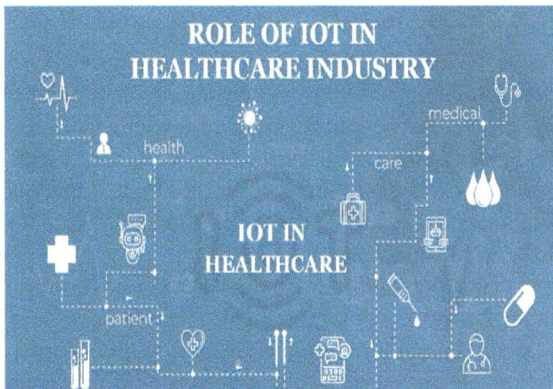

*Figure 11.2   Different roles of IoT in health industry [7]*

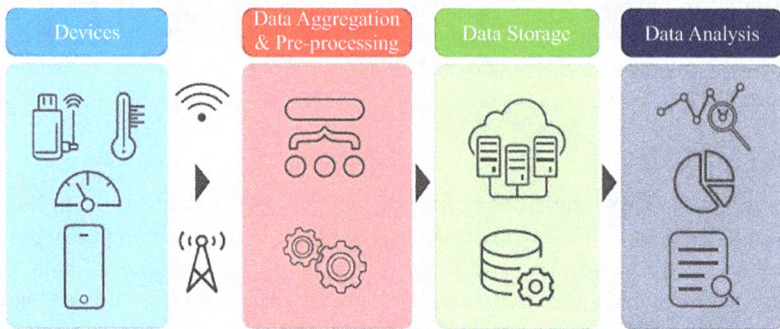

*Figure 11.3    The four stages of IoT solution for health monitoring [9]*

**Phase 1:** The first step entails the deployment of sensors, actuators, displays, detectors, video systems, etc. that are networked. These tools gather the information.

**Phase 2:** Typically, data collected from sensors and other devices is in analogue form; this form must be combined and transformed to digital form to be processed further.

**Phase 3:** Data is first processed, gathered, and pre-processed before being standard and sent to a datacenter or the Cloud.

**Phase 4:** The completed data is subjected to the proper level of analysis and control. This data may be subjected to advanced analytics to offer useful business insights for sensible decision-making. IoT is revolutionizing healthcare by guaranteeing improved patient care, improved treatment results, and lower costs. Additionally, it is enhancing performance, bettering processes and procedures, and enhancing patient satisfaction for healthcare professionals.

## 11.4.3    Healthcare on the IoT

Despite the theoretical viability of remote health monitoring, research in related fields suggests that there may be other circumstances where the benefits outweigh the disadvantages. It could be beneficial for rural inhabitants to have easier access to healthcare or to let seniors age in place for longer. In other words, it may always provide people greater power over their own health, lighten the load on healthcare institutions, and increase access to healthcare resources. Figure 11.4 displays the topology of an IoT-based health monitoring system.

There are not many drawbacks to remote health monitoring. The main disadvantages include the potential requirement for routine sensor calibration to guarantee that a person is being monitored accurately, the security risks involved with storing a lot of sensitive data in one database, and the potential for patient disconnections from healthcare services if they were outside of cellular range or their devices ran out of battery. As will be emphasized throughout the remainder of

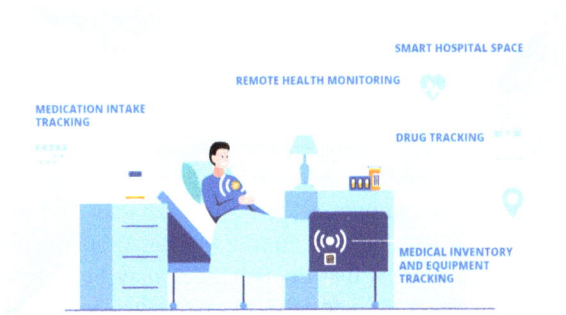

*Figure 11.4   Monitoring the structural health using IoT [15]*

this dissertation; fortunately, these problems are all fairly manageable and have previously been addressed in the literature. IoT-based solutions for remote health monitoring are quickly emerging as a viable alternative for the delivery of health-care as efforts to lessen the drawbacks continue.

Due to the numerous advantages of remote well-being nursing, investigators have begun to recognize the possibility of the IoT as a healthcare solution. Healthcare systems powered by the IoT have been created for a variety of uses, such as recovery, diabetes control, aided ambient living (AAL) for older adults, and more. Each system is securely in place, even though they were all created with various objectives in mind. Physical rehabilitation has piqued the interest of several researchers. A rehabilitation plan tailored to a person may be made using a pro-cedure that has been devised [7] based on their indications. This is achieved by comparing the affected role condition to a database of the indications, treatments, then indicators of prior patients. In 87.9% of the instances, the doctor completely accepted the scheme's suggestions and adopted the proposed course of therapy. The method necessitates that a doctor meticulously records symptoms and approves any prescribed treatments.

On the other hand, all offer mathematical methods for figuring out joint angles in physical hydrotherapy systems. permitting the tracking of increases in joint mobility during the therapy procedure [18–20]. Examines if modern IoT technol-ogy is appropriate for a system for intensive care Parkinson's disease patients. According to their study, wear sensors may be used with vision-based technology (such cameras positioned throughout the home) to monitor activity levels and gait patterns to monitor the course of Parkinson's disease. The researchers provided a useful tip on how to evaluate blood glucose levels in diabetics and suggested that machine learning may ultimately affect additional effective handling choices [19]. Individuals using this method need to physically amount their gore glucose stages at predetermined interludes. Then, two different categories of blood glucose anomalies are considered. The first is an incorrect gore glucose reading and abnormal blood glucose levels. The system then determines whether to quickly contact the patient, carers, and family members, or emergency medical personnel such as physicians, based on the severity of the aberration. Although it has been demonstrated that this strategy can be successful, automating blood-glucose readings may enhance its efficiency [20].

A heart attack detecting system was integrated [21] using readily available components and a recognizable antenna. Heart activity is processed and tracked using an ECG sensor and a microprocessor. These data are sent over Bluetooth to the user's smartphone, where they are further evaluated and displayed via a user application. The authors suggest that the technique may be enhanced by creating tools to predict cardiac attacks. Since respiratory rate has been shown to help with heart attack prediction [22], measuring it may result in further improvements. Wearable vision-based (camera-based), ambient, and activity sensors are used in the SPHERE [23] system, which is still under development. Elderly and chronically ill people will be able to remain in the comfort of their own homes while having their medical requirements assessed thanks to this paper.

## 11.5    Three revolutions

Three revolutions that are significant to modern healthcare are briefly discussed.

### 11.5.1    *Internet-based revolution*

Every aspect of our lives is significantly impacted by the Internet, which today connects several networks and a large area. Future networks will make use of a range of instruments with sophisticated sensing capabilities. These networks will comprise physically connected computers and multimodal data from social, biological, cognitive, and semantic networks. Building future net-centric communities will require making use of these interconnected networks.

The IoT is sometimes described as being made up of these specialized gadgets and its network, which will continually sense, monitor, and understand their surroundings (IoT). The Internet of Everything (IoE), which is the combination of IoT and social networks, will have a big impact on how healthcare is provided in the United States. Furthermore, IoE developments will support tele-medicine [24,25]. Figure 11.5 shows the uses of HIoT services.

### 11.5.2    *The revolution of omics*

The Humanoid Genome Development has been providing us a relatively accurate plot of the humanoid genome, which is the subject of the scientific discipline of genomics. The plotting led to the growth of an extensive diversity of DNA summarizing techniques. A person's whole genetic profile might soon be delivered quickly and cheaply, thanks to advances in technology. The growing fields of proteomics and metabolomics. An effort on Precision Medicine in the United States placed a lot of emphasis on integrating different "omics" to comprehend a biological system. Essentially, this integration includes gathering sizable datasets that

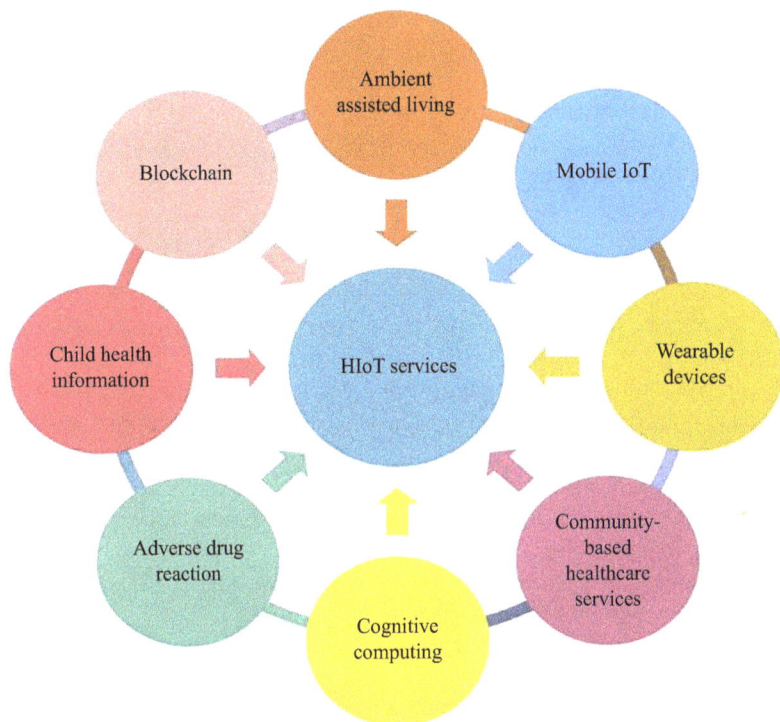

*Figure 11.5   Widely used HIoT services [24]*

characterize and count constituent parts of a certain organic scheme, then computationally analyzing them to discover dynamic and functional relationships. It is
believed that no molecule in life functions alone. Causes and effects may interact in
several different ways. To appreciate these interactions and how they impact the
biological system, a significant combination of experimental data and theoretical
knowledge is required.

## 11.5.3   Revolutions in AI

The goal of AI is to create computer programs that are intelligent in a similar way
to how humans think. This means that AI is very interested in studying how people
solve problems and implementing (or imitating) these techniques into computer
systems [26]. There has been a significant advancement in this field since the
1950s, when the word "AI" was first used. The growth of knowledge-based systems, also referred to as "the first wave or revolution," dominated the 1980s [27].
The development of multi-layered neural networks in the 2000s, made possible by
developments in computer technology, significantly improved machine learning for
particular types of issues. A "second revolution or wave" has just occurred.
Knowledge structures and neural networks will be combined in the "third wave,"
which has already begun. The third revolution will accelerate the modernization of

the medical industry. Numerous applications in the healthcare industry employ AI extensively [28,29].

To deliver complete healthcare, the technologies must function in context and would need to be organized into a system. We suggest Leroy Hood's [30] P4 medicine concept, developed at the Institute of Systems Biology, to the P9 notion to plot the junction among demands of health treatment and then upcoming well-being maintenance organization. I developed the P9 idea with Ramesh Jain from the University of California, Irvine. The P9 health concept contains, among other things, the following components:

1. **Personalized.** Making each patient's therapy unique entails personalized medicine.
2. **Predictive.** Based on information from electronic health records (EHRs) and genetic information, we must remain able toward control a person's risk of developing a certain disease.
3. **Preventive.** Technologies for decision analysis and machine learning can be used to create methods to avoid the emergence of disease rather than treating a disease after it has already affected a person.
4. **Participatory.** The patient should take a proactive role in the evaluation and management of their remedial disorder.
5. **Persistent.** Well-being attention must remain available 24/7, anywhere, and at any time.
6. **Precise.** Decision-analytic techniques can be employed once data and information have been obtained to pinpoint the origin of a disease and suggest the most effective course of treatment.
7. **Privacy-preserving.** To guarantee that processing of patient data reduces issues for patients, appropriate precautions should be applied.
8. **Protective.** We must safeguard the security of data and computer systems and take safety precautions to prevent any harm to patients by whatever means.
9. **Reasonably priced.** The price of medical care should be reasonable.

### 11.5.4   IoT benefits for healthcare

- Monitoring offered by IoT, unnecessary doctor visits, hospital stays, and readmissions are significantly reduced in cost.
- It provides total transparency and allows clinicians the authority to base their choices on the best information available.
- Quicker disease symptom-based diagnosis of illnesses at an early stage or even before they emerge is facilitated by constant patient monitoring and current data.
- Continuous proactive medical treatment is made feasible via health monitoring.
- A major challenge for the healthcare industry is the management of drugs and medical equipment. Due to connected devices, they may be used efficiently and at a cheaper cost.
- Data from IoT devices non-individual aids in improved executive then similarly ensures even healthcare actions with compact error, waste, and system costs.

## 11.6 Conclusion

The present evaluation looked at several HIoT system aspects. This chapter provides a comprehensive analysis of the construction, mechanisms, and communication of an HIoT organization. Additionally covered popular objects are the IoT-based healthcare services that are currently offered and under investigation. These concepts have enabled clinicians to display and identify a range of well-being situations, assess a range of healthiness indicators, and offer analytical facilities in isolated areas. The healthcare sector has changed as a result, moving after being predominately focused on hospitals to one that is more patient-centric. In addition, we went over several HIoT applications and current developments in each. The difficulties and problems related to the development, production, and usage of the HIoT are discussed. The challenges determination helps as the basis for future development and research goals in the next years. Additionally, readers have access to in-depth, current knowledge about HIoT devices if they want to begin or further their studies in the related field.

## References

[1] W. Almobaideen, R. Krayshan, M. Allan, and M. Saadeh. Internet of Things: geographical routing based on healthcare centers vicinity for mobile smart tourism destination. *Technol. Forecast. Soc. Change,* 123, pp. 342–50, 2017.

[2] Z. Ali, M.S. Hossain, G. Muhammad, and A.K. Sangaiah. An intelligent healthcare system for detection and classification to discriminate vocal fold disorders. *Fut. Gener. Comput. Syst.,* 85, pp. 19–28, 2018.

[3] G. Yang, L. Xie, M. Mantysalo, *et al.* A health-IoT platform based on the integration of intelligent packaging, unobtrusive bio-sensor, and intelligent medicine box. *IEEE Transact. Indust. Inform.,* 10(4), pp. 2180–2191, 2014.

[4] Y. Yan. A home-based health information acquisition system. *Health Inform. Sci. Syst.,* vol. 1, p. 12, 2013.

[5] J. Jeong, O. Han, and Y. You. A design characteristics of smart healthcare system as the IoT applications. *Indian J. Sci. Technol.,* 9(37), pp. 1–8, 2016, ISSN 0974-6846.

[6] A. Kulkarni and S.R. Sathe. Healthcare applications of the Internet of Things: a review. *Int. J. Comput. Sci. Inf. Technol.,* 5(5), pp. 6229–6232, 2014.

[7] Y.J. Fan, Y.H. Yin, L.D. Xu, Y. Zeng, and F. Wu. IoT-based smart rehabilitation system. *IEEE Trans. Ind. Informat.,* 10(2), pp. 1568–1577, 2014.

[8] S.M.R. Islam, D. Kwak, H. Kabir, M. Hossain, and K.-S. Kwak. The Internet of Things for health care: a comprehensive survey. *IEEE Access,* 3, pp. 678–708, 2015.

[9] D.V. Dimitrov. Medical Internet of Things and big data in healthcare. *Healthcare Inform. Res.,* 22(3), pp. 156–163, 2016. http://www.ncbi.nlm. nih.gov/pmc/articles/PMC4981575/

[10]    P. K. Schwab. *The Fourth Industrial Revolution: What It Means, and How to Respond*. Cologny, Switzerland: World Economic Forum, 2016.

[11]    Smart Parking. SmartEye, SmartRep, and RFID Technology Westminster City Council London, 2017. http:// www.smartparking.com/keep-up-to-date/ case-studies/3-500-vehicledetection-sensors-and-epermit-technology-in-the-city-of-westminsterlondon

[12]    University of New England. SMART Farm, 2017. http://www.une.edu.au/ research/research-centres-institutes/smart-farm

[13]    Sensus. Smart WaterSmarter at Every Point, 2017. www.sensus.com/internet-of-things/smart-water

[14]    H. El-Sayed and G. Thandavarayan. Congestion detection and propagation in urban areas using histogram models. *IEEE Internet Things J.*, to be published.

[15]    C.A. Tokognon, B. Gao, G. Tian, and Y. Yan. Structural health monitoring framework based on Internet of Things: a survey. *IEEE Internet Things J.*, 4 (3), pp. 619–635, 2017.

[16]    K.M. Alam, M. Saini, and A.E. Saddik. Toward social Internet of vehicles: concept, architecture, and applications. *IEEE Access*, 3, pp. 343–357, 2015.

[17]    S. Tan, D. De, W.-Z. Song, J. Yang, and S.K. Das. Survey of security advances in smart grid: a data driven approach. *IEEE Commun. Surveys Tuts.*, 19(1), pp. 397–422, 2017.

[18]    R.C.A. Alves, L.B. Gabriel, B.T.D. Oliveira, C.B. Margi, and F.C.L.D. Santos. Assisting physical (hydro)therapy with wireless sensors networks. *IEEE Internet Things J.*, 2(2), pp. 113–120, 2015.

[19]    C.F. Pasluosta, H. Gassner, J. Winkler, J. Klucken, and B.M. Eskoer. An emerging era in the management of Parkinson's disease: wearable technologies and the Internet of Things. *IEEE J. Biomed. Health Inform.*, 19(6), pp. 1873–1881, 2015.

[20]    S.-H. Chang, R.-D. Chiang, S.-J. Wu, and W.-T. Chang. A contextaware, interactive M-health system for diabetics. *IT Prof.*, 18(3), pp. 14–22, 2016.

[21]    G. Wolgast, C. Ehrenborg, A. Israelsson, J. Helander, E. Johansson, and H. Manefjord. Wireless body area network for heart attack detection [education corner]. *IEEE Antennas Propag. Mag.*, 58(5), pp. 84–92, 2016.

[22]    M.A. Cretikos, R. Bellomo, K. Hillman, J. Chen, S. Finfer, and A. Flabouris. Respiratory rate: the neglected vital sign. *Med. J. Austral.*, 188(11), pp. 657–659, 2008.

[23]    N. Zhu, T. Diethe, M. Camplani, *et al.* Bridging e-health and the Internet of Things: the SPHERE project. *IEEE Intell. Syst.*, 30(4), pp. 39–46, 2015.

[24]    A. Sheth, U. Jaimini, K. Thirunarayan, and T. Banerjee. Augmented personalized health: how smart data with IoTs and AI is about to change healthcare. In *IEEE 3rd International Forum on Research and Technologies for Society and Industry (RTSI)*. IEEE, 2017.

[25]    A. Sheth, U. Jaimini, and H.Y. Yip. How will the Internet of things enable augmented personalized health? *IEEE Intell. Syst.*, 33(2018), pp. 89–97, 2018.

[26]   S. Russell and P. Norvig. *Artificial Intelligence: A Modern Approach*, 4th ed. *Pearson Education Inc.*, Prentice Hall, 2020.

[27]   R.D. Sriram. *Intelligent System for Engineering: A Knowledge-Based Approach.* Berlin: Springer, 1997.

[28]   R.D. Sriram and S.K. Reddy. Artificial intelligence and digital tools: future of diabetes care. *Clin. Geriatr. Med.* 36(3), pp. 513–525, 2020.

[29]   E.J. Topol. High-performance medicine: the convergence of human and artificial intelligence. *Nat. Med.,* 25(1), pp. 44–56, 2019.

[30]   L. Hood and M. Flores. A personal view on systems medicine and the emergence of proactive P4 medicine: predictive, preventive, personalized and participatory. *N. Biotechnol.,* 29, pp. 613–624, 2012. https://doi.org/10.1016/j.nbt.2012.03.004

*Chapter 12*

# Integrated and intelligent cloud service platforms for transition from Healthcare 1.0 to 4.0

*S. Lavanya[1], N.M. Saravanakumar[2], A.M. Ratheesh Kumar[3] and Tu Nguyen[4]*

## Abstract

Hospital records, patient medical records, test findings, and Internet-of-Things devices are just a few examples of the sources used in the healthcare sector. The public healthcare data is also produced in great quantities by the biomedical research field. To produce useful information, effective administration and analysis are necessary. By creating new opportunities for contemporary healthcare, effective data management, analysis, and interpretation may completely alter the game. That is precisely the reason why a variety of sectors, including the healthcare sector, are moving aggressively to transform this potential into better services and financial benefits. Modern healthcare institutions may revolutionize medical therapies and personalized medicine with a strong integration of biological and healthcare data. This chapter introduces various modern devices used in healthcare sectors for a variety of purposes.

**Keywords:** Cloud apps; Healthcare 1.0; IoT; mHealth apps; Wearable devices

## 12.1    Introduction

Healthcare devices are the pioneers in the fastest-growing sectors of the current market. Health services include medical professionals, organizations, and ancillary healthcare workers who are responsible for offering healthcare services to the needy people such as patients, families, communities, and populations. These

[1]Department of Artificial Intelligence, M. Kumarasamy College of Engineering (autonomous affiliated under Anna University), Karur, India
[2]Department of Information Technology, Karpagam College of Engineering (affiliated under Anna University), Coimbatore, India
[3]Department of Information Technology, Sri Krishna College of Engineering and Technology (affiliated under Anna University), Coimbatore, India
[4]Department of Computer Science, College of Computing and Software Engineering, Kennesaw State University, Marietta, GA, USA

services include hospital, diagnostic, primary, palliative, long-term, preventive, rehabilitative, emergency, and other home care services [1–5]. There are different services and providers who can improve patient-centeredness, accessibility, and quality of healthcare is discussed as follows.

## 12.2    Types of services

Many people seek out primary care, outpatient treatment, and emergency care when they are unwell or generally feeling under the weather for a variety of medical conditions [6–8]. However, there are many medical services that are focused on certain diseases or problems. These health services include:

- Mental healthcare
- Laboratory and diagnostic care
- Substance abuse treatment
- Dental and prenatal care
- Preventive and pharmaceutical care
- Physical and occupational therapy
- Nutritional support
- Transportation, etc.

## 12.3    Types of providers

The providers of health services are primary care physicians, pharmacists, nurses, and specialists. The healthcare evolution cycle is as in Figure 12.1.

## 12.4    Related works

According to a Markets & Markets analysis from 2017, the Internet of Things (IoT) healthcare industry will grow to $158.07 billion by 2022. The plot's credibility and effectiveness are immediately important given how drastically healthcare is changing and how much it also helps people's health. The issues in the healthcare industry are really significant. Due to the increase in chronic illnesses among individuals, most of the world's healthcare systems are currently experiencing a

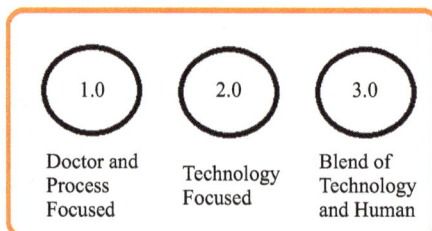

*Figure 12.1    Healthcare Evolution Cycle 1.0 to 3.0*

number of problems [9]. In parallel, there is a need for healthcare to be more affordable. The combination of technology and healthcare serves as a cure-all for all such problems. Approximately 76% of physicians think that technology has the ability to advance medical treatment.

Technology also enables people to take an active role in keeping track of their wellbeing. As a result, this union results in affordable, efficient patient care and happiness. Fernandez and Pallis [10] emphasized the importance of using IoT in 2014 to have true data-driven healthcare. According to studies in [11], the IoT healthcare system is expected to expand as a provider of various technical options for the industry. A smart gateway along with fog computing was also shown by the researchers for use in a variety of applications, including healthcare [9]. Computing is now being used in a number of life-threatening tasks where time is of the essence to improve patient care and monitoring.

For instance, in the treatment of chronic obstructive pulmonary disease [12], mild dementia, stroke mitigation [13], and ECG feature extraction [14], the performance of the system was empirically tested by the researchers after they installed a fog-based cloud-based architecture [15]. Some individuals also developed devices or systems using the fog computing technique. SOA-FOG, a privacy-aware security model, a secure monitoring, and alert-generating architecture are the other numerous examples. There have also been established healthcare frameworks and systems for chikungunya, energy-efficient systems, patient monitoring [16], etc.

Kaur *et al.* have conducted numerous studies in energy efficiency, difficulties with fog deployment in healthcare 4.0, many improvements in ECG monitoring system, as well as the detection and management of illnesses spread by mosquitoes [17]. A similar pattern was seen in 2019 as well. For the benefit of cancer patients, a fog computing-based architecture was suggested. To provide an assessment against all recognized vulnerabilities in healthcare situations, a research based on vulnerability assessment was also carried out that year. Similar to this, a blockchain-related computing framework was created for remote patient monitoring to recognize human activity. Researchers have also highlighted distributed machine learning (ML) as a potential area for further study.

Many aspects of manufacturing systems and the research of healthcare systems are similar. The other industrial sectors like manufacturing, healthcare delivery have undergone several revolutions throughout the years. We use what we know about the progression from industry 1.0 to 4.0 to define analogous various stages to depict the move from Healthcare 1.0 to 4.0. The core patient–clinician interaction is described in Healthcare 1.0. A patient will go to a clinic and engage with a doctor and other healthcare professionals there. The clinician (or care team) consults with the patient, conducts tests, makes a diagnosis, and then prescribes drugs, develops a treatment plan for the ailment, and arranges follow-up appointments. This model has been practiced for hundreds of years [7,8,18,19].

Along with substantial developments in health, life science, and biotechnology, many new medical devices and instruments have been developed, manufactured, and tested and are being used more often in the delivery of healthcare. Hospitals and other care facilities are increasingly using imaging test equipment (like MRI, ultrasound, and CT scan), monitoring tools (like pulse oximeter, arterial lines), surgical and life support tools (like da Vinci robot chest tubes) to support diagnosis, treatment, and monitoring. This change is referred to as Healthcare 2.0.

Since the last ten years, electronic health or medical records (EHR or EMR) have been used to coordinate patient care among units and departments of healthcare organizations. These health information technologies have significantly impacted clinical and operational processes. Many manual operations have been computerized and digitalized, and the EHR has a number of time-stamped activities [20–24].

The development of computer networks has also made telehealth and remote care possible, and certain in-person contacts are starting to be replaced by electronic visits (such as communication between a patient and their doctor through a patient portal). The continuing COVID-19 epidemic has caused an increase in demand for telehealth and virtual visits. All of these have caused the delivery of healthcare to undergo several revolutionary modifications. This revolution falls under the category of Healthcare 3.0.

The fourth healthcare revolution and Industry 4.0 are now coemerging. In such a case, the process of delivering healthcare becomes a cyber-physical system equipped with wearables, radio-frequency identification (RFID), IoT, and different medical devices, intelligent sensors, medical robots, etc., which are integrated with cloud computing, big data analysis, artificial intelligence (AI), and decision support techniques to achieve smart and interconnected healthcare delivery [25–29]. As a result, the paradigm of "Healthcare 4.0" develops, which is characterized by a ubiquitous, intelligent, and networked healthcare community.

Growing automation is a component of Healthcare 4.0, which is evolving similar to Industry 4.0. People's involvement is the most obvious and important distinction between Industry and Healthcare 4.0. Patients (and carers) and physicians are more jointly responsible for patients' health monitoring, symptom reporting, and collaborative decision-making for planning the treatment and care in the context of Healthcare 4.0. Patients as well as professionals will be at the center of Healthcare 4.0 as they take on more crucial responsibilities.

## 12.5   Methodology

Healthcare 1.0 concentrates on limited awareness about healthcare among people and they were called and processed through manual records, fixed set of procedures, non-experimental treatments. The time period was dominated by technical advancements and the doctors used the traditional approach to treatment. Every step of the procedure, from admission to post-treatment formalities, requires a significant amount of manual labor, which caused the medical business to transition from the Healthcare 1.0 era to 2.0.

When Healthcare 2.0 was first launched in the 2000s, it was more concerned with computer technology than with human engagement. It focuses on pharmacy, digital platforms, diagnostics, single specialty care, patient-focused health and wellness services, and medical technology with a particular emphasis on care quality. The phrase "technology as an enabler for the industry" was used to describe this period from its inception. But in late 2010, a revised definition was released that is SaaS, a new cloud digital technology through smartphones which are concentrated on user experience. An interlinkable technology allows other applications and tools to be integrated with the existing technology and was helpful to the patients [30–32]. Data-driven is a way in which the statistics is created, analyzed, and presented to make a quick decision.

Healthcare 2.0 encouraged streamlined processes and fewer human efforts. A medical sector that heavily relies on empathy lacks personal connections. Establishing a human connection in every process along with healthcare technology leads to the increasing popularity of various mobile health applications and service-based apps. These programs are intended to serve as a liaison between patients and medical professionals. The focus of this mobile healthcare technology is on the use of AI, ML, digital services, etc.

In the 3.0 age, technology is used to care for patients rather than practitioners, which saves time. The gap between consumers and their healthcare professionals is closed by this technology and applications. An mHealth app is The Foundation of Healthcare 3.0. It is employed by the sector as a bridge between patients and physicians or as a tool for physicians to communicate difficult procedures to their staff and patients. Keeping the industry's fusion of technology and people alive, every process is going transparent and smooth with various mHealth apps. Ranging from low-end applications to FemTech solutions and mHealth apps, all the applications involving technologies improve millions of lives. A few elements of digital medical devices serve as evidence that technology is enabling the healthcare sector from the views of users, physicians, and hospitals [33,34].

The features are

1.  Manual records management
    The most time-consuming and demanding jobs at a hospital or healthcare facility are the maintenance of patient files. Tasks such as keeping track of medical records, and extracting the record within a while during an emergency are easy and it is the foundation for introducing a mobile app for patient records management.
2.  Cost saving
    There are many other situations, such as choosing the hospital, the patient onboarding procedure, the instructions or handbook for post-care that is provided to each patient, costs, etc., that are totaled up on the hospital's expenditure sheet.
3.  Time saving
    mHealth apps are used in streamlining the processes to a great extent in spending with hospital formalities and getting their appointments. This app saves a lot of time.
4.  Reduced workload
    There are a few tasks such as creating and managing persons databases, sending care flyers, hospital on boarding, and managing appointments that will be reduced with the help of mHealth applications.

5. Fraud management
The frequency of medical fraud was decreased, which was one of the largest contributions made by mHealth apps. Thanks to these types of medical technology, the patient and the hospital administration may now communicate openly about health practice and financial information.

6. Improved health through IoT
It is now much simpler for people to keep track of their health and determine when they need to visit a doctor. A big thanks to apps that remind users to take their medications, drink water, check their heart rate and cholesterol levels, and even keep track of their sleep. Additionally, it has sparked a fresh revolution in the medical industry.

7. e-Prescription
This enables doctors to write prescriptions with all the necessary information and deliver them to their patients. It uses digital technology to enhance practitioner communication. Anyone can include a built-in pharmacy lookup tool to check whether or not certain medications are sold locally.

8. Dashboard management
Many mHealth apps have features that enable users to make use of simple dashboards. It has user monitoring information, recovery progress information, and a visual health record that both patients and doctors may access right away. It displays a patient's health in a visual style; therefore the dashboard's vibrant and colorful images are really helpful.

The mHealth market has been segmented into a number of categories based on the numerous services provided by fitness and health applications in terms of the individual income generation. Numerous studies have shown that mobile applications would be used extensively in the healthcare industry, acting as a bridge between patients and their physicians and vice versa.

Some of the mHealth Apps are the following:

(A) WebMD App
This WebMD software, which is accessible on both Android and iPhone, allows users to monitor their symptoms, real-time access to medicine information, medical assistance, and hospital location. It provides rapid access to first-aid information in offline mode and gets you ready to discuss your health with your doctor.

(B) App-Health: ePeople
It is now the most widely used application for managing medical records. This software not only monitors your weight, blood pressure, heart rate, and amount of activity but it also allows you to follow the whereabouts of loved ones who are separated from you.

(C) Doctor on demand
It links local patients with physicians so that patients do not have to wait a long time for a doctor when they enquire about their availability. It facilitates scheduling appointments well in advance and contacting a doctor right away.

(D)   GOLD COPD

It provides a way to manage chronic obstructive pulmonary disease (COPD). It enables medical professionals to conduct a COPD assessment test and examine patients. The doctors can effectively forecast the severity and course of COPD, record the patient's health state, and monitor illness symptoms.

(E)   Dr. Pad

This software is a management tool that enables healthcare providers to keep track of all patient information, including personal data, visit and prescription histories, medical histories, medical reports, and other health-related information. It is also possible to keep and retrieve data related to other tests, such as blood tests, X-rays, ultrasounds, screens, and other patient files.

The two dominant platforms in use today include a number of apps that serve as tools for the healthcare sector. The first is the creation of healthcare mobile apps for Android, and the second is the creation of healthcare mobile apps for iOS. The Android interface is advantageous for mobile health apps if you want them to provide information for free or to operate around databases. If the app should be secured, then one must choose iOS as Apple. Applications for Apple and Android have various options and potential for development. The global market for Mobile Apps in healthcare sector was estimated around US$4.2 Billion for the year 2020 during COVID-19 crisis and is further reconsidered to reach US$20.7 Billion by 2027. Its growing rate of CAGR is 25.5% over the period 2020–2027.

## 12.5.1   *Technology influence on Healthcare 4.0*

The revolution in Industry 4.0 relies on smart machines which allow users to make decisions without human involvement and get access to large amounts of data. Industry 4.0 technologies help a lot in the era of Healthcare 4.0 and it refers to a wide range of possibilities to improve healthcare with a new and innovative vision. The objective is to provide patients with better, more cost-effective and value-added healthcare services. The technologies are IoT, cloud, AI, data analytics, etc.

1.   Remote patient monitoring

The IoT-based application and gadget for healthcare known as remote patient monitoring allows patients who are physically or psychologically unable to enter a healthcare institution to automatically provide metrics like blood pressure, heart beat rate, sugar level, temperature level of a body, and many more. Thanks to these facilities so that patients can avoid visiting service providers often.

The information gathered by the medical IoT devices will be sent to a software program so that either patients or healthcare professionals may access it. Many different algorithms may be used to analyze the data and treat patients, suggest therapies, or produce alarms. Keeping the security of the personal data acquired by these IoT devices secure is a significant concern.

2.   Glucose monitoring system

In the United States, more than 30 million people have diabetes. By offering continuous and automated monitoring, the glucose monitoring equipment that these diabetic people utilize enables them to deal with their issues. It does away with the need to manually preserve health records and notifies patients when their blood sugar levels are abnormal.

3. Heart-rate monitoring

   Regular heart rate monitoring cannot prevent sudden changes in the heart rate. Patients must continually be hooked up to equipment as a result of the traditional continuous cardiac monitoring systems used in hospitals, which limit their movement. With the introduction of new, miniature IoT devices in Healthcare 4.0, patients are now free to move around, and their heart rates are continuously monitored. The most recent technology can give accuracy rates of up to 90%.

4. Hygiene monitoring

   When patients enter hospital rooms, many hospitals and other primary healthcare facilities advise them to adequately sanitize their hands. It reminds staff to replace the sanitizer liquid in the device and provides instructions on how to sanitize effectively to reduce a potential danger.

5. Depression and mood monitoring

   As a conventional method, depression can be analyzed by visiting a physiologist on a regular frequency. Information about depression symptoms and general mood cannot be predicted more accurately by the psychology specialist and it is difficult for them to analyze and anticipate sudden mood swings all the time continuously. Additionally, sufferers would not appropriately describe their emotions. The well-known IoT gadget known as "Mood-Aware" can address, gather, and analyze information on blood pressure, eye movement, and heart rate in patients. It accurately maintains track of all other reasons for concern.

6. Connected inhalers

   Heart attacks frequently occur as a result of patient diseases like COPD or asthma. Patients can track the frequency of attacks with the assistance of the linked inhaler. It gathers information from the surroundings to assist healthcare experts in determining what precipitated an attack. When patients leave their inhalers at home, it can warn them. Inhaler makes the patient to suffer in case of its improper usage.

7. Connected contact lenses

   Passive, unobtrusive data collection is used by smart contact lenses. Micro cameras that were patented by Google are integrated within it, enabling users to shoot images while wearing it.

8. Robotic surgery

   The surgery is easily performed by a tiny, Internet-connected robot that has been implanted within a mortal body. The surgeries were done by small robotic bias to minimize the extent of the lacerations needed to perform surgery. It leads to a less invasive process and quick recuperation in some cases. These biases are pity in nature and dependable enough to perform surgeries with minimum dislocation.

9. Automated IV pumps

   This automated device controls the tablets and drips given to cases. It allows nurses to change the drip situations and specifics given to the cases.

Additionally, patients can raise their own regulated amount of painkillers with the help of the tone pumps. If a quick adaption is required in a critical scenario, it aids nurses in hastening the procedure. Since there are several types of automated IV pumps used in hospitals, training and education are simple to complete. Many nursing seminaries provide instruction and knowledge about new software and technology that employs these feathers of bias.

10. Portable monitors

    Professionals in the nursing field can use this technology to monitor patients' vital signs such respiration rates, ECGs, $SPO_2$ levels, and oxygen saturation. It sends the data back to a cloud-based central monitoring platform. If there is an emergency, the medical staff will be informed by alarm notification. This enables them to continuously monitor patients from any location, and the portable monitor's alarm warning can assist save lives in the hospital. Nursing students are taught the value of life and how to use a variety of equipment using these tools in the educational setting.

11. Smart beds

    It enables specialists to monitor a patient's mobility, weight, and even vital signs. The monitoring of patients' comfort and safety over a prolonged stay is greatly aided by smart beds. The device for continuous in-room monitoring offers frequent updates and notifications on a patient's activity. It aids in the discovery of numerous patterns that might result in an accurate diagnosis.

12. Wearable devices

    Smartphone applications and wearable technology are revolutionizing the healthcare sector. People can improve their health by using devices that monitor heart rates, exercise, sleep, breathing, and other factors. As more individuals own iPhones, nurses may take use of technologies and applications that enhance patient care. For instance, with nothing more than their smartphones, nurses and doctors may see heart rates and receive breathing sounds with the Steth IO smartphone stethoscope. The fact that the data is transmitted directly from the gadget itself helps nurses reduce the risk of human error. It enables quicker record keeping and aids patients and staff in maintaining regular health monitoring.

13. EHRs

    EHRs are taking the place of outdated paper filing methods. The caretaker team, which consists of doctors, patients, and trusted staff members, is able to utilize the information entered into computer systems as needed. Even though HIPAA regulations ensure that healthcare organizations preserve the confidentiality and safety of electronic records, safety issues for EHRs are being reduced by new technologies like blockchain and cryptography.

14. Centralized command centers

    Centralized command centers promise ways for clinicians to manage technology, resources, and capacity. This is accomplished via real-time updating software tools like dashboards. Nurses and doctors may be actively aware of the availability of rooms, OR schedules, and which individual patients require extra treatment before being discharged if there are no glitches during the transfer of care. Everyone is able to work more efficiently and assist patients better as a result. As a consequence, everyone is able to work more productively and provide patients with better care.

15.  Telehealth and apps

A recent and important component of healthcare is telehealth. Patients can virtually video chat with a doctor or nurse in hospitals and clinics to describe their symptoms or to show the doctor items like lumps or rashes. Patients benefit from speedy diagnoses without having to leave the comfort of their own home thanks to this. They can acquire a prescription for medication, receive medical guidance, and learn if they need to visit for additional examinations or diagnosis. It saves both time and resources for patients as well as healthcare professionals. It stops sick people from visiting public locations and potentially exposing other sufferers. This helps patients save time and stress while saving resources in clinics. Using apps can help with mental health difficulties. Users who use mindfulness apps can better understand their energy and mental wellness. They are reminded to make time for these crucial wellness-related activities.

16.  Nursing education

The introduction of new clinical healthcare technology is both exhilarating and revolutionary, and it greatly aids nursing education. It presents difficulties for nurses who must learn about the new technology and use it to their jobs to develop their careers. With the continuous improvement in the healthcare industry, the process of both nurses and patients elevates to the next level in medical care.

Figure 12.2 shows the technology intervention in Healthcare 4.0 and these devices are integrated with cloud and other next-generation computing techniques like robotics, IoT, big data analytics, etc.

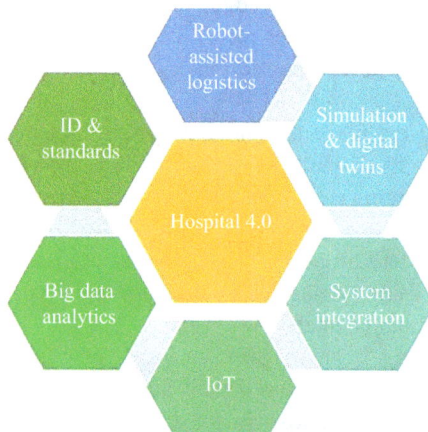

*Figure 12.2    Technology intervention in Healthcare 4.0. Source from Ref. [35].*

"Machine as a Service" is logistics with robot assistance. What is not a robot in today's world? Automated guided vehicle/autonomous mobile robot (AGVs/AMRs), self-driving robots transporting items, robots for picking medication, machines for laundry and washing, pneumatic tube systems, automated dispensing devices for medicine, uniforms, etc.

Along with clinical simulation, goods logistics related to, for instance, the design and capacity estimation of sterile service departments and the logistics design of AGV systems have also been simulated in the industry. In the future, we will be able to gather real-time data using RFID and sensors and upload it online to our digital twin, a virtual replica of our logistics system.

We require a connection between the systems supporting our logistics flows from the ERP system to the PLC level, including integration layers such as MES, to allow smooth administrative data flows mirroring the physical movements in real time, transactions, and traceability. The IoT gives us one of many platforms for connecting people, things, and processes that are tied to processes, events, times, and locations, giving us the groundwork for event-based traceability. Objects will be easily recognizable, localizable, and able to take detours that are more suited to their intended destination.

Big data analytics, which gathers information from chips and sensors, has the potential to forecast consumer demand for goods through data mining and enhance the efficiency of the supply chain more generally and stock management in particular. Identification and standards will be the prerequisite for all the above. It recognizes who, what, where, and when across departments, hospitals, and trading partners in a uniform and standardized manner.

All the above devices are used at maximum in the healthcare services and the security part of the devices plays a major role in healthcare since these devices are connected to the cloud technologies. The data acquired by various IoT devices used for diverse purposes must be securely secured by the device creators, managers, and suppliers. A large portion of the information gathered by medical devices is utilized as authenticated health information as defined by HIPAA. Data security from unmonitored devices is achieved by developing secure hardware and software. The managers may monitor device activity to spot abnormalities, separate susceptible from mission-critical devices, and conduct risk assessments once the IoT devices have been identified, regulated, classed, and protected under the appropriate terms and conditions.

## 12.6 Results

The results infer that the healthcare transitions from 1.0 to 4.0 gives tremendous benefits toward healthcare sectors integrated with modern technologies and tools in the current era. A few examples represent the influence of technology in healthcare sectors including IoT, AI, virtual reality, sensor and wearable devices, RPA, big data, cyber security, 5G, Edge and Fog computing, and so on. The global spending on IOT devices till 2027 is referred in Figure 12.3.

AI and virtual reality play an important role in technological development in healthcare which shows extreme improvement in the global market as shown in Figures 12.4 and 12.5.

Healthcare sector concentrates more on wearable technologies to monitor patient's health and other vital signs on and off the environment. Figure 12.6 indicates the technology intervention in medical treatments.

Most crucial things that every enterprise concentrates more are big data and its security threats. The analysis done on it gives useful information to make smatter decisions to drive business in a successful way. One has to protect these big data from breaches for strong decisions. The market analysis of both is presented in Figures 12.7 and 12.8.

Enterprise IoT market 2019–2027

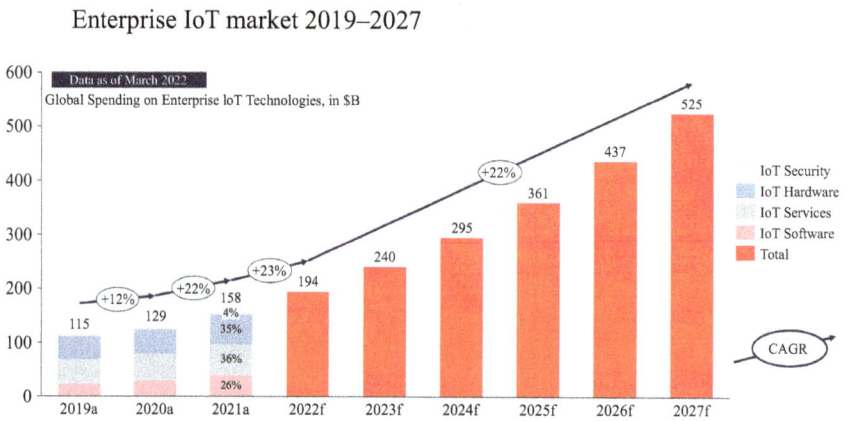

*Figure 12.3    Global market of IoT in healthcare*

ARTIFICIAL INTELLIGENCE IN HEALTHCARE MARKET SIZE, 2021 TO 2030 (USD BILLION)

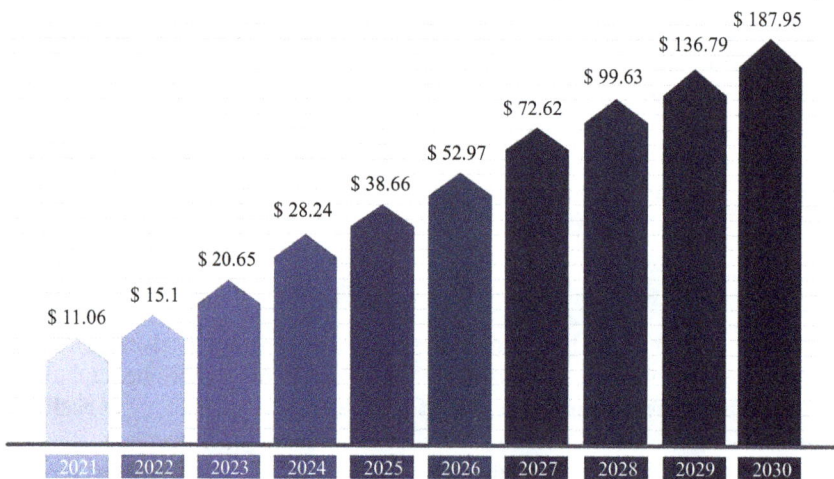

*Figure 12.4    Market of AI in healthcare*

Virtual Reality in Healthcare Market Size, 2022–2032

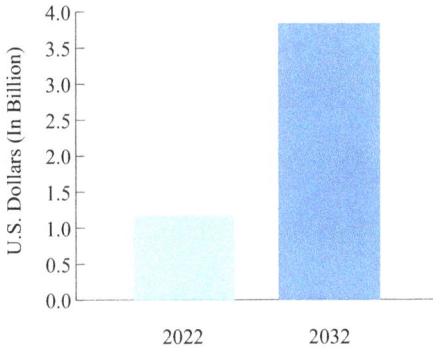

*Figure 12.5 Global market of virtual reality in healthcare*

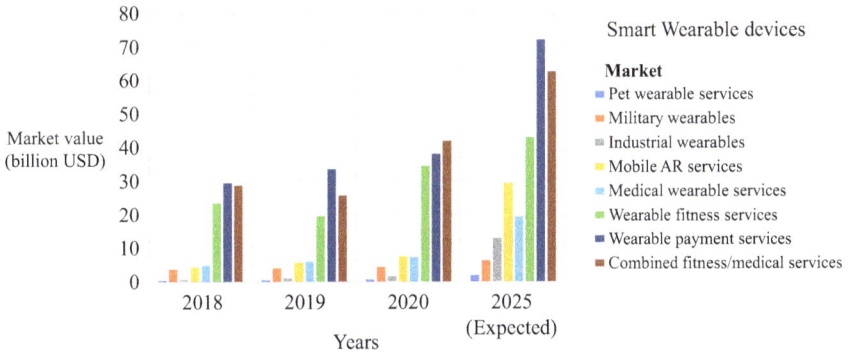

*Figure 12.6 Global market of sensor and wearable devices in healthcare*

Big Data Analytics in Healthcare Market Size, 2022 To 2030 (USD Billion)

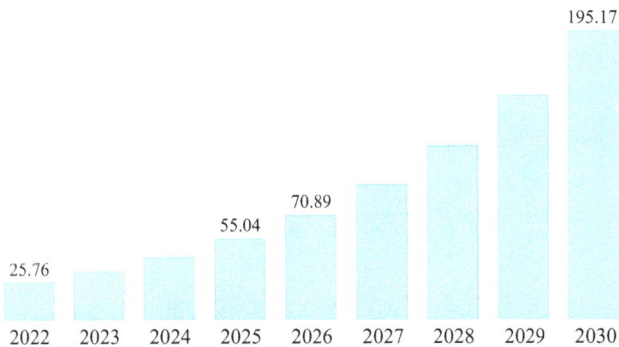

*Figure 12.7 Big data analytics in healthcare*

Healthcare Cyber Security Market
Share, by Threat Type, 2022 (%)

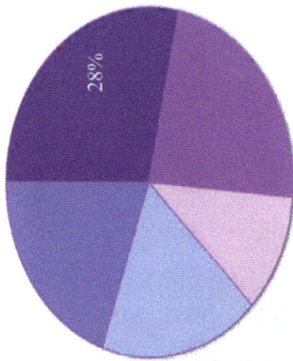

28%

- Malware
- DDOS
- Spyware
- Advanced Persistent Threat
- Other Threat Types

15.2
Total Market Size (USD Billion), 2022

17.1%
CAGR 2022–2032

Global Healthcare Cyber Security Market
share, by end use, 2021 (%)

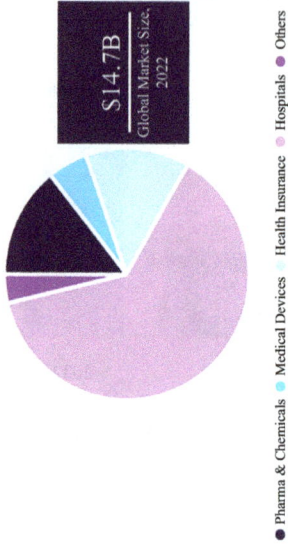

$14.7B
Global Market Size, 2022

● Pharma & Chemicals  ● Medical Devices  ● Health Insurance  ● Hospitals  ● Others

*Figure 12.8  Cyber security in healthcare*

## 12.7    Conclusion

In conclusion, technology intervention in healthcare services offers more benefits toward medical professionals. Still there is a lot of scope for improvement in this field that automates every work done by humans. All the innovations are involved with integrated technologies to make smarter decisions and work independently. Health systems engineering is presented with a wide range of opportunities and challenges by Healthcare 4.0. The following recommendations are made to take advantage of the opportunities and get through the challenges that stand in the way of attaining connected and smart healthcare.

To create a shared vision, a variety of stakeholders must be included, including those from engineering, health sciences, education, enhancing the delivery of healthcare, and health and healthcare technology. It requires a lot of cooperation, contact, and communication among many fields.

Second, various technologies and methods need to be applied. The use of quantitative approaches, such as modeling, simulation, computation, and optimization techniques, should be integrated with the use of qualitative methods, such as survey, human-centered design, evaluation, and field observations. Combining quantitative and qualitative methodologies as well as combining different methods and data sets should be prioritized. A significant supplement to modeling is also the use of empirical research and experimental projects like virtual reality, medical simulation, and pilot studies, especially before, during, and after the adoption of new practices. This will make it possible for continuous learning and healthcare improvement.

Third, the hardware and software components of the loop should be linked together. To ensure efficient connectivity and secure use of smart technologies, the suggested socio-technical approach makes human–machine or human–technology interactions crucial. Finally, in both research and practice, the focus of connected and smart healthcare should be on people, including patients, family members, and healthcare professionals. Addressing gaps and inequities is crucial, as is ensuring that Health Treatment 4.0 is built to lessen and ameliorate these injustices and give everyone access to high-quality, safe treatment. It is essential that the public health sector participate and make an effort to guarantee that the socioeconomic determinants of health are given more attention.

## References

[1]    Li, J. and Carayon, P. (2021). *Health Care 4.0: a vision for smart and connected health care. IISE Transactions on Healthcare Systems Engineering*, 11, 1–14. 10.1080/24725579.2021.1884627.

[2]    Kaur, J., Verma, R., Alharbe, N., Agrawal, A. and Khan,R. (2020). Importance of fog computing in Healthcare 4.0. In *Fog Computing for Healthcare 4.0 Environments* (pp. 79–101). Springer. Doi:10.1007/978-3-030-46197-3_4.

[3]  Luz Tortorella, F., Fogliatto, F.S., Kurnia, S., Thürer, M., and Capurro, D. (2022). Healthcare 4.0 digital applications: an empirical study on measures, bundles and patient-centered performance. *Technological Forecasting and Social Change*, 181, 21780. ISSN 0040-1625, https://doi.org/10.1016/j.techfore.2022.121780.

[4]  Gutema Robi, Y. and Sitote, T.M. (2023). Neonatal disease prediction using machine learning techniques. *Journal of Healthcare Engineering*, 2023, Article ID 3567194, 16 pages. https://doi.org/10.1155/2023/3567194.

[5]  Abid Haleem, M.J., Singh, R.P, and Suman, R. (2022). Medical 4.0 technologies for healthcare: features, capabilities, and applications. *Internet of Things and Cyber-Physical Systems*, 2, 12–30. ISSN 2667-3452, https://doi.org/10.1016/j.iotcps.2022.04.001.

[6]  Li, J. and Carayon. P. (2021). Health Care 4.0: a vision for smart and connected health care. *IISE Transactions on Healthcare Systems Engineering*, 11(3), 171–180.

[7]  Al-Jaroodi, J., Mohamed, N., and Abukhousa, E. (2020). Health 4.0: on the way to realizing the healthcare of the future. *IEEE Access*, 8, 211189–211210.

[8]  Mwanza, J., Telukdarie, A., and Igusa, T. (2023). Impact of industry 4.0 on healthcare systems of low- and middle-income countries: a systematic review. *Health and Technology*, 13, 35–52. https://doi.org/10.1007/s12553-022-00714-2.

[9]  Aazam, M. and Huh, E.-N. (2014). Fog computing and smart gateway-based communication for cloud of things. In *2014 International Conference on Future Internet of Things and Cloud*. Washington, DC: IEEE.

[10] Fernandez, F. and Pallis, G. C. (2014). Opportunities and challenges of the Internet of Things for healthcare: systems engineering perspective. In *2014 Fourth International Conference on Wireless Mobile Communication and Healthcare-Transforming Healthcare Through Innovations in Mobile and Wireless Technologies (MOBIHEALTH)*. Washington, DC: IEEE.

[11] Kanth, R.K., Liljeberg, P., Westerlund, T., *et al.* (2014). Information and communication system technology's impacts on personalized and pervasive healthcare: a technological survey. In *2014 IEEE Conference on Norbert Wiener in the 21st Century (21CW)*. Washington, DC: IEEE.

[12] Fratu, O., Pena, C., Craciunescu, R., and Halunga, S. (2015). Fog computing system for monitoring mild dementia and COPD patients—Romanian case study. In *2015 12th International Conference on Telecommunication in Modern Satellite, Cable and Broadcasting Services(TELSIKS)*. Washington, DC: IEEE.

[13] Cao, Y., Chen, S., Hou, P., and Brown, D. (2015). FAST: a fog computing assisted distributed analytics system to monitor fall for stroke mitigation. In *2015 IEEE International Conference on Networking, Architecture and Storage (NAS)*. Washington, DC: IEEE.

[14] Jiang, T.N., Rahmani, M., Westerlund, A.-M., Liljeberg, T., and Tenhunen, H. (2015). Fog computing in healthcare Internet of Things: a case study on ECG feature extraction. In *2015 IEEE International Conference on Computer*

and Information Technology; Ubiquitous Computing and Communications; Dependable, Autonomic and Secure Computing; Pervasive Intelligence and Computing. Washington, DC: IEEE.

[15] Chakraborty, S., Bhowmick, S., Talaga, P., and Agrawal, D.P. (2016). Fog networks in healthcare application. In *2016 IEEE 13th International Conference on Mobile Ad Hoc and Sensor Systems (MASS)*. Washington, DC: IEEE.

[16] Sood, S.K. and Mahajan, I. (2017). A fog-based healthcare framework for chikungunya. *IEEE Internet of Things Journal*, 5(2), 794–801.

[17] Mahmoud, M.M.E., Rodrigues, J.J.P.C., Saleem, K., Al-Muhtadi, J., Kumar, N., and Korotaev,V. (2018). Towards energy-aware fog-enabled cloud of things for healthcare. *Computers & Electrical Engineering*, 67, 58–69.

[18] Kotzias, K., Bukhsh, F.A., Arachchige, J.J., Daneva, M., and Abhishta, A. (2022) Industry 4.0 and healthcare: context, applications, benefits and challenges. *IET Software*, 17, 195–248. https://doi.org/10.1049/sfw2.12074.

[19] Popov, V.V., Kudryavtseva, E.V., Kumar Katiyar, N., Shishkin, A., Stepanov, S.I., and Goel, S. (2022). Industry 4.0 and Digitalisation in Healthcare. *Materials*, 15(6), 2140. https://doi.org/10.3390/ma15062140

[20] Nwobodo-Anyadiegwu, E., Tambwe, D.B., and Lumbwe, A.K. The integration of Industry 4.0 in healthcare quality improvement. In *2022 IEEE 28th International Conference on Engineering, Technology and Innovation (ICE/ITMC) & 31st International Association for Management of Technology (IAMOT) Joint Conference*, Nancy, France, 2022, pp. 1–6, doi:10.1109/ICE/ITMC-IAMOT55089.2022.10033265.

[21] Li, J. and Carayon, P. (2021). Health Care 4.0: a vision for smart and connected health care. *IISE Transactions on Healthcare Systems Engineering*, 11(3), 171–180. doi:10.1080/24725579.2021.1884627.

[22] Saravana Kumar, N.M., Eswari, T., Sampath, P., and Selvaraj, L. (2015). Predictive methodology for diabetic data analysis in big data. *Procedia Computer Science*, 50, 203–208. 10.1016/j.procs.2015.04.069.

[23] Ramalho, F., Neto, A., Santos, K., and Agoulmine, N. (2015). Enhancing ehealth smart applications: a fog-enabled approach. In *2015 17th International Conference on E-Health Networking, Application & Services (HealthCom)*. Washington, DC: IEEE.

[24] Gu, L., Zeng, D., Guo, S., Barnawi, A., and Xiang, Y. (2015). Cost efficient resource management in fog computing supported medical cyber-physical system. *IEEE Transactions on Emerging Topics in Computing*, 5(1), 108–119.

[25] Masip-Bruin, X., Marín-Tordera, E., Alonso, A., and Garcia, J. (2016). Fog-to-cloud computing(F2C): the key technology enabler for dependable e-health services deployment. In *2016 Mediterranean Ad Hoc Networking Workshop (Med-Hoc-Net)*. Washington, DC: IEEE.

[26] Azimi, I., Anzanpour, A., Rahmani, A.M., Liljeberg, P., and Salakoski, T. (2016). Medical warning system based on Internet of Things using fog computing. In *2016 International Workshop on Big Data and Information Security (IWBIS)*. Washington, DC: IEEE.

[27]   Monteiro, A., Dubey, H., Mahler, L., Yang, Q., and Mankodiya, K. (2016). Fit: a fog computing device for speech tele-treatments. In *2016 IEEE International Conference on Smart Computing (SMARTCOMP)*. Washington, DC: IEEE.

[28]   Elmisery, A.M., Rho, S., and Botvich, D. (2016). A fog-based middleware for automated compliance with OECD privacy principles in internet of healthcare things. *IEEE Access*, 4, 8418–8441.

[29]   Ahmad, M., Amin, M.B., Hussain, S., Kang, B.H., Cheong, T., and Lee, S. (2016). Health fog: a novel framework for health and wellness applications. *The Journal of Supercomputing*, 72(10), 3677–3695.

[30]   Ahsan, M.M. and Siddique, Z. (2022). Industry 4.0 in Healthcare: a systematic review. *International Journal of Information Management Data Insights*, 2(1), 100079.

[31]   https://doi.org/10.1016/j.jjimei.2022.100079.

[32]   https://appinventiv.com/blog/role-of-mhealth-apps-in-healthcare-evolution-from-1-0-3-0/.

[33]   https://medicalnotes.co/issue-40/.

[34]   https://www.linkedin.com/pulse/hospital-10-20-3040-future-logistics-claus-fabricius.

[35]   Alia, O., Abdelbakib, W., Shresthac, A., *et al.* A systematic literature review of artificial intelligence in the healthcare sector: benefits, challenges, methodologies, and functionalities. *Journal of Innovation & Knowledge*, 8(1), 100333. doi:10.1016/j.jik.2023.100333.

*Chapter 13*

# Trending technologies in patient-centric Healthcare 4.0

*Neha Singh[1], Shilpi Birla[1], Neeraj Kumar Shukla[2] and Shaminder Kaur[3]*

## Abstract

Over the years, healthcare has shifted its approach from doctor centric to patient centric. Recently, the focus has been not only on disease treatment but also on developing prevention-oriented medicine with remote accessibility and capabilities. This requires not only to have real-time capabilities but also to automate the process from patient data management to disease prediction to its treatment to post care. Industrial Revolution 4.0 has been driven by the adoption of cyber-physical systems with the help of technological developments in mobile Internet speed, cloud technology, artificial intelligence (AI)-enabled automation, and data analytics. The objective of this chapter is to review these Industry 4.0 technologies at play which are crucial to improve performance, productivity, efficiency, and security of healthcare services without sacrificing reliability or accessibility. It can only be achieved with patient-centric smart hospitals that are automated on every step right from patient admission to data management to discharge procedures for effective management of the crowd so that the patients are served efficiently. The hospitals are not only required to manage patients but also require optimal utilization of the medical equipment, physical assets and services, not only for the admitted patients but also for extensive care of discharged patients in real-time remotely at their comfort. Mobile wearable sensors are greatly useful for tracking self-health which can be integrated into hospital systems and practitioners can observe the patients' vital parameters remotely to actively intervene in emergencies. Science and technology have advanced to increase the life span of humans which requires critical maintenance of human organs and sometimes, even replacement. The availability of human organs for donation is limited but bioprinting of human organs is a breakthrough that will definitely save the life of many critically ill patients. In such cases, skilled practitioners can extend their services to remote

[1]Department of Electronics and Communication Engineering, Manipal University, Jaipur, India
[2]Department of Electrical Engineering, King Khalid University, Abha, Saudi Arabia
[3]Department of ECE, Chitkara University, Punjab, India

locations with the use of cloud services and augmented reality devices with high capabilities. With the introduction of these new technologies in different realms of healthcare for automation and monitoring, a large set of heterogeneous data is collected with needs to be securely saved, accessed, and used. This data is also useful for scientific studies not only for improving disease prediction, for hospital management and remote patient care but developing new trends and equipment.

**Keywords:** Healthcare; Artificial intelligence; IoT and wearables; Bioprinting; Data privacy; Medical data

## 13.1    Introduction

The fourth industrial revolution, or Industry 4.0, integrates big data analytics and cloud technology with high mobile Internet speed and artificial intelligence (AI) in manufacturing as well as distribution of products for automation and optimal industrial production. The industrial processes are optimized based on the data generated, collected, and shared between different participants in the production cycle. This not only requires the sensors and control systems to be smart and independent but also requires a reliable and safe communication between different entities for efficient monitoring, diagnosis, and analysis. The requirements of industry 4.0 have been met by employing the latest AI techniques for developing self-learning intelligent machines that can interconnect and make decisions without human intervention. Also, AI together with cloud computing, big data analytics, and high-speed mobile Internet has revolutionized healthcare sector too. Healthcare 4.0 converges the physical and biological worlds with the digital world targeting improvement in healthcare services. AI has been used in medicine in different areas from disease diagnosis, treatment plans to patient monitoring, and hospital management. The main objectives [1] of healthcare 4.0 are providing real-time collection, diagnosis, tracking, and response solutions by integrating monitoring and diagnostics in real-time with AI support for an effective patient-centric system. The digital transformation with multiple touchpoints for patients helps profile patients and understand their anatomy with possible forecasting of critical illness in the future, monitor the patients remotely, and provide treatment. The implementation of such an efficient healthcare system requires to address the main aspects in each phase, as shown in Figure 13.1.

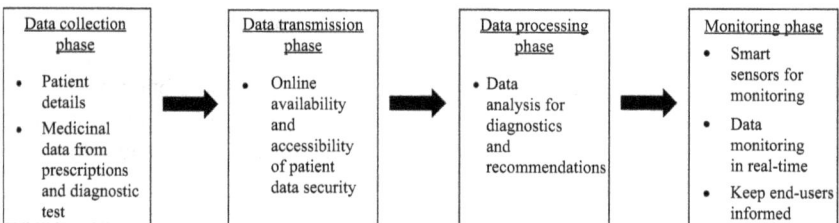

*Figure 13.1   Addressing the main aspects of healthcare system*

## 13.2  Expectations and challenges of Healthcare 4.0

The basic principles of healthcare are accessibility, availability, affordability and acceptability, and appropriateness of health services. Healthcare not only deals with diagnosis and treatment of diseases but it also involves drug development, hospital administration, and management. A resilient healthcare system should be able to provide:

  (i)    remote consultations
 (ii)    remotely aided surgical and clinical procedures
(iii)    real-time medical care
 (iv)    digital non-invasive care
  (v)    real-time and networked medical emergency support
 (vi)    collaborative sharing of patient data and information on digital platforms

For example, hospitals are required to plan and schedule shifts of healthcare workers and patient visits; schedule examinations on the medical testing equipment; store data securely that is readily accessible, plan and schedule surgeries, track patients, and provide remote services when required. The review of literature over the period of 2015–2019 in [2] identified the important challenges in adopting the research solutions by healthcare industry. Some of the major challenges are lack of quality data, increasing heterogeneous data sources, interoperability, scalability, and rapidly changing demands. It is clear from this study that there is a need of performing more practical implementation in research pertaining to Healthcare 4.0 along with standardization of data. However, while implementing Healthcare 4.0, hospitals need to look at the technical challenges as identified in [3].

Operational and security challenges while performing a case study on a proposed smart healthcare system are identified in [4]. Some important operational challenges as identified in the study are regulatory policies of the government, compatible network resources and networks, interoperability of different types of devices, device and information confidentiality and security, device cost and compliance, data management and ownership, connectivity and security of communication channels, power management of the sensors and devices. The security concern at each of the core, distribution, and access levels has been emphasized for any communication channel. The authors of [4] assert the need of using secure and encrypted formats for patient health records for secure storage and transmission.

This chapter presents some trending technological developments that address these challenges and develop healthcare systems which can plan, schedule, observe, predict, and learn in the context of patient care.

## 13.3  AI

A large range and variety of data is generated with respect to the health of patients as well as in general which can be utilized for providing better healthcare services. The data is available from the personal and electronic patient records at clinics and hospitals, electronic prescription of medicines, data from health applications on smartphones and watches and many more paths. For the management and analysis of such largely collected data, AI has been exploited phenomenally in every phase of healthcare, from hospital planning to management, from drug development to testing, from patient data recording to management to remote access, from acquiring medical data and prediction of diseases to treatment planning. Thus, AI has opened doors for a wide range of possibilities to utilize industry 4.0 technologies in healthcare and medicine for better, cost-effective, and efficient patient care [5].

The availability of low-cost efficient sensors for capturing a wide range of patient medical data which is securely accessible for remote monitoring and computations with the help of cloud technology has induced the concept of Internet of Medical Things (IoMT). AI has the ability to analyze this enormous data, using machine learning (ML) and data analytics tools, which is useful for not only creating medical database but also for training the models based on the available data for its precise analysis and evaluation of patient state for improved clinical decisions. Critical analysis of the collected medical data helps medical practitioners to predict and spot indicators for critical diseases and issues.

AI has been used a crucial component of intelligent automation in industry by analyzing structured and unstructured data to develop a knowledge base for formulating predictions. Hospitals serve as the main provider of healthcare to the population by managing the resources with well-planned referral network for efficient response to the medical needs of the population. AI automates many repetitive functions across the hospitals and facilities which not only increases the efficiency of the system but, simultaneously makes more time for the employees to focus on more strategic initiatives for patient-centric care. Data of in- and out-patients for their appointment schedules, diseases, medicines, and proactive requirements of the patient and hospital management tends to create a lot of data to be handled, saved, secured, and shared. Forecasting the number of inpatients using data science technologies can help to improve hospital services like assigning patient beds and discharging [6]. Another important part of hospital management is scheduling operating rooms efficiently for which the application UCHealth is identified to schedule operating rooms optimally for improved hospital revenue [6]. Also, in emergency department of hospitals, the crowd can be managed by rerouting patient traffic to different medical examinations if predictive modeling is used to estimate the waiting time and duration of each patient's journey through the department.

Another application of AI that helps hospitals to reduce patient inflow is the chatbots which are designed to save patients' unnecessary trips to doctors and healthcare centers by guiding and resolving general queries of the patients [2]. These chatbots can explain medical symptoms for disease diagnosis, treatment options, and hospital processes to patients who otherwise have no or limited medical knowledge [6].

AI has also been implemented in the pharmaceutical industry as well not only for automated processes and high productivity but for drug discovery and development. AI is employed for quick identification of drug response markers in the subjects for clinical trials, development of viable drug targets more cheaply and efficiently, and prediction of chemical properties of drugs.

Wide healthcare data at multiple networked hospitals together with the requirement of management and accessibility of hospital assets explores the use of blockchain technology which was initially used for decentralized money-related exchanges. It has reformed and eased interoperability of hospitals with high data accuracy for reliable and consistent data sharing within the network. The authors of [7] explore the use of blockchain technologies for improving healthcare system frameworks.

AI has changed the face of healthcare for the betterment but because the implementation of these techniques is opaque, in the sense that the optimal results are received without knowing the process, more research is required toward explainable implementation of such systems. Real-time analysis of the largely collected data set for better interpretation and hence judgment about patient care and needs has helped in developing a sustainable, service-oriented healthcare system with real-time capabilities, remote access, and mobility.

## 13.4   Wearables and IoT technologies

Sensors are employed in hospitals and labs in many positions, for example, in refrigerators to maintain temperature for storing blood or other samples, or for monitoring medical data like temperature, blood pressure, sleep patterns, heartbeat, etc. for coma patients or patients away from hospitals recovering from critical and life-threatening diseases. Wearables provide the ability to monitor the status of a patient throughout the day remotely without confining the patient in the hospital boundary. Based on the sensed and monitored data clinicians can follow up the patients' recovery, send alerts, and interact with the patients if any complication or problem is sensed. This reduces the burden on the medical staff in the hospitals, saves hospitalization charges for the patient as well as allows the hospital facilities to be made available to other needy patients. The main use of AI techniques is to manage and analyze data which is nowadays received not only from the hospital labs and machines but wearable sensors too.

Moreover, early detection of illness symptoms by smart monitoring can result in the prevention of many fatal health conditions by providing timely treatment. Smartwatches and smartphones are nowadays used by a large population to monitor their own health status, especially after the COVID-19 pandemic. People are more aware of their health and hence track their health routines while measuring important body parameters.

Not only for patient monitoring but the latest wearables are targeted to help people having sensory impairments. For example, external or implanted hearing impairment devices help in improving low sensing in ears; a wireless glove is used to interface with a mobile phone to recognize hand signals of deaf people and communicate with the help of a voice interface [8]. The use of multimodal wearables for elderly people who are suffering from dementia is surveyed in [9].

Downsizing of sensors together with high processing power of computers has enabled interlinking of multiple sensors and devices, resulting in a big network of connected devices, generally referred to as IoT. It enables interoperability between machines, sharing of information, and migration of data for improved delivery of healthcare. The sensors are continually monitoring and hence producing enormous data, which generally is now referred to as Big Data. The authors of [10] combined cloud computing to IoT to reduce the time of execution to the stakeholders' request for enhancing the healthcare system performance, optimized storage of medical records and providing a real-time data retrieval mechanism for those applications. Cloud computing enables the applications to run remotely on shared physical devices rather than on-site machine. The model used in [10] has four major components: sensors/wearables to provide patient health data, stakeholders' (patient or clinician) requests, cloud broker, and network administrator. Cloud broker is accountable for sending and receiving requests to the cloud which contains multiple resources to execute the requests. Network administrator optimally selects the virtual machine in the cloud to reduce the time of execution for the requests.

A smart healthcare system that utilizes the concept of IoT for Saskatchewan, a Canadian province is presented in [5]. The implemented model targets to cover four services:

(i)    business analytics and cloud services for monitoring and updating dashboards at medical places and billing services
(ii)   cancer care services to monitor and provide intensive care for cancer units
(iii)  emergency services to cater to emergency services like ambulance, disaster management, accident safety, etc.
(iv)   operational services for pharmacies and medicine inventory management at hospitals

Hierarchical architecture is used for implementing communication network. Different healthcare providers are connected through cloud services using mesh topology so that all points are connected to one another, and information is shared among all units.

## 13.5    Augmented reality and virtual reality

With the strength of AI and cloud computing, tools exploiting augmented reality (AR) and virtual reality (VR) are another trend setters for automation of healthcare industry as well as medical education and training. AR/VR tools and techniques allow us to construct realistic situations for learning and experience by overlaying digital augmentation on the real-life environment. Implementing AR and VR for medical applications requires precise real-time integration, registration, and interaction of real and virtual worlds. The study in [11] identified VR to be ideal for surgical trainings, pain management, etc. as it allows virtual interaction of the user with the real-time medical environment to make better medical decisions when actual case arises. However, it requires considerable effort and care to reap maximum benefits of using AR and VR in medicine.

An important application of AR/VR devices is in medical education for the study of human anatomy [11,12]. Technological advancements make the learning content available with easy access at any time and place for the students making their studies interesting and interactive with audio and visual aids even outside the classroom sessions. A study is presented in [12] to prove effectiveness of using fully immersive AR and VR-based 3D environments to replace cadavers for the study of human anatomy during medical studies. This will provide more time for the students to study applied clinical work. Moreover, transforming 2D images into 3D using AR and VR technologies helps students to understand the relative placement of human organs in the body structure. The study evaluates the effect of using VR, AR, or tablet for content delivery on student perception based on the scores obtained with ANOVA test and Kruskal–Wallis H-test. This study in [12] showed equal effectiveness of the three modes of learning under study, thereby suggesting the use of AR and VR technology for equally effective medical studies.

AR and VR tools can be used by doctors, and nurses to plan, analyze, and practice complicated surgeries, performed in multiple steps and crucial variations, virtually before performing on patients [13]. This will help them train better at handling some important medical issue(s) during surgeries. For example, VR is also used to train nursing staff for handling patients with mental illness issues by using VR simulations for clinical training in mental health nursing [14]. These simulations enable the nursing students to experience to virtually interact and communicate with patients for identifying clinical symptoms and learn management of patients with such problematic symptoms. The usefulness of employing a 360-degree video simulation of patients suffering from schizophrenia is studied in [14] for training the nursing staff.

Another important application of AR is assisted and image-guided surgery [15]. These assisted surgeries enhance surgical accuracy and increased accessibility to minimally invasive techniques. An AR-enabled glass or a head-mounted device can be used to display vitals of the patient to the surgeon during the medical procedure. This will save time for the surgeon to toggle between different instruments for checking patient's vitals. The patient experience and the quality of healthcare delivery are enhanced through interactions between the real-world and virtual objects enabled by head-mounted displays, wearables, and mobile apps.

The authors of [16] proposed a real-time monitoring system by integrating AR with steady-state visually evoked potentials (SSVED) based brain–computer interface (BCI). This facilitated hands-free remote data collection and display for a real-time monitoring. The system presented in [16] used visual stimuli for navigating the AR menu, displayed on an AR glass that contains real-time medical data of patients. The accuracy of the developed system is reported as 70% with a delay of 4 sec due to Android application to receive the parameters. The architecture of the system design proposed and tested in [16] is shown in Figure 13.2.

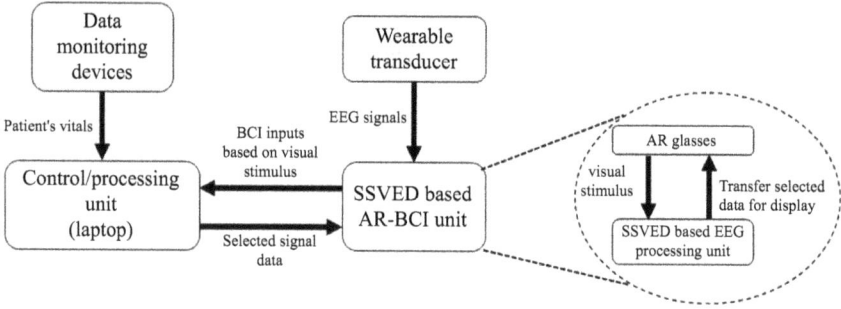

*Figure 13.2    Architecture of AR-BCI-based monitoring system [16]*

## 13.6    Healthcare data privacy and security

The enormous medical data collected through sensors in the IoT setup needs to be carefully processed using big data tools and techniques and stored on cloud for easy and secure access through Internet to remote locations for telemedicine, etc. Some important requirements while handling cloud-based healthcare data have been highlighted in [17,18] as mutual-authentication and access control, anonymity and non-traceability of the patient identity, privacy, integrity and confidentiality of patient records, network and system security, and attack resistance.

Data security is a crucial part of any smart healthcare system as this data is vulnerable to cyberattacks due to the involved personal and financial information. The security of healthcare data involves measures to guarantee the confidentiality and availability of electronically protected health information. If access to medical records and lifesaving medical devices is somehow lost, effective delivery of care to patients will not be possible. Hackers may not only steal but may alter the data intentionally or intentionally which can have serious effects on patients' treatments and hence health.

The healthcare architecture can be considered to have three layers [17], front-end layer, communication layer, and back-end layer. The front end encompasses the sensors used for reading and monitoring patient data. Owing to the small size of sensors with constrained computing capacity, this layer requires less computationally intensive security measures with even smaller communication overhead [19]. This data generated by front-end is communicated to the back-end through communication or data management layer which handles and standardizes diverse data obtained from medical sensors and store, process, and interpret the vital parameters to be sent to back-end layer. Confidentiality of patient data is the major security concern for this layer. Data encryption is generally implemented for secure storage and transfer of data on this layer. The back-end layer encompasses the medical practitioners who have authorized access to the data on cloud. Authorization of identified practitioner and verification are the main security concerns for this layer.

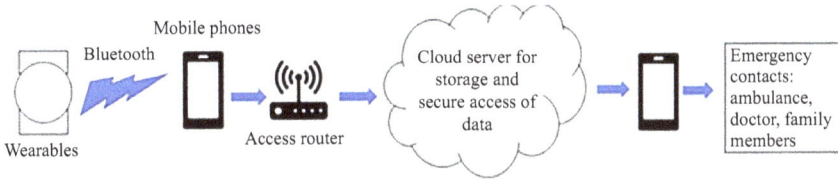

*Figure 13.3    A biometric-based access authentication system [21]*

The author of [20] presented a big data intelligence architecture using a meta-cloud redirecting architecture that interacts with the data centers on cloud for improved overall effectiveness and providing optimal alternative solutions to the end-users. The collected data is stored in different data centers based on their level of privacy as sensitive, critical, or normal by encrypting the storage path rather than the big data itself. To avoid any instance of losing data, multiple copies are stored on the cloud, this will consume more space.

Another secure scheme for accessing the electronic health records of any patient is proposed in [21]. The scheme uses biometrics for authentication to access the data, with less computational and communication costs. The architecture as used in [21] is shown in Figure 13.3.

Not only for medical data of patients but, big data analytics is used for clinical, operating and business models too. Data of in- and out-patients for their appointment schedules, diseases, medicines, and proactive requirements of the patient and hospital management tends to create a lot of data to be handled, saved, secured, and shared.

A permission-based secure system for sharing patient electronic healthcare record (EHR) using blockchain technology is presented in [7]. The use of immutable ledger technology provides system security. All the participants need to register on the blockchain network to obtain a private key. If the patient permits, the respective doctor, or lab participant can read and update his records in the EHR ledger network. The network is entirely secure because all transactions are added to the previous hash with a timestamp, allowing any participant to query the necessary data across the network.

## 13.7    Bioprinting

Bioprinting combines material science with life sciences. It utilizes cells, proteins, biological molecules, and biomaterials for precise printing of biological tissues and organ structures in three dimensions [22]. It has attracted the interest of researchers and the healthcare industry due to its ability to have precise control over positioning various tissue constituents like cells, scaffolds, and biological molecules for regenerating tissues and organs. Simultaneous printing of multiple cells, biomaterials, and biological molecules is also possible. Before printing any organ for the patient suitable medical imaging modality is chosen to generate a 3D view of

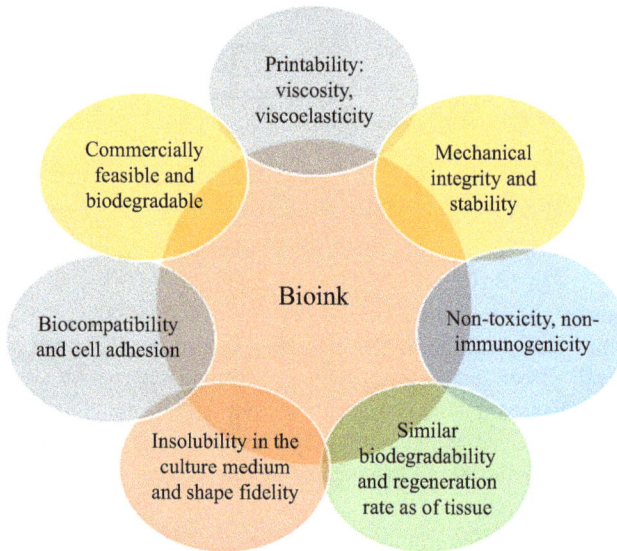

*Figure 13.4    Properties of bioink*

defected tissue or organ. Computerized tomography (CT) scans and magnetic resonance imaging (MRI) are useful for generating volumetric 3D view of the organs [23]. This information is used to develop the printing commands using computer-aided design/manufacturing (CAD/CAM) tools for choice of material and motion commands, for layer-by-layer printing of tissue using selective biomaterial.

Achieving mechanical, chemical, and morphological properties of the fabricated organs or tissues that are like real organs and tissues is the biggest challenge in organ fabrication. The biomaterials used for bioprinting, referred to as bioinks, address these properties. Some important properties of bioinks [24–26] are shown in Figure 13.4.

Many natural and synthetic materials like ceramics, polymers, elastomer, hydrogels, and lipids are generally used as bioinks. Based on the need of scaffolds for supporting the regenerative tissues while printing, the bioinks are classified as scaffold-free and scaffold-based [24]. The differences between the two types of bioinks are shown in Table 13.1.

Bioprinting has been used for printing bones and muscles [29], skin [25], heart valves [23], myocardial tissue [23], blood vessels [29], and nerves [29] too. Recently, a full-sized human heart model is developed using Freeform Reversible Embedding of Suspended Hydrogel (FRESH) printing of alginate as biomaterial to resemble the elasticity of cardiac tissue [30]. The method employed for printing these organs and tissue, however, is not always the same. The basic steps [29] for bioprinting are such that, initially, suitable medical imaging modalities are used to acquire clear data for the model to be printed. The second step is to choose the

*Table 13.1   Differences between scaffold-free and scaffold-based bioinks*

| Scaffold-free bioinks | Scaffold-based bioinks |
|---|---|
| Printing is performed in bioreactors [27] using cell sheets, isolated single cells, or spheroid cell aggregates | Contain hydrogels, microcarriers, or decellularized matrix compounds-loaded cells |
| Produce living structures using cells only which produce their own matrix and architecture | Grow, proliferate, and interact in three dimensions similar to natural tissue |
| Suitable for fabrication of nerve tissue, blood vessels, and cardiac patches | Important properties [28]: pseudoplasticity, quick gelation |
| Scaffold used to create the vessels degrade with time | Examples [28]: alginate, collagen, gelatin, hyaluronic acid, ExtracelTM, fibrin, polyethylene glycol and Pluronic® F127 |

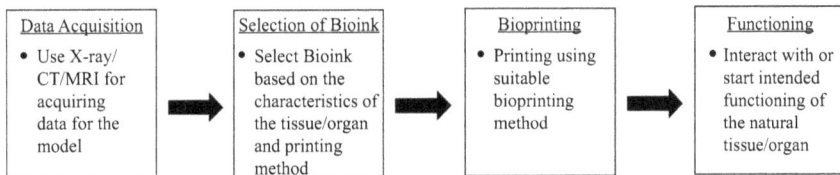

*Figure 13.5   Steps for bioprinting*

appropriate bioink to reflect the required natural properties of the bioprinted tissues and organs. Using the selected ink and the input from the first step, the tissue or organ is printed layer-by-layer. Lastly, physical and chemical stimulation is performed to make printed material interact or starts the intended functioning of the natural tissue/organ. The steps for bioprinting are shown in Figure 13.5.

Bioprinting technologies are generally classified as jetting-based and extrusion-based bioprinting [23]. Sometimes these may be combined, which is referred to as Integrated bioprinting.

Jetting-based or droplet-based bioprinting is low-cost contactless printing by deposition of bioink droplets of picoliter volume on a substrate, generally for resolutions in the range of 20–100 μm. Bioink droplets can be generated using different approaches like thermal method, piezoelectric actuators, pneumatic pressure, and focused laser [29]. These droplets can be produced continuously or drop-on-demand; however, drop-on-demand is used more due to the issue of decontamination of the ink due to recirculation and avoid wasting of unwanted drops of ink continuous process [29]. Due to the small size of bioink droplets, the processing time is long, and these methods use bioinks with low viscosity. Some examples of materials suitable for jetting-based bioprinting are thrombin, $CaCl_2$, saline, and fibrogen. It is difficult for these printed structures to maintain their shape and withstand stress.

Extrusion-based bioprinting [29] or direct ink writing prints with extrusion-based continuous filaments drawn from the nozzle of a syringe. The extrusion system to draw long filaments is driven by either pneumatic, piston or screw to push the bioink out of the nozzle. Pneumatic-driven methods use air pumps for pushing the material from the nozzle while the others use the mechanical motion of piston and the screw for the same. Pneumatic-driven bioprinting method is more suitable for hydrogels while bioinks with high viscosity work well with piston-driven and screw-driven systems. The design of the screw needs to be precise to avoid any damage to the cells in the bioink due to pressure. The syringe loaded with bioink is moved precisely using software based on the demand of the tissue/organ to be printed [29]. Printing of blood vessels uses two nozzles of different diameters as inner and outer nozzles to print hollow tubular structures or structures with different biomaterials in core and covering, coaxially.

Bioprinting is used for printing bionic skin substitutes [25] for wound management using natural as well as synthetic polymer materials. Natural materials are biocompatible and biodegradable but have long gelation times and insufficient mechanical properties. Synthetic polymers, on the other hand, offer controllable mechanical and chemical properties and lack biocompatibility. Some natural biomaterials like collagen, gelatin, linear polymer from brown algae, alginate, and some synthetic materials like polylactic acid, polycaprolactone, poly-glycolic acid, poly lactic-*co*-glycolic acid (PLGA), as well as GelMA are commonly used for skin bioprinting [25,31]. Natural and synthetic biomaterials are combined to form composite materials that exploit advantages of each type. An example of such composite biomaterial is polymeric blend of polycaprolactone with gelatin [25]. Various skin tissues like dermis, hair follicle, full-layered skin, blood vessel containing skin, sweat glands, and melanocytes-containing skin are printed [31].

3D tumor models are printed for cancer research [32–35] for understanding cancer biology. Co-printing different types of bioinks is used to replicate tumor microenvironment, including the immune cells, cancer cells, and stromal tissue for understanding and analyzing its behavior as a means of preclinical trials. Dual hydrogel-based bioinks are used in [33] for printing breast cancer models for the study of resistance to drugs. The model had cancer cells in the middle with adipose-derived mesenchymal stem/stromal cells (ADMSC) around it, which promote cancer progression. The authors of [33] successfully studied the drug resistance with different scenarios with the help of bioprinted models. Different methods for printing 3D models for cancer research are studied in detail in [34] using spheroid cultures, biopolymer scaffolds, organ-on-chip models, and ex vivo tissue slices. Selection of the most suitable modality for these models is also presented in [34].

Bioprinting also finds great application in pharmaceutical industry for screening of drug efficacies, toxicities or metabolisms, and drug delivery. It is suggested in [36] that 3D bioprinting should be used in preclinical phase to reduce the cost and time. The authors of [37] exploited high water retainment, nontoxicity, biocompatibility, and biodegradability properties of hydrogels to use them as a drug carrier and as a dressing material for wounds and burns. The material of drug carriers is carefully chosen to target cancer cells either actively or passively, while minimally affecting the normal tissues. The authors of [37] use alginate hydrogels in submicron dimensions to physically encapsulate and hold the drugs required for the treatment of localized cancer. These hydrogels respond differently based on pH, temperature, and/or enzyme in targeted sites, which makes them selective. Alginate hydrogel shrinks and produces a viscous acidic gel that prevents the encapsulated drug to be released at low pH. On passing through high pH, it gets converted to a soluble viscous gel, thereby releasing the encapsulated drug.

The main challenges for success of bioprinting for better healthcare [22,35] lie in the development and choice of bioinks with multifunction properties and highly precise printing processes for delivering survivability. The bioinks should be able to hold the structure after printing with effective and efficient crosslinking and integrate with microfluidic devices for long term. Moreover, the selection of appropriate bioink is very crucial in studies related to critical diseases and their treatment, as the selected ink should be able to mimic the true nature of the diseased cells and organs for accurate results. Another challenge for bioprinting is the lack of ability to obtain an effective and integrated vascular network for transport of oxygen and nutrients [38].

## 13.8  Conclusion and future trends

Industry 4.0 has revolutionized healthcare industry too with a wide implementation of AI for data collection, analysis, decision making, and automation. Smart wearable devices, IoT, cloud-based data storage, and analytical capabilities are implemented in the healthcare industry for better and effective patient-centric systems. Sharing patient data and information collaboratively on digital platforms is now possible with interconnected medical emergency support. Earlier the medicine and its dose for a patient was at the doctor's discretion but now the treatment is based on smart analysis of various medical data captured from the patient. Implementation of Healthcare 4.0 technologies has been found mainly in disease identification and treatments for in-hospital patients. At the same time, remote consultations and remotely assisted surgical and clinical procedures have been made possible. Remote monitoring of patients after discharging them from the hospital needs to be strengthened for quick and efficient treatment in case of emergencies post-hospitalization.

AI has been instrumental for Healthcare 4.0 in terms of precise and efficient medical diagnosis and decisions, telemonitoring and telemedicine, office operations, and data handling. The recent COVID-19 pandemic highlighted the challenges of access, quality, and cost of healthcare as hospitals struggled to test and treat the overwhelming influx of patients, and public health officials worked to prevent the spread of disease. After the outbreak of COVID-19, although telemedicine has gained momentum, however, it is generally limited to online consultations. Sharing medical information captured from imaging instruments needs to be made digital with more ease of access to patients and practitioners remotely.

AI has contributed much towards making healthcare remotely accessible with wearables, IoT techniques, and interactive user interfaces with AR/VR abilities.

The future of healthcare industry requires the ethical use of AI to imitate human intelligence and skills for exploiting advanced digital technologies to make services more efficient and effective for all stakeholders. The challenge lies in making AI-based devices and services self-explainable, emotionally intelligent, and secure. Moreover, the communication as well as transfer of medical data should be secure thereby preventing data breaches. Emotional intelligence will provide a humane touch and improve patient satisfaction and recovery and improved healthcare system.

# References

[1]   Chanchaichujit J, Tan A, Meng F, and Eaimkhong S. *Healthcare 4.0: Next Generation Processes with the Latest Technologies.* Singapore, Palgrave Macmillan; 2019.

[2]   Haleem A, Javaid M, Singh RP, and Suman R. Medical 4.0 technologies for healthcare: features, capabilities, and applications. *Internet of Things and Cyber-Physical Systems.* 2022;2:12–30.

[3]   Rehman MU, Andargoli AE, and Pousti H. Healthcare 4.0: trends, challenges and benefits. In *Proceedings of Australasian Conference on Information Systems*, 2019; Perth Western Australia.

[4]   Tortorella GL, Fogliatto FS, Vergara AMC, Vassolo R, and Sawhney R. Healthcare 4.0: trends, challenges and research directions. *Production Planning & Control: The Management of Operations.* 2020; 31(15): 1245–1260.

[5]   Onasanya A, Lakkis S, and Elshakankiri M. Implementing IoT/WSN based smart Saskatchewan Healthcare System. *Wireless Networks.* 2019; 25:3999–4020.

[6]   Yang Y, Siau K, Xie W, and Sun Y. Smart health: intelligent healthcare systems in the metaverse, artificial intelligence, and data science era. *Journal of Organizational and End User Computing.* 2022; 34(1):1–14.

[7]   Tanwar S, Parekh K, and Evans R. Blockchain-based electronic healthcare record system for healthcare 4.0 applications. *Journal of Information Security and Applications.* 2020; 50:1–13.

[8]   Rghioui A and Oumnad A. Challenges and opportunities of Internet of Things in healthcare. *International Journal of Electrical and Computer Engineering.* 2018; 8(5):2753–2761.

[9]   Yang P, Bi G, Wang X, Yang Y, and Xu L. Multimodal wearable intelligence for dementia care in Healthcare 4.0: a survey. *Information Systems Frontiers.* 2021; 1:1–18.

[10]  Elhoseny M, Abdelaziz A, Salama AS, Riad AM, Muhammad K, and Sangaiah AK. A hybrid model of Internet of Things and cloud computing to manage big data in health services applications. *Future Generation Computer Systems.* 2018; 86:1383–1394.

[11]  Hsieh MC and Lee JJ. Preliminary study of VR and AR applications in medical and healthcare education. *Journal of Nursing and Health Studies.* 2018; 3(1):1–5.

[12]   Moro C, Stromberga Z, Raikos A, and Stirling A. The effectiveness of virtual and augmented reality in health sciences and medical anatomy. *Anatomical Sciences Education.* 2017; 10(6):549–559.

[13]   Li L, Yu F, Shi D, *et al.* Application of virtual reality technology in clinical medicine. *American Journal of Translational Research.* 2017; 9(9):3867–3880.

[14]   Lee Y, Kim SK, and Eom MR. Usability of mental illness simulation involving scenarios with patients with schizophrenia via immersive virtual reality: a mixed methods study. *PLoS One.* 2020;15(9): 1–13.

[15]   Vavra P, Roman J, Zonca P, *et al.* Recent development of augmented reality in surgery: a review. *Journal of Healthcare Engineering.* 2017; 1:1–10.

[16]   Arpaia P, Benedetto ED, and Duraccio L. Design, implementation, and metrological characterization of a wearable, integrated AR-BCI hands-free system for health 4.0 monitoring. *Measurement.* 2021; 177:1–11.

[17]   Hathaliya JJ and Tanwar S. An exhaustive survey on security and privacy issues in Healthcare 4.0. *Computer Communications.* 2020; 153:311–335.

[18]   Rizk DKAA, Hosny HM, and El-Horbaty ESM. SMART hospital management systems based on Internet of Things: challenges, intelligent solutions and functional requirements. *International Journal of Intelligent Computing and Information Sciences.* 2022; 22(1):32–43.

[19]   Avinashiappan A and Mayilsamy B. Internet of Medical Things: security threats, security challenges, and potential solutions. In: Hemanth DJ, Anitha J, and Tsihrintzis GA., (eds.), *Internet of Medical Things.* Springer; 2021. p. 1–16.

[20]   Manogaran G, Thota C, Lopez D, and Sundarasekar R. Big data security intelligence for Healthcare Industry 4.0. In: *Cybersecurity for Industry 4.0.* Springer; 2017. p. 103–126.

[21]   Hathaliya JJ, Tanwar S, Tyagi S, and Kumar N. Securing electronics healthcare records in Healthcare 4.0: a biometric-based approach. *Computers and Electrical Engineering.* 2019; 76:398–410.

[22]   Sun W, Starly B, Daly AC, *et al.* The bioprinting roadmap. *Biofabrication.* 2020; 12(2):1–33.

[23]   Seol YJ, Kang HW, Lee SJ, Atala A, and Yoo JJ. Bioprinting technology and its applications. *European Journal of Cardio-Thoracic Surgery.* 2014; 46(3): 342–348.

[24]   Mobaraki M, Ghaffari M, Yazdanpanah A, Luo Y, and Mills DK. Bioinks and bioprinting: a focused review. *Bioprinting.* 2020; 18:1–16.

[25]   Weng T, Zhang W, Xia Y, *et al.* 3D bioprinting for skin tissue engineering: current status and perspectives. *Journal of Tissue Engineering.* 2021; 12:1–28.

[26]   Khoshnood N and Zamaniain A. A comprehensive review on scaffold-free bioinks for bioprinting. *Bioprinting.*2020; 19:1–44.

[27]   Alblawi A, Ranjani AS, Yasmin H, Gupta S, Bit A, and Rahimi-Gorji M. Scaffold-free: a developing technique in field of tissue engineering. *Computer Methods and Programs in Biomedicine.* 2020; 185:1–29.

[28]    Ozbolat IT. Scaffold-based or scaffold-free bioprinting: competing or com-plementing approaches? *Journal of Nanotechnology in Engineering and Medicine.* 2015; 6(2):1–20.

[29]    Gu Z, Fu J, Lin H, and He Y. Development of 3D bioprinting: from printing methods to biomedical applications. *Asian Journal of Pharmaceutical Sciences.* 2020; 15:529–557.

[30]    Mirdamadi E, Tashman JW, Shiwarski DJ, Palchesko RN, and Feinberg AW. FRESH 3D bioprinting a full-size model of the human heart. *ACS Biomaterials Science & Engineering.* 2020; 6(11):6453–6459.

[31]    Vijayavenkataraman S, Lu WF, and Fuh JYH. 3D bioprinting of skin: a state-of-the-art review on modelling, materials, and processes. *Biofabrication.* 2016; 8:1–31.

[32]    Knowlton S, Onal S, Yu C H, Zhao JJ, and Tasoglu S. Bioprinting for cancer research. *Trends in Biotechnology.* 2015; 33(9): 504–513.

[33]    Wang Y, Shi W, Kuss MA, *et al.* 3D Bioprinting of breast cancer models for drug resistance study. *ACS Biomaterials Science & Engineering.* 2018; 4 (12):4401–4411.

[34]    Kang Y, Datta P, Santhanam S, and Ozbolat I. 3D Bioprinting of tumor models for cancer research. *ACS Applied Bio Materials.* 2020; 3(9): 5552–5573.

[35]    Datta P, Dey M, Ataie Z, Unutmaz D, and Ozbolat IT. 3D bioprinting for reconstituting the cancer microenvironment. *NPJ Precision Oncology.* 2020; 4(18):1–13.

[36]    Peng W, Datta P, Ayan B, Ozbolat V, Sosnoski D, and Ozbolat IT. 3D bioprinting for drug discovery and development in pharmaceutics. *Acta Biomaterialia.* 2017; 57:26–46.

[37]    Abasalizadeh F, Moghaddam SV, Alizadeh E, *et al.* Alginate-based hydro-gels as drug delivery vehicles in cancer treatment and their applications in wound dressing and 3D bioprinting. *Journal of Biological Engineering.* 2020; 14(8):1–22.

[38]    He P, Zhao J, Zhang J, *et al.* Bioprinting of skin constructs for wound healing. *Burns & Trauma.* 2018; 6(5):1–10.

# Index